Long-Term Care of Kidney Transplant Patients

Long-Term Care of Kidney Transplant Patients

Edited by

SUNDARAM HARIHARAN

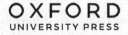

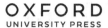

OXFORD
UNIVERSITY PRESS

Oxford University Press is a department of the University of Oxford. It furthers
the University's objective of excellence in research, scholarship, and education
by publishing worldwide. Oxford is a registered trade mark of Oxford University
Press in the UK and certain other countries.

Published in the United States of America by Oxford University Press
198 Madison Avenue, New York, NY 10016, United States of America.

Library of Congress Cataloging-in-Publication Data
Names: Hariharan, Sundaram, editor.
Title: Long-Term Care of Kidney Transplant Patients / [Edited by] Sundaram Hariharan.
Description: New York, NY : Oxford University Press, [2024] |
Includes bibliographical references and index.
Identifiers: LCCN 2024006259 (print) | LCCN 2024006260 (ebook) |
ISBN 9780197697320 (paperback) | ISBN 9780197697344 (epub) |
ISBN 9780197697351 (other) Subjects: MESH: Kidney Transplantation |
Long-Term Care | Transplant Recipients Classification: LCC RD575 (print) |
LCC RD575 (ebook) | NLM WJ 368 | DDC 617.4/610592—dc23/eng/20240216
LC record available at https://lccn.loc.gov/2024006259
LC ebook record available at https://lccn.loc.gov/2024006260

DOI: 10.1093/med/9780197697320.001.0001

Printed by Marquis Book Printing, Canada

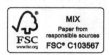

Contents

Contributors

Richard J. Baker, MB, BChir, PhD, FRCP
Consultant Nephrologist
Renal Transplant Unit
St. James's University Hospital
Leeds, UK

Steven J. Chadban, MD
Professor of Medicine
Kidney Centre, Charles Perkins Centre
University of Sydney
Department of Renal Medicine
Royal Prince Alfred Hospital
Camperdown, Australia

Jeremy Chapman, MD, FRCP,
FRACP, FAHMS
Editor in Chief Transplantation Journals
Department of Renal and Transplantation
Medicine
Westmead Hospital
University of Sydney, NSW, Australia

Aravind Cherukuri, MD, PhD
Associate Professor of Medicine
University of Pittsburgh Medical Center
Pittsburgh, PA, USA

Craig P. Coorey, BSc(Adv), MD
Clinical Lecturer
Faculty of Medicine and Health
University of Sydney
Department of Renal Medicine
Royal Prince Alfred Hospital
Camperdown, Australia

Marta Crespo, MD, PhD
Associate Professor of Medicine
University of Hospital Affiliation Hospital
del Mar University Pompeu Fabra,
Barcelona
Barcelona, Spain

Daniel Cukor, PhD
Director, Behavioral Health
The Rogosin Institute
New York, NY, USA

Raja S. Dandamudi, MD
Assistant Professor
Washington University School of
Medicine
St. Louis Children's Hospital
St. Louis, MO, USA

Vikas Dharnidharka, MD
Professor of Pediatrics
Washington University School of
Medicine in St. Louis
St. Louis Children's Hospital
St. Louis, MO, USA

Mona D. Doshi, MD
Professor of Transplant Nephrology
University of Michigan
Ann Arbor, MI, USA

Ty B. Dunn, MD, MS
Professor of Surgery
Surgical Director
Kidney and Pancreas Transplantation
Center for Advanced Care
Froedtert Hospital
Milwaukee, WI, USA

John Gill, MD
Professor of Medicine
University of British Columbia
St Paul's Hospital
Vancouver, BC, Canada

Gaurav Gupta, MD
Professor of Medicine and Surgery
Division of Nephrology and Hume-lee
Transplant Center
Virginia Commonwealth University
Richmond, VA, USA

Sundaram Hariharan, MD
Emeritus Professor of Medicine
University of Pittsburgh
Pittsburgh, PA, USA

Allyson Hart, MD, MSc
Associate Professor of Medicine
Hennepin Healthcare and University of
Minnesota
Minneapolis, MN, USA

Britta Höcker, MD
Professor of Pediatrics and Pediatric
Nephrology
Zentrum für Kinder- und Jugendmedizin
Universitätsklinikum Heidelberg
Heidelberg, Germany

George T. John, MD, FRACP
University of Queensland
Royal Brisbane and Women's Hospital
Brisbane, Australia

Rajiv Khanna, PhD
Professor
QIMR Berghofer Medical Research
Institute
Herston, Australia

Krista L. Lentine, MD, PhD
Professor of Medicine
Saint Louis University
SSM Health Saint Louis University
Hospital
St. Louis, MO , USA

Chien-Jung Lin, MD, PhD
Assistant Professor of Medicine
Saint Louis University
SSM Health Saint Louis University
Hospital
St. Louis, MO, USA

Rajil B. Mehta, MD
Associate Professor of Medicine and
Surgery
University of Pittsburgh Medical Center
Pittsburgh, PA, USA

Sumit Mohan, MD, MPH
Professor of Medicine & Epidemiology
Department of Medicine
Division of Nephrology
Columbia University
New York, NY, USA

Michele Molinari, MD, MHS
Professor of Surgery
University of Pittsburgh Medical Center
Pittsburgh, PA, USA

Maarten Naesens, MD PhD
Professor of Medicine
KU Leuven
Leuven, Belgium

Sandesh Parajuli, MD
Associate Professor of Medicine
University of Wisconsin School of
Medicine
Madison, WI, USA

Chethan M. Puttarajappa, MD
Associate Professor of Medicine
University of Pittsburgh Medical Center
Pittsburgh, PA, USA

Hamid Rabb, MD
Professor of Medicine
Johns Hopkins Hospital
Baltimore, MD, USA

Natasha M. Rogers, MD, PhD
Professor of Nephrology and
Transplantation Medicine
Westmead Institute for Medical Research
University of Sydney, NSW, Australia

Nida Saleem, MBBS, FCPS (Nephrology)
Department of Renal and Transplantation
Medicine
Westmead Hospital, NSW Australia
College of Medicine and Public Health,
Flinders University
Centre for Kidney Research, Kids
Research Institute
The Children's Hospital at Westmead,
NSW, Australia

Carrie Schinstock, MD
Associate Professor of Medicine
Mayo Clinic
Rochester, MN, USA

Adnan Sharif, MD MBChB FRCP (Edin)
Transplant Nephrologist and Honorary
Associate Professor
University Hospitals Birmingham and
Queen Elizabeth Hospital
Birmingham, UK

Akhil Sharma, MD
Assistant Professor of Medicine and
Surgery
Pittsburgh, PA, USA

Puneet Sood, MD
Professor of Medicine and Surgery
University of California, San Francisco
San Francisco, CA, USA

Jennifer L. Steel, PhD
Professor of Surgery, Psychiatry, and
Psychology
University of Pittsburgh
Pittsburg, PA, USA

Angus W. Thomson, PhD, DSc
Professor of Surgery and Immunology
Professor of Clinical & Translational
Science
University of Pittsburgh School of
Medicine
Pittsburgh, PA, USA

Brahm Vasudev, MD
Associate Professor of Medicine
Division of Nephrology
Medical College of Wisconsin
Milwaukee, WI, USA

Christine M. Wu, MD
Associate Professor of Medicine
Renal and Electrolyte Division
University of Pittsburgh Medical Center
and VA Pittsburgh Healthcare Nephrology
Pittsburgh, PA, USA

Germaine Wong, MBBS, FRACP,
MMed, PhD
Department of Renal and Transplantation
Medicine
Westmead Hospital, NSW Australia
College of Medicine and Public Health,
Flinders University
Centre for Kidney Research, Kids
Research Institute
The Children's Hospital at Westmead,
NSW, Australia

Abbreviations

AA	systemic amyloid A
AAV	associated vasculitis
ABMR	antibody-mediated rejection
ACC	American College of Cardiology
ACEi	angiotensin-converting enzyme inhibitors
ACKD	acquired cystic kidney disease
ACOG	American College of Obstetricians and Gynecologists
ACS	acute coronary syndrome
ADR	annual data report
AHA	American Heart Association
aHUS	atypical hemolytic uremic syndrome
AKI	acute kidney injury
ALERT	assessment of lescol in renal transplantation
AMR	antibody-mediated rejection
ANCA	Anti-Neutrophil cytoplasmic antibody
anti-PLA2R	anti-phospholipase A2 receptor
ANZDATA	Australia New Zealand Data
APC	antigen presenting cell
ARB	angiotensin receptor blockers
ARNI	angiotensin receptor/neprilysin inhibitor
AST	American Society of Transplantation
ATN	acute tubular necrosis
AVF	arteriovenous fistula
AZA	azathioprine
BAL	bronchoalveolar lavage
BCC	basal cell cancer
BCMA	B cell maturation antigen
BCR	B cell receptor
BKV	BK virus
BKVN	BK virus nephropathy
BMI	body mass index
C3GN	complement 3 glomerulonephritis
CABG	coronary artery bypass surgery
CAD	coronary artery disease
CAKUT	congenital anomalies of the kidney and urinary tract
CAR	chimeric ag receptor
CAR	chimeric antigen receptor
CCB	calcium channel blocker

CDC	Centers for Disease Control
CDC	complement-dependent cytotoxicity
CFH	complement factor H
CIT	cold ischemia time
CKD	chronic kidney disease
CMV	cytomegalovirus
CNI	calcineurin inhibitor
COPD	chronic obstructive pulmonary disease
COVID-19	coronavirus disease-2019
cPRA	calculated panel reactive antibody
CRRT	continuous renal replacement therapy
CSA	cyclosporin A
CTA	computed tomography angiography
CTLA-4	cytotoxic T-lymphocyte antigen-4
CVD	cardiovascular disease
CVP	central venous pressure
DAPT	dual antiplatelet therapy
DBD	donation after brain death
DC	dendritic cell
DCD	donation after cardiac death
DCGL	death-censored graft loss
DCGS	death-censored graft survival
DD-cfDNA	donor-derived cell-free DNA
DD	deceased donor
DGF	delayed graft function
DM	diabetes mellitus
DN	diabetic nephropathy
DPP-4	dipeptidyl peptidase-4
DSA	donor-specific antibody
DWFG	death with a functioning graft
EBV	Epstein-Barr virus
EC	emergency contraception
ECG	echocardiogram
ED	erectile dysfunction
eGFR	estimated glomerular filtration rate
EHR	electronic health record
ESC	European Society of Cardiology
ESKD	end-stage kidney disease
FBS	fasting blood sugar
FC	facilitating cell
FDA	Food and Drug Administration
FSGS	focal segmental glomerulosclerosis
FSH	follicle stimulating hormone
GBM	glomerular basement membrane

GFR	glomerular filtration rate
GLP-1	glucagon-like peptide 1
GLP	glucagon-like peptide
GN	glomerulonephritis
GR	glucocorticoid receptor
GVHD	graft versus host disease
HbA1c	hemoglobin A1c
HLA	human leukocyte antigen
HPV	human papillomavirus
HSCT	hematopoietic stem cell transplant
HTN	hypertension
HZV	herpes zoster virus
ICI	immune checkpoint inhibitor
IDO	intragraft indoleamine dioxygenase
IDSA	Infectious Disease Society of America
IFN	interferon
Ig	immunoglobulin
IGAN	immunoglobulin A nephropathy
IGKV	kappa variable cluster
IGKVID-13	Ig kappa variable 1D-13
IGLL1	Ig lambda-like polypeptide 1
IGRA	interferon gamma release assay
IL	interleukin
IL2-RA	interleukin 2 receptor antagonist
IPA	invasive pulmonary aspergillosis
IS	Immunosuppression
KAS	kidney allocation system
KDIGO	Kidney Disease Improving Global Outcomes
KDPI	Kidney Donor Profile Index
KPCOP	Kidney and Pancreas Community of Practice
KPD	kidney paired exchange
KT	kidney transplant
KTA	kidney transplant alone
KTR	kidney transplant recipient
LD	living donor
LH	luteinizing hormone
LV	left ventricle
MACE	major adverse cardiovascular events
MCC	Merkel cell cancer
MCP	membrane-cofactor protein
MELD	Model for End-Stage Liver Disease
mHAgs	minor histocompatibility antigens
MI	myocardial infarction
MIC	minimum inhibitory concentration

MMF	mycophenolate mofetil
MMR	measles-mumps-rubella
MN	membranous nephropathy
MOHAN	Multi-Organ Harvesting Aid Network
MPA	mycophenolate acid
MPGN	membranoproliferative glomerulonephritis
MPGN	membranoproliferative GN
mTORi	mammalian target of rapamycin inhibitor
NAAT	nucleic acid amplification testing
NAPRTCS	North American Pediatric Transplant Collaborative Study
NHP	non-human primates
NICE	National Institute of Health and Clinical Excellence
NK	natural killer
NKF	National Kidney Foundation
NKR	National Kidney Registry
NMSC	nonmelanomatous skin cancer
OPTN	Organ Procurement and Transplantation Network
PCI	percutaneous coronary intervention
PCP	primary care provider
PCR	polymerase chain reaction
PH	pulmonary hypertension
PIR	paired immunoglobulin like-receptor
PJ	*Pneumocystis jirovecii*
PJP	*Pneumocystis jirovecii* pneumonia
PLA2R	anti-phospholipase A2 receptor
PML	progressive multifocal leukoencephalopathy
PRA	panel reactive antibody
PTA	pancreas transplant alone
PTH	parathyroid hormone
PTLD	post-transplant lymphoproliferative disease
PTSD	post-traumatic stress disorder
QFT	QuantiFERON-TB GOLD
RAAS	renin-angiotensin-aldosterone-system
RCC	renal cell cancer
RV	right ventricle
SAB	single antigen bead
SCC	squamous cell carcinoma
SDoH	social determinants of health
SES	socioeconomic status
SGLT-2	sodium-glucose cotransporter 2
SGLT2-i	sodium-glucose cotransporter-2 inhibitor
SLE	systemic lupus erythematosus
SLKT	simultaneous liver and kidney transplantation
SMFM	Society for Maternal-Fetal Medicine

SPKT	simultaneous pancreas and kidney transplantation
SRTR	Scientific Registry of Transplant Recipients
STEMI	ST-elevation myocardial infarction
TB	tuberculosis
TBI	total body irradiation
TCMR	T-cell-mediated rejection
TCR	T-cell receptor
TFH	T follicular helper cell
TGF-β	transforming growth factor beta
TGF4	Transforming growth factor beta
THSD7A	anti-thrombospondin type-1 domain-containing 7
TLI	Total lymphoid irradiation
TMA	thrombotic microangiopathy
TMP/SMZ	trimethoprim/sulfamethoxazole
TNF-α	tumor necrosis factor-alpha
TNF	tumor necrosis factor
TOLS	Treg-rich organized lymphoid structures
Treg	regulatory T cells
UNOS	United Network for Organ Sharing
US	ultrasound
USPSTF	US Preventive Services Task Force
USRDS	United State Renal Data System
UTI	urinary tract infection
UV	ultraviolet
UVA	ultraviolet A
VCZ	voriconazole
VEGF	vascular endothelial growth factor
VZV	varicella zoster virus
WHO	World Health Organization
WIT	warm ischemia time

About the Editor

Sundaram Hariharan is an Emeritus professor of medicine at the University of Pittsburgh Pennsylvania, USA. His research interest is in the fields of kidney and pancreas transplantation. He has published over 200 peer-reviewed articles on various topics centered around transplantation and has participated in numerous clinical trials. His scientific contributions cover a variety of renal transant topics, and publications that have been cited extensively over last 30 years include "Recurrent and De Novo Diseases after Renal Transplantation," "Long-Term Kidney Transplant Survival," "Surrogate Markers for Renal Transplant Outcome," and "BKV Infection after Renal Transplantation." Over the past decade his research interest has been on identification, pathogenesis, and treatment of subclinical acute T-cell-mediated rejection and subclinical inflammation in renal transplant recipients with a goal of treating them and improving long-term allograft survival. In 2021 he published an important review article in *NEJM* titled "Long-Term Survival after Kidney Transplantation." He is an associate editor for the Journal Transplantation. He has been recognized as a leader in clinical transplantation in both the national and international scene.

Preface

Sundaram Hariharan

An introduction to long-term survival after kidney transplantation!
It gives me a great pleasure and privilege to write and edit *Long-Term Care of Kidney Transplant Patients*. I entered the kidney transplant field in 1983, the year cyclosporine was approved for clinical use in the United States. The introduction of cyclosporine resulted in a new era for kidney transplantation with marked reduction in rates of acute rejection leading to better short-term survival.[1] Improvement in long-term survival was first noted in 2000,[2] and further steady improvements over next 20 years were confirmed in 2021.[3] It is difficult to ascertain specific reasons for improvements in long-term survival, but with advances over four decades, there are several potential factors:

- Introduction of potent immunosuppressive agents such as mycophenolate mofetil and tacrolimus in mid-1990s, additional agents such as sirolimus in 2002, and belatacept in 2012;
- Concurrent technological advances with newer platforms for testing for human leucocyte antigens (HLA), HLA antibodies, and T and B crossmatch techniques;
- Introduction of sensitive and specific nucleic acid amplification testing for the diagnosis and management of viral infections;
- Effective use of antiviral agents for the prevention and treatment of viral infections;
- Standardization of kidney biopsy findings through Banff classification;
- Consensus in the overall management of kidney transplant patients;
- Changes in organ allocation; and
- Successful introduction of living-donor-paired exchange transplants.

Improvements in long-term survival have resulted in a robust increase in the number of kidney transplant patients across the globe. I have been fortunate to care for kidney transplant patients for over 40 years—it has been my life's work. I have enjoyed managing these patients and have continuously sought to improve my knowledge and contribute to scholarly work in the field. That is why I took on the task of writing and editing this book with experienced renowned authors from all over the world. I believe this book will help clinicians, trainees, researchers, and eventually thousands of patients across the globe. The purpose of the book is to provide comprehensive information on all aspects of long-term management of kidney transplant patients, with the goal of improving patient outcomes.

The book begins with chapters on current long-term survival rates after kidney transplantation and the phases of kidney transplantation. These are followed by a chapter on transplant wellness, addressing the importance of immunization against pathogens, family planning, reproductive health, cancer screening, travel, and return to work after transplantation. These issues are critical for patients to be healthier, be productive, and contribute to the society in a meaningful way. Subsequent chapters address immunosuppressive medications, immunological and nonimmunological factors impacting outcome, and alloimmune injury to allograft—short and late T-cell-mediated rejection and antibody-mediated rejection. Subsequent chapters focus on various late post-transplant events like cardiovascular and metabolic diseases, infections, tumors, and recurrent and de novo glomerular diseases. Other chapters address specific populations, including multiorgan transplantation patients—combined kidney with liver, and kidney with pancreas—and transplantation in children. The importance of psychological and behavioral issues after transplantation and the social determinants of health are addressed in dedicated chapters. A separate chapter on management of failing and failed transplant kidney provides clinicians insight into understanding how to manage these patients as well. The final chapter is dedicated to transplant tolerance, which remains the "Holy Grail" of transplantation. Thus, this book provides all aspects of long-term care of kidney transplant patients. All chapters address the topics in depth and provide current thinking with a balanced approach toward managing various post-transplant clinical events that impact long-term survival.

This book is a valuable resource for all clinical transplant physicians and surgeons, primary care physicians, and various specialists who are caring for kidney transplant patients. It will also benefit other healthcare providers such as pharmacists, psychologists, advanced nurse practitioners, pharmaceutical and diagnostic companies, and agencies involved in kidney transplantation.

Many of the chapters highlight unmet needs relevant to certain post-transplant events that influence survival. Chapters provide clinicians and researchers with opportunities to investigate and advance the science by performing studies that can alter the trajectory of specific post-transplant diseases, which will improve long-term kidney survival further until we achieve the Holy Grail—transplant tolerance.

I dedicate this book to all my kidney transplant patients from whose malady I have grown and learned. I hope that I have given the best of me by caring for them.

I anticipate that there will be further improvements in the long-term outcome of renal transplant patients, and I encourage all readers to explore this book and provide input that can be used to improve future editions.

Thank you!

References

1. Merion RM, White DJ, Thiru S, Evans DB, Calne RY. Cyclosporine: five years' experience in cadaveric renal transplantation. *N Engl J Med*. 1984;*310*(3):148–154.
2. Hariharan S, Johnson CP, Bresnahan BA, Taranto SE, McIntosh MJ, Stablein D. Improved graft survival after renal transplantation in the United States, 1988 to 1996. *N Engl J Med*. 2000;*342*(9):605–612.
3. Hariharan S, Israni AK, Danovitch G. Long-term survival after kidney transplantation. *N Engl J Med*. 2021;*385*(8):729–743.

1

Long-Term Survival after Kidney Transplantation

Brahm Vasudev and Sundaram Hariharan

Kidney transplantation is performed to improve long-term survival!

Introduction

Kidney transplantation is the best option for renal replacement therapy for end-stage kidney disease (ESKD) because it can restore kidney function and improve the quality and quantity of recipients' lives. In the United States, over three decades the number of kidney transplant (KT) performed from deceased donors (DDs) and living donors (LDs) have increased, but not enough to keep up with demand—most patients must wait for a few years for a DDKT. The success of KT is a function of patient survival and the transplanted organ's long-term survival. The survival rates of KT recipients have progressively improved over the years due to improvements in pretransplant processes, better surgical techniques, advances in immunosuppressive therapies, and prevention and treatment of post-transplant cardiovascular disease (CVD), infections, and tumors. In addition, over the years, advances in technology, including improved platforms for human leukocyte antigen (HLA) and antibody testing and cross-match techniques, legislative changes, better communication through the electronic health record (EHR) system, and the introduction of telemedicine have had a positive impact on patient care. This chapter provides an overview of the importance of long-term KT survival, current survival rates, pre- and post-transplant factors that affect KT survival, and methods to improve survival rates further.

Importance of Long-Term Graft Survival

The availability of cyclosporine in the early 1980s marked a turning point for KT recipients. Prior to this breakthrough, both short-term and long-term survival rates were significantly low. However, over the past four decades, there has been remarkable progress in improving the survival rates for KT recipients.[1-3] Enhancing long-term KT survival rates benefits patients, the healthcare system, researchers, and healthcare workers. It greatly improves the quality of life for patients by restoring normal kidney functions, eliminating the need for dialysis, and extending their lifespan. Recipients not only experience better physical and emotional health, improved sleep patterns, and increased social and economic benefits but also enjoy a higher quantity of life. Moreover, transplantation is cost-effective in the long run compared to long-term dialysis treatment. By reducing the financial burden on patients and the healthcare system, long-term KT survival rates have substantial economic implications. Lastly, long-term KT survival rates positively impact the transplantation landscape. They decrease the necessity for repeat transplantations, thus increasing the availability of organs for other patients in need. This not only saves lives but also alleviates the financial strain on both patients and the healthcare system.[4]

Kidney Transplant Survival Rates

The short-term and long-term survival rates of KT from both LDs and DDs have improved over the past four decades due to a multitude of interventions in kidney donors, KT candidates, and KT recipients (Figure 1.1). Due to improved overall medical care, patients with chronic kidney disease (CKD) live longer and develop ESKD at an older age, a common clinical issue facing before and after KT. Over the last few decades, donor interventions, pretransplant immunologic and nonimmunologic interventions, post-transplant interventions, and a variety of socioeconomic interventions have all played a vital role in improving KT survival rates.[4] This has been achieved despite the fact that, over the years, there has been an increase in recipient variables that are unfavorable to improving KT outcomes, including more older KT recipients or transplanting recipients who have one or more risk factors for poorer outcomes like diabetes, smoking, cardiac disease, elevated body mass index (BMI), longer dialysis vintage and a higher degree of HLA sensitization, increasing donor age, or transplanting DD kidneys from donation after circulatory death or with a higher Kidney Donor Profile Index (KDPI) score representing lower quality of the transplanted kidneys.[5,6]

The 10-year kidney graft survival among recipients of DD transplants in the United States has improved from 42% in 1996–1999 to 54% in 2008–2011. In addition, the 10-year patient survival in that same time frame increased from 61% to 67%. However, the long-term transplant survival rates among DD and

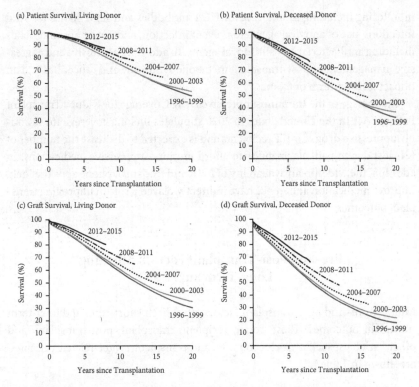

Figure 1.1 Graft and patient survival after kidney transplantation in the United States. Shown are Kaplan-Meier estimates of patient survival (Panels A and B) and graft survival (Panels C and D) after transplantation of grafts from living donors (Panels A and C) and deceased donors (Panels B and D), with the data grouped in 4-year cohorts from 1996 to 2015. There were gradual improvements in patient and graft survival from the 1996–1999 period to the 2012–2015 period.

LD transplant recipients in the United States are lower than among transplant recipients in Canada, Europe, Australia, and New Zealand.[4]

Reasons for Improving Kidney Transplant Survival Rates

Some of the key factors responsible for the improvement in transplant outcomes are the availability of virtual and physical crossmatching techniques before transplant, the option of a paired-exchange LDKT, induction immunosuppression protocols based on risk for rejection, optimal immunosuppression post-transplantation, a decline in clinical acute rejection rates, post-transplant monitoring including monitoring for HLA antibodies and surveillance for viral infections, use of antiviral agents to prevent infection, and newer antimicrobials including antibacterial and antifungal agents. In addition, aggressive and aggressive management of post-transplant metabolic syndrome and cancer has had an impact on long-term outcomes.

The passage of the Immunosuppressive Drug Coverage for Kidney Transplant Patients Act in the United States in 2020 stipulates lifelong coverage for immunosuppressive drugs for KT recipients and is expected to decrease the number of KTs lost due to patients' inability to afford immunosuppressive medications. In addition, the widespread availability of EHR and free smartphone apps that help improve medication adherence have indirectly played a role in improving transplant outcomes.

Pre- and Post-Transplant Factors Affecting Long-Term Survival

Multiple pre- and post-transplant factors affect both short-term and long-term transplant outcomes. These donor, recipient, transplant, post-transplant, and other variables, such as socioeconomic and transplant center-related variables, are shown in Table 1.1.

Donor Variables

Multiple donor-related factors can impact long-term KT survival. These include the age of the donor, the donor's underlying medical conditions, and the nature of the donor's kidney's surgical anatomy. In addition, the quality of the donor's kidney is measured using the KDPI, and a higher KDPI number is associated with decreased kidney transplant survival.[6]

Recipient Variables

Multiple recipient-related factors can impact long-term KT survival. Recipient-related post-transplant factors affecting survival include increasing age, presence of diabetes, higher BMI, longer pretransplant dialysis duration, degree of HLA mismatch, and degree of sensitization measured by panel reactive antibody measured immediately prior to transplant.[7,8] Sensitization occurs via blood transfusions, pregnancies, and prior transplants. Other comorbid conditions impacting survival are previous history of CVD, a history of cancers, and native

Table 1.1 Select Donor, Recipient, Transplant, and Post-Transplant Variables Impacting Long-Term Survival

Variable types	Select variables
Donor	Age, DCD organs, higher KDPI
Recipient	Extremes of age, African American race, obesity
	ESKD due to diabetes, c3GN, aHUS, FSGS
	Dialysis vintage
	Comorbidities from CVD, COPD, cancer, pulmonary HTN, limited functional status
Transplant	HLA mismatch, sensitization (pregnancy, blood transfusion, prior transplant), Combined kidney with pancreas, liver, and heart transplant
Post-Transplant	Prolonged WIT, prolonged CIT, DGF, acute rejection
Other	Socioeconomic factors, nonadherence, limited financial and social support, substance abuse, and transplant center–related factors

Abbreviations: C3GN: complement 3 glomerulonephritis, CIT: cold ischemia time, COPD: chronic obstructive pulmonary disease, CVD: cardiovascular diseases, DCD: donation after circulatory death, DGF: delayed graft function, FSGS: focal segmental glomerulosclerosis, HLA: human leucocyte antigen, HTN: hypertension, aHUS: atypical hemolytic uremic syndrome, KDPI: Kidney Donor Profile Index, WIT: warm ischemia time

kidney diseases with a high chance of recurrences, such as FSGS, c3GN, and aHUS. Recipients who are seronegative for cytomegalovirus (CMV) or Epstein-Barr virus (EBV) upon receiving an organ from a seropositive donor for CMV or EBV are at high risk for these infections post-transplant. Patients who do not adhere to their medication regimen or who experience medication side effects are also at increased risk of graft failure. Infections, CVD, and other medical complications post-transplant can negatively impact graft survival. These are discussed extensively in Chapter 5, "Immunological and Nonimmunological Factors Affecting Kidney Transplant Outcomes."

Socioeconomic Variables

Socioeconomic factors in transplant recipients include limited health literacy, poor social and family support, limited access to the transplant center or healthcare workers, financial barriers, and various cultural factors. These factors can hinder patients from getting listed for transplantation and from accessing good post-transplant care, thus influencing outcomes. Other variables including adherence to medications, follow-up care, and avoidance of high-risk behavior such as smoking, alcohol, and drug use are critical to optimizing long-term transplant outcomes. These are discussed extensively in Chapter 13, "Social Determinants Impacting Transplant Outcomes."

Transplant Center–Related Variables

Transplant center-related factors like the skill set of both the surgical and medical team, protocols to optimize postoperative recovery from surgery, availability of immunosuppressive medications, and surveillance protocols for monitoring allograft function, alloimmune injury, viral infections, tumors, metabolic disease, and CVD are all critical in improving long-term transplant survival.

Methods to Further Improve Kidney Transplant and Patient Survival Rates

The leading causes of KT failure in the first year of transplantation include vascular complications, technical issues, acute rejection, and recurrent disease. Beyond the first year of transplant, chronic alloimmune injury is the leading cause of KT loss. The leading cause of death with a functioning KT in the first year after transplantation is CVD, followed by infection and cancer. Beyond the first year, cancer is the leading cause of death, followed by CVD and infection. Efforts to improve KT outcomes thus need to focus on preventing and managing alloimmune injury, CVD, infection, and cancer.

Donor Interventions

Various donor interventions are critical to improving long-term survival. Some of the key elements are promotion of LD-paired exchanges to avoid ABO incompatible or positive crossmatch transplants, promotion of LD transplants to avoid or minimize time on dialysis, judicious use of kidneys with high KDPI, use of hepatitis C kidneys from DD followed by early treatment, use of HIV-positive donor kidneys for HIV-positive candidates, use of Hep B-positive kidneys from DD in appropriate candidates and institution of post-transplant antiviral therapy. LD-paired exchanges are also being considered to avoid high-risk CMV and EBV recipients. The use of APOL1 risk alleles testing in Black donors and recipients is being explored at the current time.

Pretransplant Recipient Interventions

Various recipient interventions are critical as well to improve long-term survival. Some of the key elements include early referral for KT; education of candidates to improve transplant-related healthcare literacy; promoting preemptive KT; aggressive management of hypertension, diabetes, obesity, and dyslipidemia; review of immunization records; serologies and administration of appropriate vaccinations; age-appropriate cancer screening; evaluation for occult infections in candidates at risk; serological HLA testing; performing transplants with 1 or 2 HLA-DR match for younger recipients; and use of eplet-matched transplants to decrease sensitization. In addition, the use of virtual crossmatching to reduce cold ischemia time (CIT) and delayed graft function (DGF), avoiding CMV D+ R- transplants if possible and avoiding transplantation in ESKD patients with limited survival.[9]

Post-Transplant Recipient Interventions

Individualized and protocol-based post-transplant surveillance labs and kidney histology to monitor for allograft function, alloimmune injury, immunosuppressive drug levels, and viral infections are beneficial. The use of belatacept in appropriate patients—besides lack of nephrotoxicity, its monthly infusion offers directly observed therapy, thereby improving medication and laboratory adherence. Other monitoring—such as circulating Donor Specific Antibody (DSA) and the use of surveillance biopsies—can also be helpful. The use of noninvasive biomarkers in patients to identify alloimmune injury is being explored.[10] It is prudent to prevent and treat T-cell- and antibody-mediated rejection and develop targeted therapies for recurrent glomerulonephritis.

Socioeconomic Interventions

Many socioeconomic interventions have the potential to improve long-term KT outcomes. These include mandatory reporting of long-term KT survival data (5 to 10 years) by transplant centers to the regulatory agencies, continued education to improve healthcare literacy, use of smartphone apps to improve adherence, provision of social support to patients at risk of nonadherence, improving access to transplant centers, the option of televisits, continued involvement of the referring nephrologist in post-transplant care, and ensuring that recipients have access to immunosuppressive medications.

Conclusion

Long-term KT survival has slowly and steadily improved despite the increase in unfavorable risk factors among both donors and recipients. As medical care is becoming more standardized and more accessible, multiple donor, recipient, and socioeconomic interventions have been put in place in transplant centers to improve the quality of both pre- and post-transplant patient care. The availability of the non-nephrotoxic immunosuppressive medication belatacept is beneficial in select KT recipients. In the United States, the number of transplant nephrologists has increased over the years. Most transplant centers also have advanced practice providers to help provide care to pre- and post-transplant patients, thus improving access to care. Further advancement in the field of biomarkers to detect alloimmune injury can also help improve long-term KT survival. Newer novel therapies such as antiviral agents, adoptive T cell therapy, and newer treatments for acute and chronic T-cell- and antibody-mediated rejection and desensitization are in the pipeline and are expected to improve the long-term KT survival further.

Acknowledgment

We acknowledge and thank the *New England Journal of Medicine* for permitting us to include Figure 1.1 in this chapter from Hariharan et al., "Long-Term Survival after Kidney Transplantation," *N Engl J Med*. 2021;385:729–743.

References

1. Hariharan S, Johnson CP, Bresnahan BA, et al. Improved graft survival after renal transplantation in the United States, 1988 to 1996. *N Engl J Med*. 2000;342:605–612.
2. Sola E, Gonzalez-Molina M, Cabello M, et al. Long-term improvement of deceased donor renal allograft survival since 1996: a single transplant center study. *Transplantation*. 2010;89:714–720.
3. Zolota A, Solonaki F, Katsanos G, et al. Long-term (≥25 years) kidney allograft survivors: retrospective analysis at a single center. *Transplant Proc*. 2020;52:3044–3050.
4. Hariharan S, Israni AK, Danovitch G. Long-term survival after kidney transplantation. *N Engl J Med*. 2021;385:729–743.

5. Kleinsteuber A, Halleck F, Khadzhynov D, et al. Impact of pre-existing comorbidities on long-term outcomes in kidney transplant recipients. *Transplant Proc.* 2018;50:3232–3241.
6. Molinari M, Kaltenmeier C, Liu H, et al. Function and longevity of renal grafts from high-KDPI donors. *Clin Transplant.* 2022;36(9):e14759.
7. Jankowska M, Bzoma B, Małyszko J, et al. Early outcomes and long-term survival after kidney transplantation in elderly versus younger recipients from the same donor in a matched-pairs analysis. *Medicine (Baltimore).* 2021;100:e28159.
8. Liese J, Bottner N, Büttner S, et al. Influence of the recipient body mass index on the outcomes after kidney transplantation. *Langenbecks Arch Surg.* 2018;403:73–82.
9. Puttarajappa CM, Tevar A, William Hoffman W, et al. Virtual crossmatch for deceased donor kidney transplantation in the United States: a survey of histocompatibility lab directors and transplant surgeons. *Hum Immunol.* 2023;84(3):214–223.
10. Puttarajappa CM, Mehta R, Roberts MS, Smith KJ, Hariharan S. Economic analysis of screening for subclinical rejection in kidney transplantation using protocol biopsies and non-invasive biomarkers. *Am J Transplant.* 2021;21(1): 186–197.

2

Kidney Transplantation with Transplant Phases

Chethan M. Puttarajappa and Sumit Mohan

Clinical phases with key events after kidney transplantation!

Introduction

Kidney transplantation offers a great opportunity to improve an end-stage kidney disease (ESKD) patient's quality of life and mortality risk. Long-term success, however, requires overcoming several challenges along the post-transplant journey. These challenges vary with time after transplant and often require a multifaceted approach to ensure that recipients obtain optimal care leading to substantial benefit from their transplantation.[1] This chapter will highlight key challenges faced by patients and healthcare providers as they navigate these different post-transplant phases, which we have demarcated here as early, middle, and late phases. The chapter will highlight immunological, medical, and social factors that pose a risk for poor graft and patient outcomes and discuss opportunities for mitigating these risks and thus improving long-term outcome.

Transplant Phases

Barriers to improving long-term kidney transplant (KT) outcomes change with time after transplant, and are often a combination of surgical, medical, social, and psychosocial issues. We have highlighted key issues by categorizing the post-transplant period into three arbitrary but useful time phases:

- Early phase: Within 1st year after transplantation),
- Middle phase: Between 1 and 5 years after transplantation and
- Late phase: >5 years after transplantation.

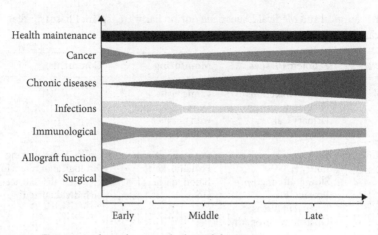

Figure 2.1 Post-transplant phases with clinical domains.

These phases reflect a gradual shift (Figure 2.1) from a focus on surgical complications, early acute rejections, and opportunistic infections (such as BK virus and cytomegalovirus [CMV]) toward chronic disease management and health maintenance (for diabetes mellitus [DM], hypertension [HTN], cardiovascular disease [CVD], cancer screening, and vaccinations) and culminating finally with a focus on caring for a patient with a failing KT and/or end-of-life issues. The overarching role of social determinants of health, including socioeconomic status, health literacy, and medical nonadherence, across the three phases will also be highlighted.

Early Phase (<1 Year Post-Transplant)

This early post-transplant period is a busy phase with patients requiring very close monitoring and active management in several key domains (Table 2.1). Depending on the type of transplant (living vs. deceased donor KT) and recipient characteristics, patients can experience widely varying post-transplant course with regard to surgical complications, the level of renal function, physical functioning, immunological events, infections, medication side effects, and psychosocial issues. Adverse events and complications in this early phase can have a lasting impact on patient and allograft outcomes.

Table 2.1 Surgical and Medical Issues Seen during Early Transplant Phase (<1 Year Post-Transplant)

	Problems/Issues	Monitoring	Comments
Surgical	Wound infections Hematomas Urinary leak Vascular thrombosis	Clinic visits Ultrasonography with doppler Fluid chemistry	
Renal function	Perfusion injury (DGF Slow graft function) Lower GFR Recurrent disease Obstructive uropathy	Serum creatinine Proteinuria Blood markers for GN	Utility of monitoring serological markers in recurrent disease needs to be individualized
Alloimmune-injury	TCMR ABMR Mixed rejections	Serum creatinine Proteinuria DSA Protocol renal biopsy DD-cfDNA Gene expression	Cost-effectiveness data on routine DSA monitoring is lacking, Utility of DD-cfDNA and gene expression markers have not been adopted uniformly.
Hematological parameters	Leukopenia Anemia (bone marrow suppression, hemolysis, Parvovirus B19) Post-transplant erythrocytosis	Blood counts Hemolysis labs Parvovirus B19 NAAT	Leukopenia often peaks around 30–90 days; Hemolytic anemia, though rare, can occur due to drug-induced TMA or from dapsone-related hemolysis
Infections	BKV CMV Recurrent UTIs Vaccinations	BKV NAAT (blood/urine) CMV NAAT (blood)	Screening or treatment of asymptomatic UTI is not recommended.
Cancer	PTLD (EBV+)	EBV NAAT (Blood)	EBV monitoring may benefit high-risk EBV recipients; Role of monitoring and preemptive therapy has not been established.
Others	Hypertension Electrolyte disorder Tertiary hyperparathyroidism New onset of diabetes	BP measurement Electrolytes Serum PTH, Vit D, Calcium, phosphorus FBS, HbA1c	Periodic monitoring will detect abnormalities

Abbreviations: ABMR: antibody-mediated rejection, BKV: BK virus, CMV: cytomegalovirus, DD-cfDNA: donor-derived cell-free DNA, DGF: delayed graft function, DM: diabetes mellitus, DSA: donor-specific antibody, EBV: Epstein-Barr virus, FBS: fasting blood sugar, HbA1c: hemoglobin A1c, NAAT: nucleic acid amplification testing, PTH: parathyroid hormone, PTLD: post-transplant lymphoproliferative disorder, TCMR: T-cell-mediated rejection, TMA: thrombotic microangiopathy, UTI: urinary tract infection.

Surgical Complications

Surgical complications such as wound infections, lymphoceles, perinephric hematomas, urinary leak, and obstructive uropathy add to significant morbidity, delay recovery, increase morbidity, lower quality of life, and increase healthcare costs. Comorbid conditions including DM, obesity, and frailty can significantly increase the risk for these events. Measures targeted at key risk factors that are potentially modifiable, such as obesity and frailty, need to be systematically evaluated prior to transplant, thereby creating a potential opportunity for appropriate intervention. Additionally, patients and caregivers should be provided education and support, if recovery from transplant is delayed, when patients need prolonged wound care management and additional procedures.

Renal Function

Incidence of delayed graft function (DGF) remains quite high, particularly among deceased donor KT (DDKT) recipients. Though often related to donor risk factors, some recipient characteristics such as obesity, systemic hypotension, and long dialysis vintage increase DGF risk. These factors also increase the risk of prolonged DGF,[2] which prolongs hospital length of stay, increases costs, and in some studies has been shown to be associated with inferior longer term graft function and survival. While DGF is often a result of donor disease and ischemic Acute Kidney Injury (AKI), physicians may wish to perform an allograft biopsy to rule out early recurrence of the original renal disease and/or rule out any underlying alloimmune injury. Biopsy may be particularly challenging among patients with obesity, who are at higher risk for DGF since they also have higher incidence of wound complications and concomitant CVD necessitating use of anticoagulants/antiplatelet agents. Continuation of dialysis and close monitoring may be particularly challenging for patients residing farther from transplant centers and will vary among different healthcare settings. Patients and family members will require emotional support and education, particularly in situations with prolonged DGF that may require continued dialysis treatments coupled with frequent visits to the transplant center, additional procedures, and sometimes changes to non-calcineurin-inhibitor-based immunosuppression regimens.

Contrarily, patients experiencing robust and rapid recovery of renal functions often experience significant changes and fluctuations in fluid status, blood pressure (BP), and electrolytes. Close monitoring with frequent labs, regular clinic visits, and home monitoring of BP and weight, and blood sugar among diabetic recipients, will allow for timely interventions (e.g., changes in antihypertensives and diuretics, electrolyte replacements, insulin, etc.) and reduce risk of adverse events and rehospitalizations.

Along with renal functions, patients should be regularly monitored for proteinuria. This will allow for early diagnosis of recurrent disease among those at risk for early recurrent kidney disease, such as focal segmental glomerulosclerosis (FSGS) and complement-mediated glomerular diseases. This will also allow for recognizing recurrence among those with unclear ESKD etiology and among patients whose native disease may have been attributed empirically to HTN. While routine monitoring of serological markers such as anti-neutrophil cytoplasmic antibody (ANCA), complements, or anti-phospholipase A2 receptor (anti-PLA2R) antibody is not universal, abnormal proteinuria and/or suboptimal renal functions should prompt evaluation for trends and levels of these serological markers of disease activity. While therapy remains suboptimal for diseases that recur aggressively in the early post-transplant period, the rapidly evolving landscape of sodium-glucose cotransporter 2 (SGLT-2) inhibitors and novel targeted renal therapeutics (e.g., FSGS, immunoglobin A nephropathy, lupus, ANCA-associated vasculitis) offer promise of significantly improving the management of these recurrent glomerular diseases. These are further discussed in Chapter 11, "Recurrent and De Novo Diseases after Transplantation."

Alloimmune Issues and Immunosuppression

Though wide variation exists in immunosuppression (IS) protocols across the world, in general, most patients are maintained on a combination of calcineurin inhibitor (CNI) and an antimetabolite (mycophenolate mofetil or azathioprine) with or without prednisone. Regular monitoring for therapeutic CNI drug levels in the early post-transplant phase is key to ensuring adequate level of IS. While the protocols vary across centers, generally it is reasonable to aim for tacrolimus trough levels of 8–12 ng/mL in the first 6 months followed by 6–10 ng/mL (6–12 months). If using cyclosporine, trough levels of 200–300 ng/mL (0–6 months) and 150–200 ng/mL (6–12 months) are reasonable provided there are no serious infections or side effects. Monitoring for mycophenolic acid (MPA) trough levels is not recommended given their poor correlation with drug exposure and clinical events. However, patients should be closely monitored for side effects that may require mycophenolate dose adjustments such as gastrointestinal issues, poor appetite, weight loss, and leukopenia. Patients should be regularly educated about potential side effects and the importance of medication adherence. Offering emotional support when side effects adversely impact quality of life is important so that patients are forthcoming when they are unable to tolerate medications. Finally, though the diagnosis of CNI nephrotoxicity is often one of exclusion, it is important to carefully evaluate select patients in the 1st year who might benefit from a CNI-free regimen such as one that incorporates the use of belatacept (among EBV seropositive recipients).

Despite the significant reduction in early post-transplant acute rejections over time, patients remain at heightened risk for alloimmune injury within the 1st post-transplant year. Risk is particularly high among those with preformed donor-specific antibodies (DSAs), prior transplants, and higher human leukocyte antigen (HLA) mismatch, and those receiving ABO-incompatible transplants. Increasingly, it has been recognized that subclinical rejection (both T cell mediated, and antibody mediated) makes up a significant proportion of this residual rejection risk. Both clinical and sub-clinical rejection (SCR) episodes in the early post-transplant phase have been shown to contribute to poor long-term graft outcomes.[3,4] This has led to increased interest in investigating methods for early and noninvasive detection of rejection as well as investigating newer therapies. Despite its limitations, serum creatinine remains a simple, reliable, and reproducible test for monitoring for clinical rejection episodes. However, it is a nonspecific marker of injury and is not sensitive for detecting small changes in renal impairment, which has increasingly led centers to perform protocol biopsies for identifying SCR. Given the cost, invasiveness, and potential risk of biopsies, several other novel biomarkers (such as peripheral blood DD-cfDNA and gene arrays) have been evaluated and used in select centers. These tests have not been adopted universally for routine monitoring of KT recipients due to higher cost, modest sensitivity and specificity, inability to differentiate acuity from chronicity, and lack of controlled studies showing improved outcomes. In addition, some of the markers are nonspecific injury markers and not alloimmune injury markers. Monitoring for DSAs, particularly among sensitized patients and in those with renal dysfunction can guide decision making regarding kidney biopsies.

Hematological Parameters

Anemia is common in the first few weeks owing to surgical losses, pre-existing anemia of chronic kidney disease (CKD), and bone marrow suppression from medications. When prolonged and/or severe, ruling out other etiologies such as hemolysis and parvovirus B19 infection is necessary (Table 2.2). Similarly, leukopenia occurs in around 30%–50% of KT recipients, peaks around 3 months, and generally improves/responds to antimetabolite dose reductions. Care should be

Table 2.2 Immunological and Medical Issues Seen during Middle Phase (1–5 Years Post-Transplant)

Topics	Problems/Issues	Monitoring	Comments
Renal function	GFR, CKD staging Recurrent disease	Serum creatinine Proteinuria	
Immunological events	Chronic T-cell rejection Chronic antibody-mediated rejection Acute T-cell- or antibody-mediated rejection. Mixed rejection De novo DSA	Serum Creatinine Proteinuria DSA Allograft biopsy	Rare in the absence of IS nonadherence. Routine monitoring with newer noninvasive markers is not cost-effective. Routine DSA monitoring has been recommended.
Hematological parameters	Leukopenia Post-transplant erythrocytosis	Blood counts	Anemia and leukopenia are uncommon. Rare patients may have prolonged leukopenia/neutropenia.
Infections	BKV CMV Opportunistic (other)	BKV NAAT (blood/urine) CMV NAAT	BKV infections beyond 2 years is rare. Refractory and resistant CMV infection can occur in high-risk CMV D+R- recipients
Chronic diseases	Weight gain–obesity DM HTN Cardiovascular health	FBS HbA1c	Lifestyle measures, use of newer anti-DM and antiobesity drugs, preferably in coordination with PCPs.
Vaccination and cancer screening	Periodic vaccines (inactivated) Skin cancer Native kidney cancer Other regular cancer screening	Dermatology visits for cancer screening	Ultrasound evaluation of native kidneys to detect cancer has not been uniformly adopted
Miscellaneous	Pregnancy AVF and cardiovascular disease	AVF doppler	Close monitoring of CNI levels in pregnancy. Consider echocardiography if features of heart failure/volume overload in those with large proximal AVF

Abbreviations: AVF: arteriovenous fistula, BKV: BK virus, CKD: chronic kidney disease, CNI: calcineurin inhibitor, DM: diabetes mellitus, DSA: donor-specific antibody, FBS: fasting blood sugar, HbA1c: hemoglobin A1c, HTN: hypertension, NAAT: nucleic acid amplification testing, PCP: primary care provider.

taken to not reduce valganciclovir dose, particularly among those with high-risk CMV transplants.

Infectious Disease

Kidney transplant recipients are at risk for both routine as well as opportunistic infections, which greatly increase their morbidity and mortality. Monitoring protocols should align with the changing pattern of post-KT infections. Cytomegalovirus (CMV) and BK virus infections are the most common opportunistic viral infections among KT recipients. Monitoring for CMV viremia is needed among patients being managed without prophylaxis (i.e., preemptive approach) and among high-risk CMV (D+R-) recipients after completing prophylaxis. Given the lack of effective anti-BK therapies, regular monitoring and IS reduction remains the cornerstone of preventing severe BKV infections and nephropathy. Since missed surveillance can delay timely diagnosis of CMV and BK, patients should be educated to not miss regular lab tests. Additionally, among those undergoing significant IS reduction, careful monitoring for renal function for rejections and DSA formation is necessary. Screening for hepatitis C and B and human immunodeficiency virus (HIV) infections is also necessary for those receiving kidneys from Hep B/C-positive donors or from donors considered as increased-risk donors. Finally, for the approximately 5%–10% of KT recipients who have a high-risk Epstein-Barr virus (EBV) serostatus (D+R-), monitoring for EBV viremia in the first year of transplantation is reasonable, as higher levels of viremia has been shown to correlate with the occurrence of post-transplant lymphoproliferative disorder (PTLD).[5] It should, however, be noted that a specific viremic threshold has not been established and diagnosis of PTLD is based on clinical symptoms and pathology.

Miscellaneous

Approximately 10%–20% can develop post-transplant DM and hence require close monitoring of fasting sugars and hemoglobin A1Cs during the first year. Monitoring parameters of mineral bone disease (calcium, phosphorus, and parathyroid hormone) is also necessary given the risk for tertiary hyperparathyroidism, hypercalcemia, and hypophosphatemia in the early post-transplant phase. Kidney transplant recipients of childbearing age should be counseled regarding the teratogenic risks associated with mycophenolate mofetil. They should also be advised to delay pregnancy until at least a year after transplantation. This topic is discussed in detail in Chapter 3, "Wellness after Kidney Transplantation."

Middle Phase (1–5 Years Post-Transplant)

As patients move beyond the early post-transplant phase, the focus shifts away from the immediate perioperative challenges and adaptation of functioning kidney toward the long-term consequences of under- or over-immunosuppression, and chronic medical issues related to impaired renal function and lifestyle factors (Table 2.2).

Renal Function/CKD Management

While kidney transplantation restores renal excretory and metabolic functions to a significant level, patients often have varying levels of CKD and associated manifestations. Except for patients with poor early outcomes, most patients have mild to moderate CKD during the first few years after transplantation. CKD management in the nontransplant setting is heavily focused on the use of antiproteinuric therapies (renin-angiotensin-aldosterone-system [RAAS] inhibitors) and SGLT-2 inhibitors to reduce CKD progression. In contrast, in the absence of recurrent disease and chronic antibody-mediated rejection (ABMR), significant proteinuria is uncommon and conclusive evidence for the benefits of optimizing RAAS therapy in transplant recipients is lacking. Additionally, CNI-mediated hyperkalemia, anemia, and renal impairment are major barriers to optimizing RAAS therapy. The availability of novel potassium-binding resins has been a welcome improvement in this regard and can allow for maximizing RAAS therapy when indicated. Optimal strategies for management of bone disease after transplant also remain unclear. Better renal function post-KT significantly improves the metabolic bone disease, though residual issues remain and new challenges occur in the form of chronic steroid therapy.[6] Tertiary hyperparathyroidism is common after KT and is often treated with cinacalcet but sometimes with subtotal parathyroidectomy. Impact of screening and managing secondary hyperparathyroidism and osteoporosis on long-term skeletal health of KT recipients remains poorly studied.

Alloimmune Issues and Immunosuppression

While the risk of alloimmune events persist throughout the post-transplant period, the overall incidence per unit time is significantly lower as patients move beyond the 1st post-transplant year. There however remain a subset of patients who will either have recurrent or persistent rejections and will as a result experience inferior long-term outcome. While these patients do not necessarily fit into a specific clinical phenotype, there are some common risk factors that can be used to further risk stratify patients at the one1year mark. These include a combination of biological factors (e.g., HLA mismatch, prior rejections, presence of DSAs) and behavioral/social factors that increase the risk of medication nonadherence (e.g., financial, health literacy, support systems). Current processes of care do not systematically identify patients at high risk of alloimmune events. This leads to missed opportunities to potentially modify the long-term trajectories. While the lack of effective and therapies targeted toward chronic active ABMR and resistant T-cell-mediated rejection (TCMR) is a key driver of inferior outcomes, we must also acknowledge the contribution of patients not being on optimized regimens of currently available effective IS medications. Ensuring that patients are on optimized IS will require a more personalized approach to patient management with channeling of appropriate resources (coordinator, social worker) to high-risk groups. Since resources are limited, studies should investigate cost-effective methods to provide this type of care. While it is very reasonable to reduce the frequency of clinic visits and labs as patients move beyond the 1st year, there should be systems in place to screen for patients at risk for or already deviating from a favorable post-transplant trajectory. Increased use of telehealth technologies may be beneficial in this regard. Tacrolimus trough levels should be preferably maintained at >5 ng/mL in most patients since levels <5 ng/mL have been associated with development of de novo DSAs.[7] Continued monitoring for immunosuppression-related adverse events (recurrent infections, tumors, and severe cytopenia) remains essential along with appropriate and careful dose modifications. Prospective studies evaluating best methods of preventing chronic subclinical alloimmune injury are urgently needed.

Infectious Disease

Though most BKV and CMV infections occur in the 1st-year post-transplant, late-onset BK and CMV can occur beyond the 1st year as well. While monitoring for CMV is not cost-effective beyond the 1st year (except in those with recurrent CMV), it is prudent to continue monitoring for BK beyond year 1 (2–4 times in year 2); the role of subsequent screening remains unclear. Vaccinations to prevent influenza and pneumococcal pneumonia remain essential. For patients with recurrent urinary tract infections, prophylactic antibiotic therapy should be considered.

Chronic Diseases

There is a high prevalence of chronic diseases among KT recipients due to a combination of pre-existing diseases and risk for developing de novo issues after transplantation. Effective management of these is necessary for successful transplant outcomes. This will generally require close coordination between the transplant team, primary care providers (PCPs), and other subspecialists involved. Specific issues and opportunities are noted below.

Obesity and DM

Availability of several novel effective agents for DM-2 (SGLT-2 inhibitors, glucagon-like peptide-1 [GLP-1] agonists) and obesity (GLP-1 agonists) has tremendously expanded the therapeutic options for KT recipients affected by these conditions. While effectiveness and risk data are mostly extrapolated from studies done in the nontransplant population, there is appropriate enthusiasm for their adoption to manage these conditions in KT recipients. While early experience in KT settings suggest that SGLT-2 inhibitors are safe, continued monitoring for any potential increased risk for adverse events (infections, amputations, etc.) is necessary.[8] Similarly, effective use of GLP-1 agonists for obesity management will require considerations of access to medications and cost-effectiveness among various subgroups.[9]

Hypertension, Hyperlipidemia, and Cardiovascular Disease

Despite a high prevalence of hyperlipidemia among KT recipients, there is lack of definitive data showing effectiveness of statin therapy in those without prior established CVD.[10] Nevertheless, given the high incidence of coronary artery disease (CAD) and its significant contribution to mortality among KT recipients, optimizing hyperlipidemia therapies seem prudent and is recommended by major **medical** societies. Regarding HTN, while a specific trial among KT recipients comparing less intense versus more intense BP control has not been done, observational data provides some evidence regarding potential benefit from tighter control of BP.[11] Given the risks for adverse events associated with intense BP control, until definitive studies are available, ensuring a BP goal of <130/80 seems prudent. Encouraging and educating patients to be actively involved in lifestyle management, medication and diet adherence, and home monitoring (BP and glucose levels) is important.

Vaccination and Cancer Screening

Kidney transplant recipients face unique challenges with regard to vaccine-preventable diseases and cancer screening. Patients are at higher infection risk but are also exposed to additional risk due to inability to receive live vaccines and from inadequate response to inactivated vaccines. Emerging research, particularly in the setting of the coronavirus disease-2019 (COVID-19) pandemic has offered invaluable insight into the benefits and limitations of repeated vaccination and use of monoclonal antibodies for prevention. The partial effectiveness of vaccines among transplant recipients is compounded by skepticism over their safety and effectiveness. Despite biological plausibility, there has generally been no conclusive evidence for an elevated risk of rejection in the setting of vaccination. Healthcare providers (HCPs) should continue to reinforce to patients the benefits of periodic vaccination to prevent morbidity and mortality from common infections (e.g., influenza, pneumococcal disease; COVID-19, zoster). This topic is discussed in detail in Chapter 3, "Wellness after Kidney Transplantation."

Along with routine cancer screening that is applicable to the general population, at-risk transplant recipients should undergo periodic surveillance for skin malignancies given the significantly increased incidence and contribution to morbidity/mortality. Additionally, continued education regarding the benefits of avoiding intense sunburns should occur beginning at the pretransplant phase and continuing well after transplant. This topic is discussed in detail in Chapter 10, "Cancer after Kidney Transplantation."

Pregnancy

The relatively stable middle post-transplant phase offers the best opportunity for patients interested in pregnancy. Patients should be educated about the high-risk nature of pregnancy. Pregnancies should be planned with appropriate changes to immunosuppression (switching mycophenolate to azathioprine) prior to conception. Patient will also need close follow-up with monitoring of IS levels, proteinuria, blood pressure, and renal functions. Involving obstetric teams experienced in high-risk patients will be useful. This topic is discussed in detail in Chapter 3, "Wellness after Kidney Transplantation."

Arteriovenous Fistula

Large arteriovenous fistulas (AVFs) are associated with left ventricular hypertrophy, pulmonary hypertension, and high-output heart failure. Therefore, in patients with large AVFs, periodic clinical evaluation for symptoms of heart failure is useful to identify patients who may benefit from AVF doppler study to evaluate flows and echocardiography. The decision to ligate a functioning AVF should be done using shared decision-making after considering the risks and benefits.[12] Ligation or banding can be considered in those with stable renal function, and having an AVF flow >2 L/min with or without signs of CHF/pulmonary HTN.

Late Phase (Long-Term; >5 Years Post-Transplant)

The prevalence of KT recipients with a functioning kidney continues to increase worldwide given the significant improvements in the short-term survival and the increase in number of transplants. Most patients generally are in a "stable" phase as they go beyond the first few years of their transplant journey and thus require less intense monitoring. However, there is still a need to actively monitor for several issues including identifying patients that may be having a decline in renal function or a failing kidney and/or those developing complications from long-term immunosuppression (Table 2.3). Ensuring adequate health maintenance and preventative measures and good adherence to medications and follow-up remain paramount.

Renal Function: CKD Management, Failing Allograft

As the number of patients living with a functioning transplant continues to grow, an increasing number of patients will be faced with the consequences of a failing allograft. These consequences can be varied and are dependent on the cause and rapidity of decline in renal function. Patients experiencing slowly progressive CKD are best placed for pre-ESKD planning (dialysis, retransplant, or conservative care). For such patients, education regarding the natural history, lifestyle measures, bone health, and attention to pre-ESKD planning is key to improving chances of a timely repeat transplant as well as avoiding emergent dialysis starts. However, those experiencing abrupt onset of allograft failure either due to an episode of acute kidney injury (AKI) or due to acute rejection, often in the setting of nonadherence, are at significantly higher risk of morbidity and mortality. This is due to a combination of coexisting medical issues, effects of intense immunosuppression for treatment of rejection episodes, and chronic inflammation from a failing kidney. While gradual cessation of immunosuppression after graft failure is reasonable to reduce the long-term risk of infectious complications, it does increase the risk of allosensitization and the occurrence of symptomatic allograft inflammation. This in turn negatively affects the chances of retransplantation, and frequently also necessitates allograft nephrectomy. Management of failing and failed allograft is discussed further in Chapter 17, "Management of Patients with Failing Kidney and Failed Kidney Transplant."

Immunological Events and Medication Adherence

Ensuring medication adherence remains critical as suboptimal adherence is the key driver for acute and chronic rejection among patients in this late post-transplant phase. While several methods (self-report, electronic pill bottle monitoring, therapeutic drug level monitoring, etc.) have been investigated,

Table 2.3 Immunological and Medical Issues during Late Phase (>5 Years Post-Transplant)

Topics	Problems/Issues	Monitoring	Comments
Renal function	CKD Recurrent Disease Failing allograft	Serum Creatinine Proteinuria Anemia of CKD Secondary hyperparathyroidism	CKD management Identifying late onset glomerular diseases [IGA nephropathy, Membranous Nephropathy, Diabetic Nephropathy] Transition of care to nephrology for failing and failed grafts
Immunological events	Chronic T-cell rejection Chronic Ab-Mediated Rejection De novo DSA Mixed Rejection	Serum Creatinine Proteinuria	Rare in the absence of IS non-adherence
Infections	Opportunistic (other)	Various fungal infection and TB (in select countries)	
Chronic diseases	Obesity DM, HTN, Lipidemia and Gout Cardiovascular & Cerebrovascular diseases	Metabolic profiles (HbA1c, lipids)	
Vaccination and cancer screening	Periodic vaccines (inactivated) Skin cancer Other regular cancer screening	Dermatology visits Cancer screening	
Miscellaneous	Pregnancy Terminal illness/ failure to thrive.		Palliative/conservative care options should be made available for appropriate patients

Abbreviations: CKD: chronic kidney disease, DM: diabetes mellitus, DSA: donor-specific antibody, FBS: fasting blood sugar, HbA1c: hemoglobin A1c, HTN: hypertension, IS: immunosuppression, PCP: primary care providers.

these have not translated to clinical use to the degree necessary. Also, since clinic visits and lab monitoring during this post-transplant phase occur at lower frequency, monitoring for nonadherence is challenging. Therefore, ongoing patient education regarding adherence is necessary at every encounter and the role of telehealth and/or nurse coordinator for active surveillance needs further investigation. Measures aimed at reducing IS nonadherence, if effective, can significantly reduce the risk of early allograft failures and HLA sensitization and can reduce healthcare expenses. Adherence to medical therapy is discussed further in Chapter 13, "Social Determinants Impacting Transplant Outcome."

Chronic Diseases, Cancer, and Health Maintenance

Long-term immunosuppression and CKD coexist and contribute to the high burden of chronic diseases (HTN, CVD, etc.), opportunistic infections, and cancers experienced by transplant recipients. Adequate management and appropriate preventive measures require good care coordination between patients' primary providers and the transplant teams. Patients should receive regular education and counseling regarding healthy lifestyle measures, periodic vaccinations, and cancer screening (including skin cancer). These are addressed in more detail in Chapter 3, "Wellness after Kidney Transplantation," and Chapter 10, "Cancers after Kidney Transplantation."

Miscellaneous

For patients experiencing a chronic terminal illness due to a serious infection, malignancy, or failed allograft (with no retransplant options and doing poorly on dialysis), appropriate resources should be in place to provide timely and informed care coordinated with a palliative care team. This will prepare patients and families well and limit inappropriate medical care that impairs quality of life and increases healthcare costs.

Social Support System for Each Phase

The entire journey of going through a transplant evaluation, receiving a transplant, and ensuring a successful outcome is a complex endeavor. While many patients independently manage the entire process well, most are likely to fare better if they have adequate family, financial, and social support to assist in transplant care. The nature and intensity of support will vary based on the phase patients are in. Patients in the early post-transplant phase generally need the most intensive support. A good support system is also key for patients with other limitations such as those with limited health literacy, financial constraints, and poor mobility and/or travel limitations. Support system is particularly key when considering transplant among those with intellectual disability, limited health literacy, and visual and physical disability—as they will need assistance with medication intake, labs, and clinic follow-up throughout their transplant journey.

Future Directions

Comprehensive care, solid support systems, and ongoing research are leading to better long-term survival for KT recipients. While the long-term success of a KT is dependent on several factors, adequate long-term monitoring, clinical follow-up, care coordination, and support systems are highly essential for ensuring a successful transplant outcome. While how these are achieved will vary based on the healthcare setting, studies demonstrating the most cost-effective way of doing this are needed. Table 2.4 highlights potential opportunities and research

Table 2.4 Few Novel Opportunities for Research towards Improving Care for the Transplant Patients

Topics	Suggested research opportunities
Monitoring alloimmune events	Assess whether routine monitoring with newer biomarkers: Improves transplant outcomes, Reduces need for transplant biopsies, Is cost-effective, and Has utility in late alloimmune injury.
Improving medication adherence and chronic disease management	Evaluate whether tools via EHR, telehealth, and tablet/phone are useful for identifying patients at risk for nonadherence. Evaluate providing increased post-transplant coordination and social support to optimize adherence and improving outcome.
Recurrent diseases	Assess whether monitoring serological markers is useful for Stratifying recurrence risk and Identifying patients that may benefit from targeted therapies.
Failing allograft	Identify subgroups who may benefit from lower doses of immunosuppression. Improve pre-ESKD care to facilitate higher rates of preemptive retransplantation, Avoid unplanned dialysis initiation for ESKD
Chronic diseases and health maintenance	Evaluate long-term safety and utility of SGLT-2 inhibitors in KT recipients. Examine role of GLP-1 agonists for weight loss in KT recipients
Cancer	Assess role of EBV monitoring in EBV D+R- recipients who are at risk for EBV-related PTLD Assess the role of various immunomodulatory therapy for cancers
Miscellaneous	Assess role of monitoring for pulmonary hypertension in those with patent AVF

Abbreviations: AVF: arteriovenous fistula, EBV: Epstein-Barr virus, ESKD: end-stage kidney disease, EHR: electronic health record, GLP-1: glucagon-like peptide 1, PTLD: post-transplant lymphoproliferative disorder, SGLT-2: sodium-glucose cotransporter 2.

topics geared toward improving care for transplant patients through their post-transplant course.

Conclusion

In summary, while improvements in graft and patient survival among KT recipients are laudable, much needs to be done to further improve long-term outcomes. Patients and HCPs are faced with ever-changing challenges as patients go through the different post-transplant phases (<1 year, 1–5 years, and >5 years). While intense monitoring and focus on early events remain vital, it is important that KT recipients remain under long-term effective surveillance and management in several key clinical domains (allograft function, adherence, immunological events, infections, cancer, and cardiovascular health). Ensuring this is particularly challenging as patients go beyond the early post-transplant phase. Therefore, studies investigating cost-effective ways of implementing long-term monitoring, improving medication adherence, managing chronic metabolic disease, preventing infection and cancer, and coordinating post-transplant care are highly necessary.

References

1. Hariharan S, Israni AK, Danovitch G. Long-term survival after kidney transplantation. *N Engl J Med.* 2021;385(8):729–743. https://doi.org/10.1056/NEJMra2014530.
2. Wazir S, Abbas M, Ratanasrimetha P, Zhang C, Hariharan S, Puttarajappa CM. Preoperative blood pressure and risk of delayed graft function in deceased donor kidney transplantation. *Clin Transplant.* 2022;36(9):e14776. https://doi.org/10.1111/ctr.14776.
3. Clayton PA, McDonald SP, Russ GR, Chadban SJ. Long-term outcomes after acute rejection in kidney transplant recipients: an ANZDATA analysis. *J Am Soc Nephrol.* 2019;30(9):1697–1707. https://doi.org/10.1681/asn.2018111101.
4. Mehta RB, Melgarejo I, Viswanathan V, et al. Long-term immunological outcomes of early subclinical inflammation on surveillance kidney allograft biopsies. *Kidney Int.* 2022;102(6):1371–1381. https://doi.org/10.1016/j.kint.2022.07.030.
5. Tsai DE, Douglas L, Andreadis C, et al. EBV PCR in the diagnosis and monitoring of posttransplant lymphoproliferative disorder: results of a two-arm prospective trial. *Am J Transplant* 2008;8(5):1016–1024. https://doi.org/10.1111/j.1600-6143.2008.02183.x.
6. Disthabanchong S. Persistent hyperparathyroidism in long-term kidney transplantation: time to consider a less aggressive approach. *Curr Opin Nephrol Hypertens.* 2023;32(1):20–26. https://doi.org/10.1097/mnh.0000000000000840.
7. Wiebe C, Rush DN, Nevins TE, et al. Class II eplet mismatch modulates tacrolimus trough levels required to prevent donor-specific antibody development. *J Am Soc Nephrol.* 2017;28(11):3353–3362. https://doi.org/10.1681/asn.2017030287.

8. Ujjawal A, Schreiber B, Verma A. Sodium-glucose cotransporter-2 inhibitors (SGLT2i) in kidney transplant recipients: what is the evidence? *Ther Adv Endocrinol Metab.* 2022;13:20420188221090001. https://doi.org/10.1177/20420188221090001.

9. Baig K, Dusetzina SB, Kim DD, Leech AA. Medicare part D coverage of antiobesity medications—challenges and uncertainty ahead. *N Engl J Med.* 2023;388(11):961–963. https://doi.org/10.1056/NEJMp2300516.

10. Palmer SC, Navaneethan SD, Craig JC, et al. HMG CoA reductase inhibitors (statins) for kidney transplant recipients. *Cochrane Database of Syst Rev.* 2014;2014(1):Cd005019. https://doi.org/10.1002/14651858.CD005019.pub4.

11. Ku E, McCulloch CE, Inker LA, et al. Intensive BP control in patients with CKD and risk for adverse outcomes. *J Am Soc Nephrol.* 2023;34(3):385–393. https://doi.org/10.1681/asn.0000000000000072.

12. Rao NN, Stokes MB, Rajwani A, et al. Effects of arteriovenous fistula ligation on cardiac structure and function in kidney transplant recipients. *Circulation.* 2019;139(25):2809–2818. https://doi.org/10.1161/circulationaha.118.038505.

3

Wellness after Kidney Transplantation

Christine M. Wu and Mona D. Doshi

Maintenance of good health is critical for long-term success after kidney transplantation!

Introduction to Transplant Wellness

There is a difference between being alive and living. Wellness in life is derived from positive relationships with family and friends, spiritual health, engagement in meaningful work, participation in hobbies, and ability to travel and engage with the world. Kidney transplant (KT) provides independence from dialysis and improved life expectancy with better quality of life, a term that encompasses the interdependent dimensions of physical, mental/emotional, social, spiritual, vocational, financial, and environmental health.[1] This chapter will address some important aspects of long-term wellness after kidney transplantation including (1) immunization, (2) family planning and reproductive health, (3) cancer screening, and (4) return to work after transplantation. The transplant community can help patients to maximize their quality-of-life following transplantation.

Immunization

The subject of immunization is an integral part of managing transplant patients. Vaccines remain underutilized, and vaccine preventable disease accounts for a significant proportion of morbidity and mortality in immunosuppressed KT recipients. However, immune response remains suboptimal in immunosuppressed transplant patients. A large Medicare study reports that only 18.7% of patients received an influenza vaccine within the first year of transplant. Influenza vaccination is associated with a lower rate of death (HR 0.82, $p < 0.001$) without any increase in acute rejection.[2] All medical providers should educate transplant patients and their households about vaccination, recommending and, when possible, administering vaccines to them. The benefit of immunizing close contacts to create a "safe pod" or "circle of protection" was highlighted during the COVID-19 pandemic and applies for all vaccine-preventable illnesses. This effective strategy has been demonstrated with influenza, where vaccination of healthcare providers in long-term care facilities was found to decrease the mortality risk of elderly residents.[3] A summary of vaccination for KT patients is illustrated in Table 3.1.

Guidelines for Vaccination

The Infectious Disease Society of America (IDSA) published its evidence-based *Clinical Practice Guidelines for Vaccination of the Immunocompromised Host* in 2013.[4] Updated recommendations were subsequently published in 2019 by the American Society of Transplantation Infectious Diseases Community of Practice in Clinical Transplantation.[5] Annual updates in the United States are published by the Centers for Disease Control and Prevention (CDC-ACIP), and the most recent recommendations are summarized below.

Timing and Type of Vaccination

Response to vaccination, as has been unequivocally demonstrated in the case of hepatitis B, declines with progression to chronic kidney disease (CKD) and with immunosuppression. Therefore, patients need a higher dose and/or an additional booster dose. Assessment of vaccination status should be undertaken prior to transplantation or even prior to development of end-stage kidney disease (ESKD). In the best-case scenario, transplant candidates and their household members, including pets, should receive all recommended vaccines prior to transplant—with inactivated vaccines given at least 2 weeks prior, and live attenuated vaccines at least 4 weeks prior to transplantation. For patients who did not receive vaccination prior to transplantation, live attenuated vaccines are not advised after transplantation. For inactivated vaccines, American Society of Transplantation (AST) and IDSA recommends they be given 3–6 months after transplant, except for influenza vaccination, which can be administered as early as 1 month post-transplant, based on the time of year and community risk. Household members can receive recommended inactivated vaccines at any time. If live vaccines are administered to household members, transplant patients should take appropriate precautions to limit exposure, especially to symptomatic individuals, and to monitor closely for the development of symptoms. Symptomatic infection from transmission of virus from live attenuated vaccines to immunosuppressed individuals is rare, and illness is likely to be less severe than infection from wild-type virus.

Table 3.1 Recommended Immunizations for Kidney Transplant Recipients (Adapted from IDSA and CDC-ACIP guidelines)

Infectious organism	Available vaccines, vaccine type	Administration schedule	Recommended prior to transplant	Recommended/safety after transplant*	Recommended for household contacts
Hepatitis B	Recombivax HB, recombinant vaccine (should be administered in deltoid rather than gluteal muscle)	Early CKD: 5 mcg dose at time 0, 1, and 6 months. Advanced CKD/ESKD: 40 mcg dose at time 0, 1, and 6 months. Accelerated schedule: Time 0, 7, 21 days (check anti-HBsAb titer 4 weeks after complete series for response adequacy (>10 IU/mL)	Yes	Safe, but response unlikely	
influenza	IM injection, Inactivated	Yearly in Fall season (consider geographical variability of flu season for travel)	Yes	Yes, as soon as 1 month after Transplant	Yes
influenza	Intranasal, Live attenuated	Yearly in Fall	Yes	No	Yes** if healthy, age 2–49, nonpregnant
pneumococcus	13-, 15-, 20-valent protein-conjugated (PCV13/15/20) and 23-valent polysaccharide pneumococcal vaccine (PPSV23)	PCV 13/15/20 (preferred) followed by PPSV23 after ≥ 8 weeks. If PPSV23 only previously given, PCV20 after ≥ 1 year. If any PCV only given, PPSV23 after ≥ 1 year. If PCV13 (and not PCV 15 or 20) was given, consider PPSV23 every 5–10 years or a one-time dose age ≥ 65 if more than 5 years since last dose	Yes	Yes	Yes

Vaccine	Type	Recommendations			
Meningococcus	ACWY, quadrivalent vaccination (meningococcal B vaccine is available but not yet tested in transplant population)	1st dose for ages 11–18 or any high-risk individual over 2 months of age.*** Booster after 5 years in high-risk individuals	Yes	Yes	Yes
Measles, mumps, rubella	MMR, live attenuated		Yes****	No	Yes*
Diphtheria, Tetanus, Pertussis	TDaP Td, diphtheria and tetanus toxoid (inactivated proteins) and acellular pertussis antigens	Once prior to age 18, then every 10 years (single TDaP recommended after age 18, then Td for subsequent boosters every 10 years or after serious wound)	Yes	Yes	Yes
Varicella (VZV)	Live attenuated	Seronegative adults should receive one dose with repeat if seronegative on postvaccination testing at 4 weeks	Yes****	No (Although cautious use in pediatric patients on low-dose maintenance immunosuppression can be considered.)	Yes**
Herpes zoster (HZV)	Shingrix, recombinant vaccine	Recommended for all KTR ≥ 19 years old. 2 doses given 2–6 months apart (need for revaccination if patients ≤ 50 remains unknown)	Yes	Yes	Yes
Human papillomavirus (HPV)	9-valent Gardisil 9 (currently only one available in US), quadrivalent Gardisil 4, bivalent Cervarix. inactivated	Recommended for ages 11–12, catch up through age 26 (approved in US up to age 45 but may not be covered by insurance after age 26). 3-shot series given at time 0, 1–2 months, 6 months.	Yes	Yes	Yes

(continued)

Table 3.1 Continued

Infectious organism	Available vaccines, vaccine type	Administration schedule	Recommended prior to transplant	Recommended after transplant	Recommended/safety after transplant*	Recommended for household contacts
SARS-CoV2/ COVID 19	mRNA vaccines (Pfizer and Moderna monovalent and bivalent)	1–3 doses monovalent given 4 weeks apart followed by up to 4 bivalent boosters at least 8 weeks apart	Yes		Yes	Yes
Travel vaccines						
Oral polio	Live attenuated			No	No	No
Oral typhoid	Live attenuated			No	No	Yes**
Yellow Fever	Live attenuated			No	No	Yes**
Miscellaneous childhood vaccines						
rotavirus	Live attenuated	Infants age 2–7 months	No		No	Yes**(Effort should be made to avoid diapers for 4 weeks)

*Recommended waiting time of at least 2 months post-transplant in KT recipients.

**Precautions should be taken to avoid infection of the transplant recipient and to monitor closely for development of symptoms. When possible, KT recipients should consider use of barrier protection (masks, gloves) and minimizing contact with bodily secretions of their vaccinated children during the period of active post-vaccination viral shedding.

***High risk for meningococcal infection: member of military, college freshmen living on campus, travelers to high-risk areas, properdin or terminal complement component deficiency or patients receiving complement inhibitor therapy, or anatomic/functional asplenia. Patients receiving eculizumab should receive ACYW at least 2 weeks prior to initiating therapy.

***In general, administration of live virus vaccines should be completed ≥ 4 weeks prior to transplant.

*****No current vaccines are available for prevention of CMV, EBV, BK, or HCV.

Specific Vaccination

This section addresses prevention of viral infections through vaccination for various viruses.

Hepatitis B
Vaccine efficacy diminishes with progression to ESKD and should be considered at earlier stages of CKD. An accelerated schedule (at days 0, 7, and 21) can be attempted prior to transplant if time is limited for a preemptive living kidney transplant. Higher vaccine dose (40 mcg) is recommended with ESKD. Postvaccination antibody titers are recommended at approximately 4 weeks postvaccination to assess for adequate protection (anti-HBs titer >10 IU/mL).

Influenza
Influenza vaccine can be administered as early as 1 month following transplant during influenza season. Inactivated high-dose influenza vaccination is recommended. Because of suboptimal immune response to vaccination during the early post-transplant phase, revaccination can be considered in 3–6 months based on time of year. Live attenuated vaccination with intranasal influenza vaccination is not recommended and if inadvertently given, should be managed with antivirals with revaccination using inactivated vaccine. Every effort should be made to give inactivated vaccine to household contacts, but if only live attenuated vaccine can be given, precautions should be taken to prevent infection of the transplant patient.

Pneumococcal Vaccination
Both the 13- or 15-valent protein-conjugated (PCV13 or PCV 15) and 23-valent polysaccharide pneumococcal vaccine (PPSV23) are recommended. If neither has been given pretransplant, PCV13 is recommended first, followed by PPSV23 after 8 weeks. If only PPSV23 has been given, a single repeat dose of PCV23 is recommended at least 1 year after the PPSV23 dose. A PPSV23 booster is recommended for immunosuppressed solid organ transplant recipients 5 years after the first dose. If this booster is given before age 65, a final dose of PPSV23 can be considered after age 65 and 5 years after the previous dose.

Meningococcal Vaccination
Quadrivalent meningococcal vaccination (ACYW) is recommended for all patients ages 11 to 18 years. In addition, any patients over 2 months of age who meet any of the following criteria—member of military, college freshmen living on campus, travelers to high-risk areas, properdin or terminal complement component deficiency or patients receiving complement inhibitor therapy, or

anatomic/functional asplenia—should also receive ACYW before or after transplant. ACYW should be administered at least 2 weeks prior to the first dose of eculizumab. An ACYW booster should be administered every 5 years to at-risk individuals. Serological testing for vaccine response is not available outside of the research setting. Meningococcal B vaccination may also be given to at-risk adults and adolescents with clinical discretion but has not yet been evaluated in transplant recipients.

Measles, Mumps, and Rubella Vaccination
Measles, mumps, and rubella (MMR) vaccine is a live-attenuated vaccine and is recommended prior to transplantation and not after transplant. A series of two doses, regardless of serology, is considered sufficient for immunity. In an outbreak setting, MMR vaccination may be considered for immunosuppressed KT recipients with informed consent and close follow-up.

Diphtheria, Tetanus, and Pertussis Vaccination

A single diphtheria, tetanus, and pertussis (TDaP) booster dose is recommended after age 18. Tetanus and diphtheria are recommended every 10 years or after a serious wound (puncture, cut, bite, burn, etc.).

Varicella Vaccination
Vaccination against varicella-zoster virus (VZV) should be considered prior to transplant as chicken pox can be very severe in seronegative immunocompromised adults. VZV vaccine is a live-attenuated vaccine, thus recommended *prior* to transplant in seronegative individuals and not after transplant. Seronegative adults should receive one dose of vaccine with postvaccination serologic testing, and repeat vaccination if seroconversion is not seen, at least 4 weeks prior to transplant. Postexposure prophylaxis should be considered for transplant patients without immunity.

Herpes Zoster Vaccination
Herpes zoster virus (HZV) vaccination is strongly recommended for all transplant candidates 19 years of age and older (50 years and older in the general population). Subunit vaccination can be given safely both prior to and after transplantation. Shingrix is a dead, recombinant vaccine given in 2 doses 2–6 months apart and appears to be safe.

Human Papillomavirus Vaccination
Human papillomavirus (HPV) vaccination is routinely given to children between the ages of 11–12 in the United States. Catch-up vaccination is recommended

up to age 26. It is also approved in the United States for individuals up to age 45. HPV vaccination can be given 3–6 months after transplant (3 shot series at months 0, 1–2, and 6). Three inactive HPV vaccines are FDA approved for use in the United States, but only Gardasil 9 (9-valent vaccine) is currently available.

COVID-19

Recommendations regarding COVID vaccination for KT patients continue to evolve. Both Moderna and Pfizer monovalent mRNA vaccines are recommended in a primary series up to 3 doses at least 4 weeks apart with additional periodic booster doses of the bivalent vaccine. Pre-exposure prophylaxis with Evusheld (tixagevimab-cilgavimab) was approved in the United States under emergency use authorization for those who do not tolerate vaccination or fail to mount an antibody response, for protection against COVID-19 infection in immunosuppressed KT patients. However, Evusheld appears to offer less protection against some of the newer subvariants of the Omicron strain (BA.4.6, BF.7, BA.2.75.2, BQ1, BQ1.1, etc). At this time, it is not available for use in the United States.

Cytomegalovirus Vaccination

Effective vaccination against cytomegalovirus (CMV) remains a current unmet need in kidney transplantation and is being investigated.

Vaccination prior to International Travel

Many transplant providers recommend against travel to areas at high-risk for communicable disease within the first year post-transplant. Patients should be referred to travel clinics 12 weeks prior to departure to allow adequate time for serologic testing and administration of vaccinations and boosters. Influenza seasons and strains differ between hemispheres (October–March in the Northern Hemisphere, April–September in the Southern Hemisphere, year-round in the tropics).

Live Virus Vaccines

Live virus vaccines such as nasal influenza, yellow fever, oral typhoid, oral polio, and Bacille Calmette-Guerin (BCG) are not recommended for immunosuppressed KT recipients but can, other than oral polio, be given safely to companions and close contacts to help mitigate the risk of disease transmission to KT recipients.

Vaccination for Children

Transplant recipients who interact frequently with young children (parents, grandparents, daycare workers, teachers, etc.) should be aware of the live attenuated vaccines that are administered routinely to children and the potential for viral shedding. For example, children receiving rotavirus vaccination may shed live virus in their stool for up to 4 weeks.[6] Oral polio vaccine, not given in the United States but administered internationally, is associated with risk of transmitting infection and paralytic poliomyelitis, and should be avoided for close contacts of KT recipients. Kidney transplant patients should use barrier protection (masks, gloves) and minimize contact with bodily secretions of their vaccinated children during the period of active postvaccination viral shedding.

Vaccination Summary

Table 3.1 provides a summary of vaccination. It is prudent to promote vaccination for immunosuppressed KT patients.

Family Planning and Reproductive Health

The family is the first essential cell of human society.

—Pope John XXIII

Fertility in CKD

In 1958, Edith Helm became the first woman to give birth successfully following a KT. Table 3.2 highlights reproductive health in KT patients. Advanced CKD is associated with decreased fertility and increased risk of pregnancy complications both for the fetus and mother.[7,8] The disruption of normal hypothalamic-pituitary-gonadal axis, hyperprolactinemia due to CKD, and suppressed dopaminergic activity is common, resulting in inhibition of gonadotropin secretion. In addition, levels of follicle stimulating hormone (FSH) and luteinizing hormone (LH) can be elevated in CKD without the normal midcycle LH surge, leading to anovulation. The psychological impact of CKD can result in anxiety and depression affecting libido.

Table 3.2 Reproductive Management of Female Kidney Transplant Recipients

Precontemplation management

—Review likelihood of pregnancy (fertility can be restored as early as 1 month post-transplant, regular menses by 7 months)

—Review teratogenic potential of medications

—Review risks of pregnancy to patient (worsening graft function, pre-eclampsia, eclampsia, increased rate of Cesarean delivery) and to fetus (higher rate of fetal demise, prematurity, low birth weight)

—Review need for effective birth control if pregnancy not desired

  —Online educational resources for contraception: www.cdc.gov/reproductiv ehealth/contraception/#Resources-for-consumers; who.int/health-topics/contraception#tab=tab_1

  —Consider providing emergency contraception for women at high risk of unwanted pregnancy or without ready access to healthcare

—Discuss importance of planning pregnancy with the support of transplant care providers and high-risk obstetricians

Prepregnancy planning

—Optimize health and timing

  —BP goal <140/90. ACE inhibitors and angiotensin receptor blockers should be discontinued

  —sCr <1.5, UPCR <0.5

  —wait for at least 1 year from transplant or last severe rejection or infection

—Review immunosuppression

  —stable, low doses preferred (tacrolimus, cyclosporine, prednisone, azathioprine are considered acceptable for use during pregnancy)

  —MPA is contraindicated; mycophenolate mofetil/mycophenolic acid should be discontinued at least 6 weeks before discontinuing birth control

  —mTOR inhibitors, belatacept are not recommended due to lack of available data

—Consider referral for genetic testing/counseling, discuss availability of fetal testing

—Discuss alternatives to pregnancy (adoption, surrogacy)

Pregnancy management

—BP control: optimal targe is not known; first-line agents recommended during pregnancy include labetalol, methyldopa, and calcium channel blockers.

—monthly monitoring of weight, renal function panel, urine protein, urine culture, viral serologies (BK, CMV), immunosuppression drug levels

—careful adjustment of immunosuppression especially going into 2nd trimester and postpartum; consider more frequent monitoring of levels

—stop sulfamethoxazole/trimethoprim no later than 8 week before expected delivery

—consider low-dose aspirin after 12 weeks gestational age for prevention of pre-eclampsia, although its use may outweigh benefits in Hispanic and non-Hispanic Black women

Postpartum management

—careful adjustment of immunosuppression post-delivery

—screen for depression and nonadherence

—review risks/ benefits of breastfeeding; avoid sulfamethoxazole-trimethoprim, especially in infants with G6PD deficiency

—review need to resume birth control

*Adapted from Webster P, et al. Pregnancy in chronic kidney disease and kidney transplantation. *Kidney Int.* 2017;91(5):1047–1056.

Fertility after Kidney Transplant

Fertility can recover within one month after KT Regular menses generally resumes after a median of 7 months.[9] Women of childbearing age should be counseled about the effects of immunosuppression on the unborn fetus and the effect of pregnancy on the allograft. Therefore, pregnancy needs to be planned and contraception should be highly encouraged prior to transplant. Particularly those who are not medically or psychologically ready for pregnancy should be counseled about the importance of using effective contraception early after transplant. Unplanned pregnancy rates among KTs are high (93% reported in Brazil, 88% in China), and contraceptive use low (48%).[10,11] The World Health Organization and the US CDC provide patient and provider guides to contraception in many languages on their respective websites. (www.cdc.gov/reproductivehealth/contraception/#Resources-for-consumers). In the United States, the CDC site offers links to help women locate health centers and to access services such as emergency contraception, which may be challenging as local and federal policies governing women's reproductive rights continue to evolve.

Permanent Surgical Sterilization
Permanent sterilization with tubal ligation or occlusion or partner vasectomy are highly effective but irreversible and recommended only for select patients.

Temporary Medical Sterilization
Effective long-acting but reversible options include progestin implants placed subdermally in the arm, progestin injections every 1–3 months, hormone-free copper intrauterine devices (IUDs) or hormonal IUDs. Early reluctance to consider IUDs in the transplant setting resulted from experience with the poorly designed Dalkon shield introduced in the 1980s, which was associated with high rates of pelvic inflammation and is no longer available for use. However, contraceptive failure and bacterial peritonitis are low with use of IUDs in immunosuppressed transplant patients appears to be safe based on recent series examining modern IUD use in the HIV-infected population. Hormonal IUDs have also been employed to effectively treat menorrhagia in transplant patients with uterine fibroids.[12,13]

Nonadherence to Contraception
Nonadherence translates to higher failure rates. Combined estrogen-progestin hormonal-based choices include daily oral pill, weekly transdermal patch, and monthly vaginal ring and have several benefits including regulation of menses, management of ovarian cysts, and control of acne. While most modern formulations contain lower doses, estrogen can alter metabolism of calcineurin

inhibitors, increase blood pressure, and increased risk of venous and arterial thrombosis, so it should be avoided in women with underlying risk factors such as history of hypercoagulable state, myocardial infarction or stroke, tobacco smoking, migraines, or liver disease. Progestin-only pills are taken daily and do not contain estrogen but can be associated with breakthrough bleeding and increased risk of osteoporosis with long-term use. For patients on mycophenolic acid (MPA), the recommendation is to adopt two forms of contraception due to inhibition of enterohepatic recirculation which can negatively impact the efficacy of **Oral Contraceptive Pill (OCP)**.

Barrier Methods for Contraception
Barrier methods such as condoms, diaphragms, cervical caps, and spermicides are safe but depend on user technique and adherence, and efficacy rates are suboptimal with 12%–21% of women relying solely on these methods becoming pregnant within 1 year.

Postcoital Contraception
Emergency contraception (EC) (single dose antiprogestin ulipristal, progestin levonorgestrel in single or divided doses, or placement of copper IUD) can be used up to 5 days following unprotected intercourse to delay ovulation and prevent pregnancy. EC can be prescribed to women at any time and should be considered especially for women at higher risk for unwanted pregnancy or without access to healthcare. A confirmatory follow-up pregnancy test is recommended after 2 weeks.

Summary on Contraception
Providers should be aware that falsely elevated HCG tests can be seen with CKD. The CDC and the UK Medical Eligibility Criteria for Contraceptive Use recommend any method of contraception to women with uncomplicated solid organ transplants. For complicated transplants, defined as acute or chronic graft rejection or failure, both organizations recommend initiating progestin-only contraception or continuing an IUD that is already in place but recommend against combined estrogen-progestin or placing a new IUD.

Pregnancy after Kidney Transplantation

Epidemiology of Pregnancy after Kidney Transplantation
Pregnancy successes are reported through voluntary registries, case reports, or single-center case series. A population-based study conducted using Medicare claims data found that rates of pregnancy and live birth are lower in KT

recipients.[14] Statistically lower pregnancy rates were seen in patients with ESRD due to diabetes compared to glomerulonephritis, with pretransplant dialysis duration of at least 3 years compared to preemptive transplantation, and in those treated with cyclosporine compared to tacrolimus as well as those treated with mycophenolate versus azathioprine. A significant difference in pregnancy rates was not seen between races or types of transplant (living versus deceased), or with GFR (mL/m/1.73m^2) $\geq$ 60 versus <30. The lower fertility rate may be due to a combination of incomplete restoration of hormonal function, concurrent comorbid conditions, and side effects of immunosuppressive agents and other medications as well as physician recommendation and patient choice.

Live Birth among Kidney Transplant Recipients

Most pregnancies after KT result in successful live birth, although even with "good" GFR, the incidence of pregnancy complications (hypertension and pre-eclampsia, prematurity, small for gestational age, Cesarean birth, fetal demise, decline in maternal renal function) remain higher than what is seen in the general population.[15] In contrast to the high success rates (>75%) reported in voluntary registries,[16,17] a population study in the United States utilizing Medicare insurance claims data showed a substantially lower rate of live birth and higher rates of unexpected fetal loss.[14] The fetal outcome available for 453 (85%) of 530 pregnancies, demonstrated 55.4% live births 32.7% preterm births, and 50.6% Cesarean deliveries. Therapeutic abortions accounted for only 8% of fetal losses in this study and declined sharply from 18.7% to 6.2% from 1990 to 2000. The rate of fetal loss appeared to decline with time from transplant from 55.3% of pregnancies during the first post-transplant year, to 40.2% and 37.6% during the second and third post-transplant years. The live birth rate remained substantially lower at 19/1000 compared to 70/1000 in the general population and fell in parallel with pregnancy rates, from 28.5/1000 in 1990 to 6.2/1000 in 2000. The rates of fetal losses are higher in Black KT recipients, ESRD due to diabetes, and with patients with low-income status. The high rate of overall fetal loss supports the recommendation that pregnancies following KT be managed by high-risk pregnancy specialists and transplant professionals. Unfortunately, the impact of racial and social disparity on healthcare delivery remains an unmet challenge, and women at the highest risk often have the least access to high quality specialty care.[18]

Timing of Pregnancy after Transplantation

Consensus guidelines regarding pregnancy following KT have been published and most recommend that pregnancy should be delayed for at least 1 year following KT when risk of acute rejection declines and patients are on stable maintenance immunosuppression. The European best practice guidelines recommends waiting 2 years.[19] The AST recommends waiting at least 1 year from any rejection until patients are on stable maintenance immunosuppression with adequate and stable graft function, good blood pressure control, and without active infectious concerns. Based on registry data showing accelerated loss of renal function in the setting of prepregnancy serum creatinine >1.7 mg/dL,[17] therefore, arbitrary serum creatinine levels of <1.5 mg/dL and urine protein of <0.5 g/day have been proposed as safety thresholds when counseling KT recipients regarding pregnancy.

Rejection Post Pregnancy

The effects of prepregnancy donor-specific antibodies on pregnancy management and outcomes remains to be studied. In a small, single-center series reporting pregnancy outcomes, three of eight "sensitized" patients, defined as PRA >0% (mean class I 30%, class II 8%) developed antibody-mediated rejection (AMR) leading to graft loss.[20] While pregnancy is, in general, considered an immune tolerant state, the discontinuation of MPA during pregnancy, and decline in tacrolimus drug levels (by ~20%–25%) as volume of distribution expands and GFR increases during late first- to- early second trimester of pregnancy (before decreasing in the 3rd trimester and postpartum periods) may increase the risk for kidney rejection. Drug levels should be monitored frequently, and immunosuppression should be adjusted accordingly during pregnancy and in the postpartum period.

Pregnancy and Viral Infections

Isolated publications, using old non-Polymerase Chain Reaction (PCR) techniques for diagnosing polyomavirus infection, reported a possible increase in BK reactivation during pregnancy. CMV is the leading infectious cause of congenital birth defects in the general population, occurring in approximately 1% of newborns. A case study in a KT patient reports diagnosis using PCR analysis of amniotic fluid that was successfully treated with oral ganciclovir administered to the mother resulting in the delivery of a healthy infant.[21] Routine monthly surveillance for infections during pregnancy (urine culture, viral infections) has been recommended without overt evidence.

Hypertension and Pregnancy

Blood pressure management during pregnancy in KT remains controversial. Many transplant recipients have chronic hypertension and are at increased risk of developing preeclampsia/eclampsia. In addition, diagnosis of these complications is made more difficult in the setting of preexisting hypertension and proteinuria. Urine protein levels can increase as much as threefold in normal pregnancy. Blood pressure management during pregnancy is usually more permissive, but the American College of Obstetricians and Gynecology (ACOG) recommends treatment goals in line with more stringent recommendations in nonpregnant individuals for patients with any evidence of "end organ damage."[22] The UK National Institute of Health and Clinical Excellence (NICE) recommends a blood pressure goal of <140/90 mmHg in patients with CKD.

Pregnancy outcomes for fetus and mother in the setting of CKD are markedly worse when maternal hypertension is present.[23] Whether more stringent management of hypertension in patients with CKD or in KT recipients mitigates this risk remains unproven. ACE inhibitors and angiotensin II receptor blockers are absolutely contraindicated during pregnancy due to risk of oligohydramnios. First-line choices for hypertension management in pregnancy include labetalol, methyldopa, and calcium channel antagonists. The AGOG, the Society for Maternal-Fetal Medicine (SMFM), and the US Preventive Services Task Force (USPSTF) have recommended the use of low-dose aspirin (81 mg daily) after 12 weeks of gestation for pregnant women at high risk (which includes patients with chronic hypertension of kidney disease) for preeclampsia. However, no data is available to guide aspirin use in pregnant transplant recipients.

Immunosuppressive Medications during Pregnancy

The US Food and Drug Administration (FDA) classifies most immunosuppressant medications in pregnancy as "category C—human risk not ruled out." Immunosuppressive therapy linked to fetal growth retardation and preterm delivery but generally considered to be safe for use in pregnancy include the calcineurin inhibitors tacrolimus and cyclosporine, the antimetabolite azathioprine, and steroids (Pregnancy and Lactation Final Rule, 2015). MPA is considered a teratogen (FDA "category D") and consensus guidelines recommend substituting MPA with azathioprine (with or without prednisone) in its place at least 6 weeks before attempting pregnancy. The use of MPA during pregnancy is associated with increased risk of spontaneous miscarriage during the first trimester and congenital defects including external ear malformation, cleft lip and palate, and congenital malformation of the limbs, heart, esophagus, and kidneys, likely due to inhibition of purine synthesis.[24] Any exposure to MPA during the first trimester may be harmful; hence, the FDA recommends that females of reproductive potential continue effective contraception for at least 6 weeks following discontinuation of MPA before attempting conception. MPA can also reduce the efficacy of some oral contraceptives such as levonorgestrel. Due to lack of long-term safety, use of mTOR inhibitors and belatacept is currently not recommended during pregnancy.

Timing of Delivery

Pregnant KT patients should be aware of the higher rate of Caesarean section (~50% in the United States), earlier delivery (mean gestational age at birth ~36 weeks), and smaller infant size (mean 2400 g). The rate of developmental delay in infants born to KT patients does not appear to differ significantly from what is observed in the general population.

Monitoring Postpartum Patients

As GFR declines gradually to prepregnancy levels, immunosuppression levels may require frequent dose adjustment. Blood pressure and urine protein levels should also be monitored in the postpartum period with the expectation of normalization over 8–12 weeks. Reactivation of systemic lupus erythematosus and acute kidney rejection can also occur immediate postpartum. In addition, the busy, and likely sleep-deprived, new mother should be screened for medication adherence and postpartum depression.

Breastfeeding

Transplant and obstetric organizations have published conflicting recommendations regarding breastfeeding. Because there is a theoretical risk of neonatal immunosuppression from drug secretion into breast milk, KT patients have been counseled against breastfeeding. However, registry data has not shown an increase in birth defects in infants born to mothers who continued tacrolimus through pregnancy, despite known placental transfer of drug and the negligible transfer of the drug through breastmilk compared to placental exposure. An observational cohort study performed in the United Kingdom analyzing tacrolimus levels in mothers, infants, and breast milk demonstrated low excretion of tacrolimus into breast milk and negligible drug absorption by breastfed infants.[25] Furthermore, the concentration of tacrolimus in breast milk does not appear to vary per timing and dosing of tacrolimus, so breastfeeding time need not be altered.[26] Given the substantial benefits of breastfeeding, particularly in preterm infants, women maintained on tacrolimus, cyclosporine, azathioprine, and prednisone should not necessarily be discouraged from the practice. A more cautious approach to breastfeeding may still be appropriate for mothers maintained on other medications (MPA, mTOR inhibitors, belatacept) due to lack of data.

Reproductive Health in Men

Although studies and recommendations about reproduction in KT patients largely focus on women and offspring, male KT patients also encounter reproductive health challenges. While preconception genetic counseling and testing may be of interest to some male patients, pregnancy-related issues are not generally the dominant concern for male KT patients or their healthcare providers. There is, for example, no evidence to support that MPA impacts male fertility or contributes to birth defects in their offspring.[27] However, male KT patients report high rates (~60%) of erectile dysfunction (ED), which can have a marked impact on quality of life. ED can result from pre-existing co-morbidity, altered perfusion or Foley-related trauma from the transplant surgery, adverse drug effects, psychosocial stressors, and endocrinopathies such as hyperprolactinemia and hypogonadism. Immunosuppressive medications have been demonstrated to suppress gonadal function. Cyclosporine has been shown to impact penile hemodynamics through various mechanisms including suppression of nitric oxide (NO)-mediated smooth muscle relaxation, increased TGF-β1 induced fibrosis of the corpora cavernosa, and inhibition of testosterone production. Sirolimus has been associated with decreased sperm count, motility, and viability. Therefore, male KT recipients who want to start a family should consider avoiding mTOR inhibitors. Steroids suppress the hypothalamic-pituitary axis's production and normal regulation of gonadal hormones.[28]

Restoring vitamin D, prolactin, and testosterone levels to normal may improve sexual function, and evaluating gonadal function is important in KT patients reporting ED. Phosphodiesterase-5 inhibitors (PDE5i) have been used safely and effectively in KT patients and show few significant interactions with immuno-suppressive drugs, although tacrolimus can increase the peak concentration and half-life of PDE5i, so this class of medications should be initiated with caution at lower and less frequent dosing intervals. Second- and third-line interventions such as transurethral or intracavernous therapy, topical alprostadil, vacuum con-striction devices, low-intensity shockwave therapy, or penile prostheses can also be considered in patients with stable graft function.

Cancer Screening after Kidney Transplantation

Cancer is the second leading cause of death in patients after kidney transplan-tation. Cancer rates in KT recipients are two- to threefold higher than in age-, and gender-matched individuals from general population,[29] and outcomes are inferior to that reported for general population.[30] The heightened risk for cancer is largely driven by increased susceptibility to viral infections, and the in-cidence of virally mediated cancers such as Kaposi sarcoma, skin, vulvovaginal, and post-transplant lymphoma are substantially higher in KT recipients than in the general population. The incidence of cancer of the breast, prostate, ovaries, and brain are similar to the general population, and the rates of melanoma and cancer of the colon and lung are increased twofold.[31] Data from the Australia and New Zealand Dialysis and Transplant Registry and the European and North

American Registry report that the nonmelanocytic skin cancers and genitourinary cancers are the most frequent cancers seen in KT recipients. The risk for renal cell cancer in native kidneys is associated with dialysis vintage and acquired cystic disease. Cancer types also vary based on geographical location of the patient. Patients residing in Australia, Europe, and North America are at greatest risk for skin cancer, while those from Asia and the Middle East are more likely to develop urothelial transitional cell cancer and gastrointestinal tract cancer.

It is important to educate patients and primary care providers about the increased risk of cancer and the importance of screening. Prevention remains the key to identify the disease early and minimize the risk and improve outcome of certain cancers. There are no studies supporting routine cancer screening in transplant patients, and recommendations are largely extrapolated from the general population. Cancer screening should be tailored to patients individually, considering their age, comorbidities, prior history of cancer, duration of dialysis, degree of immunosuppression, overall prognosis, and local prevalence.

Screening for Cancer

In this section we discuss cancer screening guidelines set by the US Preventative Services Task Force (**USPSTF**) and provide guidance for screening KT patients. Table 10.4 in Chapter 10, "Cancer **after** Kidney Transplantation" details cancer screening for KT recipients.

Skin Cancer
Skin cancer is the most common cancer in transplant patients and is probably related to UV radiation and HPV infection. Certain immunosuppressive regimens such as cyclosporine and azathioprine augment the carcinogenic effect. The risk of squamous cell skin cancer, melanoma, and Kaposi's sarcoma are increased severalfold compared with the general population. In addition to self-exam of the skin, an annual total body screening by a primary care physician or dermatologist is recommended. This regular surveillance allows for prompt excision of suspicious precancerous lesions.

Cervical Cancer
The risk of cervical cancer is similar to that observed in general population. Women aged 21 to 65 years are advised to undergo screening for cervical cancer with cytology (Pap smear) every 3 years. For women aged 30 to 65 years who want to lengthen the screening interval, screening with a combination of cytology and HPV testing every 5 years is recommended. For those with HPV

infection and at higher risk for cervical cancer, PAP smears can be performed more frequently.

Colon Cancer
Risk of colon cancer is two times higher than in the general population. Colon cancer screening should be performed in adults aged 50--75 with colonoscopy every 10 years, or CT colonography every 5 years, or flexible sigmoidoscopy every 5 years, and Cologuard every 3 years.

Breast Cancer
Breast cancer risk is reported to be lower than in the general population, perhaps due to screening prior to waitlisting for KT. In addition to self-breast exam, breast cancer screening with mammography is recommended once every 2 years for women aged 50–74 years. For women with family history of breast cancer, screening should start earlier; screening is not recommended for those over 75 years.

Prostate Cancer
Screening for prostate cancer is debatable in the general population; therefore the decision to screen should be made on an individual basis. Many physicians perform annual PSA screening for patients above 45 years of age.

Lung Cancer
Lung cancer screening with low-dose computed tomography is recommended for patients with a 20 pack-year history of smoking who currently smoke or who have quit within the past 15 years. Screening should be discontinued once a person has not smoked for 15 years or develops a health problem that substantially limits their life expectancy or the ability to have curative lung surgery.

Thus, post-transplant cancer remains a threat to improving KT survival. We strongly recommend cancer screening for KT patients and should be individualized based on age, race, geographic location, comorbid condition, and recipient risk factors.

Return to Work after Kidney Transplantation

> I believe that the true value of life lies in work, diligence, and innovation. After all, work is the essence of humanity.
>
> —Sheikh Abdullah

Epidemiology of Return-to-Work after Kidney Transplantation

The ability to return to work is one global measure of well-being that encompasses physical, mental, and social recovery. The National Kidney Foundation (NKF) website and most major US transplant center websites report an average back-to-work time following KT of less than 8 weeks. While the return-to-work rates among KT recipients outstrip those for other solid organ transplant recipients,[32] employment rates remain low. In a recent meta-analysis on the topic of work and KT, Kirkeskov et al. noted an employment rate of 26.3% (range 10.5%–59.7%) in the dialysis population, 36.9% (range 25%–86%) at the time of transplant, and only 38.2% (range 14.2%–85%) at 1 year following transplant.[33] Rates of employment were particularly low in studies examining patients in the United States. In an analysis of United Network of Organ Sharing (UNOS) data examining KT recipients aged 18–64 with stable graft function transplanted between 2004 and 2011, Tzvetanov et al.[34] found low rates of employment at the time of transplant which improved but remained below 50% following transplant and differed significantly based on whether the patient was covered by private or public (Medicare or Medicaid) insurance. The employment rate at the time of transplant was 23.1% with private insurance and 10% with public insurance and increased to 47% and 16% at 1 year, 43% and 12% at 5 years with private and public insurance, respectively. For patients who were not employed at the time of transplant, employment rates remained below 10%, regardless of insurance type.

Factors Correlating to Return to Work

Various studies have correlated higher rates of employment following KT to paid employment at the time of transplant, male gender, married status, younger age, lower levels of comorbidity, nondiabetic status, shorter duration of dialysis, higher educational status, managerial or intellectual work over factory or physical work, and absence of depression.[35–38]

Benefits of Return to Work

Ability to work may not only reflect, but may contribute to, an individual's well-being. One study analyzed KT graft and patient survival among the six groups to which patients self-identify on the annual follow-up questionnaire collected by UNOS (patients working full-time, working part-time by choice, working part-time due to limitations of their disease, not employed by choice, not employed due to disease, or retired). The study found that after controlling for multiple donor and recipient variables, patients who were employed had better graft and overall survival at 1 and 3 years when compared to those who were not working, even those unemployed by choice and not disease. Patients who choose to work may be intrinsically different with respect to unmeasurable characteristics such as sense of responsibility, which has implications for compliance with medication, laboratory tests, and clinic follow-up or with respect to degree of motivation which might impact lifestyle choices such as diet and exercise. Gainful employment has been shown to positively contribute to an individual's financial stability, social integration, self-esteem, and lower depression scores—all factors that are associated with mortality risk.[38] Work may facilitate access to better medical insurance coverage, which is important in obtaining immunosuppressive medications.

Recommendation about Return to Work

How can transplant providers improve the ability of transplant recipients to re-enter the workforce? Prior to transplant, encouraging patients to consider home dialysis modalities to allow more flexibility to continue working after the initiation of dialysis and limiting time on dialysis by improving access to early, or even preemptive transplant by improving rates of early diagnosis and referral; good waitlist management; and encouraging living donor transplantation are all important. In a cross-sectional study of 224 KT recipients from nine Dutch institutions, Visser et al. found that undergoing preemptive transplant was associated with a high level of employment at 12 months post-transplant (82%) compared to recipients of living but nonpreemptive transplant (65%) and to recipients of deceased donor nonpreemptive transplant (55%), with the last group receiving the most disability compensation.[39] Three months after transplant there should not be any weight lifting restrictions and patients should seek a job that does not expose them to repeated infections (see Table 3.3).

Following transplant, providers should address medical barriers such as screening for and treating anxiety and depression. Some patients require encouragement, permission, and a bolstering of confidence to combat the psychological fragility that develops in the setting of chronic illness. Educating and teaching patients skills of self-management can empower patients to return to the workplace, and a patient's perception of capability to work has been shown to predict employment.[32] The ability of some patients to return to national or international sports (basketball, swimming, rowing) is an example of a successful return to work following KT. Social, cultural, and societal expectations likely play an important role in determining rates of employment. A Japanese study revealed that

Table 3.3 Optimizing Return to Work for KTR

Pretransplant interventions

—limit time on dialysis
  —early transplant referral
  —facilitate transplant evaluation, optimize waitlist management
  —encourage and facilitate living donor transplant
—encourage home dialysis modalities that allow patients to continue to work with ESKD

Post-transplant interventions

—provide patients encouragement and reassurance to return as soon as 6–12 weeks post-transplant
—screen for depression, anxiety
—limit polypharmacy and address common side effects (insomnia, neuropathy, impaired memory/concentration, tremor, GI distress)
—educate and encourage self-management
—communicate with patient's workplace regarding reasonable expectations, advocate for a safe work environment
—advocate with local, state, and federal legislators to promote legal protections for workers with chronic illness
—educate patients about programs such as Ticket to Work and Medicare buy-in that help to offset loss of disability insurance benefits

---

of transplant recipients aged 20–64 who held paid employment at the time of transplant, 85% were employed at 12 months following transplant.[36]

The rate of return to work drops over time after transplant. Transplant providers should perhaps approach patient intervention with respect to preparing patients to return to the workplace with more urgency, as the ability to shape a patient's response to transplantation and choices regarding returning to work may diminish with time.[38] Avoiding unnecessary polypharmacy and carefully eliciting and addressing the many potential side effects of the medications prescribed to transplant patients is critical. Neuropathy, difficulty with concentration and memory, and insomnia are common, partially dose-dependent, side effects of tacrolimus. Chronic gastrointestinal discomfort or diarrhea from mycophenolate may contribute to anxiety about leaving the home. Fatigue due to anemia, poor sleep, and other side effects of antihypertensive medications may also limit a patient's ability to return to work. The availability of state-sponsored disability programs may be a disincentive toward recipient's decision to return to work, an unintended consequence.[34]

Direct communication by transplant providers to employers to support a patient's ability to return to work safely, to educate employers regarding both the benefits and risk with respect to specific work tasks after transplant, and to advocate for a supportive work environment can be helpful. The transplant medical community can also work with lawmakers to promote legal protection for workers with chronic disease to ensure there is no discrimination due to pre-existing conditions.

In conclusion, wellness after KT is critical to prolong meaningful life with a long-lasting functioning kidney. Educating patients before and after transplant is as important as discussing surgery and immunosuppressive medications.

References

1. de Brito DCS, Machado EL, Reis IA, Moreira DP, Nebias THM, Cherchiglia ML. Modality transition on renal replacement therapy and quality of life of patients: a 10-year follow-up cohort study. *Qual Life Res*. 2019;28:1485–1495.
2. Hurst FP, Lee JJ, Jindal RM, Agodoa LY, Abbott KC. Outcomes associated with influenza vaccination in the first year after kidney transplantation. *Clin J Am Soc Nephrol*. 2011;6:1192–1197.
3. Carman WF, Elder AG, Wallace LA, et al. Effects of influenza vaccination of healthcare workers on mortality of elderly people in long-term care: a randomised controlled trial. *Lancet*. 2000;355:93–97.
4. Rubin LG, Levin MJ, Ljungman P, et al. 2013 IDSA clinical practice guideline for vaccination of the immunocompromised host. *Clin Infect Dis*. 2014;58:309–318.
5. Danziger-Isakov L, Kumar D, On behalf of the AST ID Community of Practice. Vaccination of solid organ transplant candidates and recipients: guidelines from the American society of transplantation infectious diseases community of practice. *Clin Transplant*. 2019;33:e13563.
6. Anderson EJ. Rotavirus vaccines: viral shedding and risk of transmission. *Lancet Infect Dis*. 2008;8:642–649.
7. Shahir AK, Briggs N, Katsoulis J, Levidiotis V. An observational outcomes study from 1966–2008, examining pregnancy and neonatal outcomes from dialysed women using data from the ANZDATA Registry. *Nephrology (Carlton)*. 2013;18:276–284.
8. Finkelstein FO, Shirani S, Wuerth D, Finkelstein SH. Therapy insight: sexual dysfunction in patients with chronic kidney disease. *Nat Clin Pract Nephrol*. 2007;3:200–207.
9. McKay DB, Josephson MA. Pregnancy in recipients of solid organs—effects on mother and child. *N Engl J Med*. 2006;354:1281–1293.
10. Roe AH, Dutton C. Contraception for transplant patients. *Transplantation*. 2017;101:1739–1741.
11. Krajewski CM, Geetha D, Gomez-Lobo V. Contraceptive options for women with a history of solid-organ transplantation. *Transplantation*. 2013;95:1183–1186.
12. Stringer EM, Kaseba C, Levy J, et al. A randomized trial of the intrauterine contraceptive device vs hormonal contraception in women who are infected with the human immunodeficiency virus. *Am J Obstet Gynecol*. 2007;197:144 e1–8.
13. Huguelet PS, Sheehan C, Spitzer RF, Scott S. Use of the levonorgestrel 52-mg intrauterine system in adolescent and young adult solid organ transplant recipients: a case series. *Contraception*. 2017;95:378–381.
14. Gill JS, Zalunardo N, Rose C, Tonelli M. The pregnancy rate and live birth rate in kidney transplant recipients. *Am J Transplant*. 2009;9:1541–1549.

15. Deshpande NA, James NT, Kucirka LM, et al. Pregnancy outcomes in kidney transplant recipients: a systematic review and meta-analysis. *Am J Transplant.* 2011;11:2388–404.

16. Coscia LA, Constantinescu S, Moritz MJ, et al. Report from the National Transplantation Pregnancy Registry (NTPR): outcomes of pregnancy after transplantation. *Clin Transpl.* 2010:65–85. PMID 21698831.

17. Sibanda N, Briggs JD, Davison JM, Johnson RJ, Rudge CJ. Pregnancy after organ transplantation: a report from the UK transplant pregnancy registry. *Transplantation.* 2007;83:1301–1307.

18. McKay DB, Josephson MA, Armenti VT, et al. Reproduction and transplantation: report on the AST Consensus Conference on Reproductive Issues and Transplantation. *Am J Transplant.* 2005;5:1592–1599.

19. Transplantation EEGoR. European best practice guidelines for renal transplantation: section IV: long-term management of the transplant recipient: IV.5.3: cardiovascular risks. *Hyperlipidaemia Nephrol Dial Transplant.* 2002;17 Suppl 4:26–28.

20. Ajaimy M, Lubetzky M, Jones T, et al. Pregnancy in sensitized kidney transplant recipients: a single-center experience. *Clin Transplant.* 2016;30:791–795.

21. Puliyanda DP, Silverman NS, Lehman D, et al. Successful use of oral ganciclovir for the treatment of intrauterine cytomegalovirus infection in a renal allograft recipient. *Transpl Infect Dis.* 2005;7:71–74.

22. Hypertension in pregnancy. Report of the American College of Obstetricians and Gynecologists' Task Force on Hypertension in Pregnancy. *Obstet Gynecol.* 2013;122:1122–1131.

23. Bateman BT, Bansil P, Hernandez-Diaz S, Mhyre JM, Callaghan WM, Kuklina EV. Prevalence, trends, and outcomes of chronic hypertension: a nationwide sample of delivery admissions. *Am J Obstet Gynecol.* 2012;206:134, e1–8.

24. Kim M, Rostas S, Gabardi S. Mycophenolate fetal toxicity and risk evaluation and mitigation strategies. *Am J Transplant.* 2013;13:1383–1389.

25. Bramham K, Chusney G, Lee J, Lightstone L, Nelson-Piercy C. Breastfeeding and tacrolimus: serial monitoring in breast-fed and bottle-fed infants. *Clin J Am Soc Nephrol.* 2013;8:563–567.

26. Gardiner SJ, Begg EJ. Breastfeeding during tacrolimus therapy. *Obstet Gynecol.* 2006;107:453–455.

27. Lopez-Lopez I, Rodelo-Haad C, Aguera ML, et al. Administration of mycophenolic acid is not associated with malformations in descendants from kidney transplanted males. *PLoS ONE.* 2018;13:e0202589.

28. Perri A, Izzo G, Lofaro D, et al. Erectile dysfunction after kidney transplantation. *J Clin Med.* 2020 Jun 25;9(6):1991. doi: 10.3390/jcm9061991. PMID: 32630390; PMCID: PMC7356955.

29. Kasiske BL, Snyder JJ, Gilbertson DT, Wang C. Cancer after kidney transplantation in the United States. *Am J Transplant.* 2004;4:905–913.

30. Miao Y, Everly JJ, Gross TG, et al. De novo cancers arising in organ transplant recipients are associated with adverse outcomes compared with the general population. *Transplantation.* 2009;87:1347–1359.

31. Sprangers B, Nair V, Launay-Vacher V, Riella LV, Jhaveri KD. Risk factors associated with post-kidney transplant malignancies: an article from the Cancer-Kidney International Network. *Clin Kidney J.* 2018;11:315–329.

32. De Baere C, Delva D, Kloeck A, et al. Return to work and social participation: does type of organ transplantation matter? *Transplantation.* 2010;89:1009–1015.
33. Kirkeskov L, Carlsen RK, Lund T, Buus NH. Employment of patients with kidney failure treated with dialysis or kidney transplantation-a systematic review and meta-analysis. *BMC Nephrol.* 2021;22:348.
34. Tzvetanov I, D'Amico G, Walczak D, et al. High rate of unemployment after kidney transplantation: analysis of the United network for organ sharing database. *Transplant Proc.* 2014;46:1290–1294.
35. Knobbe TJ, Kremer D, Abma FI, et al. Employment status and work functioning among kidney transplant recipients. *Clin J Am Soc Nephrol.* 2022;17:1506–1514.
36. Miyake K, Endo M, Okumi M, et al. Predictors of return to work after kidney transplantation: a 12-month cohort of the Japan Academic Consortium of Kidney Transplantation study. *BMJ Open.* 2019;9:e031231.
37. De Pasquale C, Pistorio ML, Veroux M, et al. Nonverbal communication and psycho-pathology in kidney transplant recipients. *Transplant Proc.* 2019;51:2931–2935.
38. D'Egidio V, Mannocci A, Ciaccio D, et al. Return to work after kidney transplant: a systematic review. *Occup Med (Lond).* 2019;69:412–4128.
39. Visser A, Alma MA, Bakker SJL, et al. Employment and ability to work after kidney transplantation in the Netherlands: the impact of preemptive versus non-preemptive kidney transplantation. *Clin Transplant.* 2022;36:e14757.

4

Immunosuppression after Kidney Transplantation

Aravind Cherukuri and Richard J. Baker

Immunosupression cannot be achieved without immunosuppressive effects!

Introduction

Immunosuppression remains the cornerstone of medical management in kidney transplantation. Progress in the field of therapeutic immunosuppression has been the key to successful kidney transplantation and long-term allograft survival. Induction immunosuppression refers to the intense immunosuppression used in the initial days post-transplantation to circumvent early acute rejection, while maintenance immunosuppression is the lower intensity immunosuppression used for the life of the transplant to maintain allograft function and prevent rejection as the graft becomes less immunogenic. In addition, these agents are also used to reverse established rejection.

Through this chapter we provide an overview of the immunosuppression strategies that shape the management of kidney transplant (KT) recipient. We highlight the immunological pathways that cause allograft rejection and how immunosuppressive agents block these pathways with the intent of reducing the incidence of rejection. Next, we summarize the mechanisms of action and adverse effects of the commonly used agents. Finally, we discuss the immunosuppression strategies applicable to routine clinical management as well as for certain high-risk patients.

Evolution of Immunosuppression for Kidney Transplantation

Major advances have been made in the immunosuppression management of KT patients since the first successful KT between identical twins in 1954. Success of KT during the first period, from 1950 to the early 1960s, relied heavily on a perfect immunological match, transplants between HLA-identical siblings in the absence of effective immunosuppression. Immunosuppression was restricted to the use of corticosteroids, 6-mercaptopurine, or total body radiation, all of which were associated with significant morbidity and mortality, predominantly through infection. The second period from the mid-1960s to the 1980s, was defined by the widespread use of azathioprine and corticosteroids. During this era the rates of acute rejection were very high and 1-year kidney graft survival rates were around 50%.

Discovered by the Sandoz pharmaceutical company in Switzerland in 1972, the calcineurin inhibitor (CNI) cyclosporine revolutionized transplant medicine when it was introduced to clinical practice, heralding the third period, which started in the 1980s. A large Canadian multicenter clinical trial of cyclosporine usage in cadaveric KT patients demonstrated a 69% 3-year graft survival compared to 58% in those maintained on azathioprine and corticosteroids.[1] Over the next decade rates of acute rejection dropped to around 50% and 1-year graft survival was over 80%, securing cyclosporine as the mainstay for immunosuppression in KT. The modern era of KT immunosuppression began in the 1990s with the emergence of tacrolimus (also a CNI) and mycophenolic acid (MPA) which led to significant improvements in 1-year allograft survival among all organ recipients by decreasing rates of acute rejection.

The Tricontinental Mycophenolate Mofetil (MMF) Renal Transplantation Study established the efficacy and safety of MMF in comparison to azathioprine along with equivalent doses of cyclosporine and steroids, leading to the widespread use of MMF in the standard immunosuppressive regimen that we use today (the acute rejection rate in the MMF group was around 20% vs. ~40% in the azathioprine group).[2] About the same time, in 1997, the CHIB 201 International Study established that the use of basiliximab induction significantly reduced the incidence of acute rejection to around 35% compared to ~50% rejection rates without induction therapy.[3] When compared to the use of cyclosporine as the CNI, tacrolimus was shown to reduce the rate of acute rejection further, leading to its widespread adoption as the CNI of choice.[4] Subsequently, the Symphony trial established the safety and efficacy of low-dose tacrolimus with MMF and corticosteroids when compared to either cyclosporine- or sirolimus-based regimens, making this the current regimen of choice worldwide.[5] Finally, while belatacept provided a CNI-free alternative for maintenance immunosuppression, the higher rates of early acute rejection episodes with better renal function and lower rates of DSA formation, logistics of monthly infusion, and high cost thwarted its widespread clinical use. The newer once-daily formulation of tacrolimus, Envarsus, is increasingly used, as it has potential to improve adherence and has better bioavailability.[6] Figure 4.1 summarizes the timeline for the advances made in transplant immunosuppression and the pivotal clinical trials

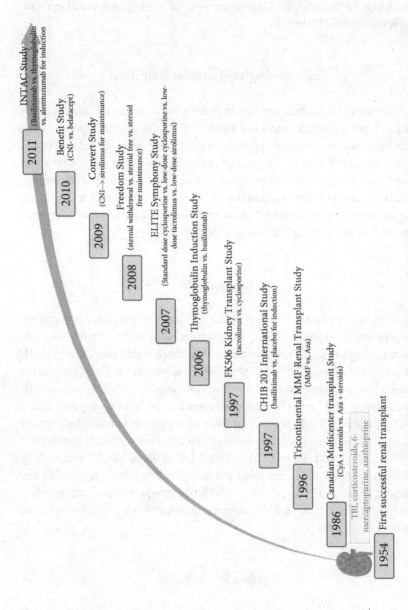

Figure 4.1 Pivotal clinical studies that influenced improvement in kidney transplant outcome.

that contributed to these innovations. While these advances in immunosuppressive strategies have markedly improved 1-year renal allograft survival, still approximately 40% of allografts are lost by 10 years and the rate of chronic graft loss has changed little over time.[7] Improving long-term allograft survival remains a major unmet need in the field.

Immunological Basis for Rejection

Kidneys transplanted between two humans are rejected unless the donor and recipient are genetically indistinguishable, as is the case in identical twins. Otherwise potent immunosuppressive medications are required for the life of the allograft. Rejection is caused by the recipient's immune response to foreign (nonself) elements ("alloantigens") present on the transplanted organ—protein or carbohydrate moieties that differ between the donor and recipient. The transplanted organ is referred to as the "allograft" and the immune response mounted against it as the "alloimmune response."

Alloantigens

Alloantigens, or transplantation antigens, are genetically encoded polymorphic proteins that are expressed on tissues and differ between individuals of the same species.[8] They can be divided into major histocompatibility antigens encoded by the major histocompatibility complex (MHC; in humans, the human leukocyte antigen [HLA] complex) and minor histocompatibility antigens (mHAgs). The terms "major" and "minor" refer to the potency of the immune response elicited by these antigens. HLAs are polymorphic glycoproteins encoded by polymorphic multigene clusters on chromosome 6 and come in two classes, class I (HLA-A, -B, -C, -E, -F, and -G) and class II (HLA-DR, -DP, and -DQ),[9] while mHAgs are defined as potentially any other polymorphic protein that is encoded anywhere in the genome.[10] In addition, ABO blood groups, which are carbohydrate moieties, serve as transplantation antigens that can be recognized by preformed antibodies in the recipient.

Antigen Presentation

The donor's mismatched MHC molecules serve as alloantigens that can be recognized by the recipient's T cells either in an intact form or after they are processed into peptides bound to the recipient's MHC molecules.[11] The first situation is peculiar to transplantation and is referred to as "direct alloantigen presentation," while the second is common with microbial antigens and is referred to as "indirect alloantigen presentation." Although it was initially thought that direct presentation occurs when donor antigen presenting cells (APCs) that accompany the graft migrate to secondary lymphoid tissues and interact with recipient T cells,[12] now it is accepted that the mechanism of direct presentation is the transfer of intact donor MHC molecules to recipient APCs.[13-15] Transfer occurs principally via exosomes shed by graft cells, including donor APCs, and is referred to as "cross-decoration" or "semidirect presentation."

Activation of the Innate Alloimmune Response

To initiate an immune response, the specialized innate immune cells known as APCs, which primarily include dendritic cells (DCs) and macrophages, need to process and present fragments of non-self-antigen to T cells in a productive fashion—that is, in a manner that leads to T cell activation, proliferation, and differentiation. To do so, APCs or their precursors, the monocytes, must first be activated to acquire antigen-presenting capacity and to upregulate costimulatory molecules and cytokines necessary for T cell activation. In mice, such activation of innate cells occurs through pattern-recognition receptors or through specific receptors such as signal regulatory protein alpha (SIRPα), which binds to CD47, and paired immunoglobulin-like receptors (PIRs), which recognize nonself MHC class I molecules. Orthologs of both mouse PIR and CD47 have been identified in humans, and they bind HLA molecules and human SIRPα, respectively, suggesting that innate recognition of allogeneic nonself could initiate alloimmune responses in humans as well.[16,17]

T Cell Activation (The Three-Signal Model)

T Cell Receptor (TCR) Engagement (Signal 1)
The principal cell of the adaptive immune system that is necessary and sufficient for allograft rejection is the T cell.[18] T cells comprise two main subsets: CD4 and CD8. CD8 T cells perform cytotoxic functions while CD4 T cells are responsible for providing help to CD8 T cells as well as other immune cells, although they can also be cytotoxic. Both CD4 and CD8 T cells recognize alloantigens (MHC-peptide complexes) via their T cell receptor (TCR). Gene rearrangement mechanisms generate an extremely diverse repertoire of TCRs that recognize virtually all possible MHC-peptide combinations with high molecular specificity. This mechanism of generating receptor diversity is one reason T cells (and

B cells) are referred to as adaptive immune cells, in contrast to APCs, which express nonrearranging, germline-encoded non-self-receptors. Engagement of the TCR by MHC-peptide, known as signal 1, triggers a signaling cascade that is required for T cell activation. Key features of this cascade are shown in Figure 4.2.[19] Note that calcineurin activation downstream of the TCR is the target of the most successful immunosuppressive therapies to date, cyclosporin and tacrolimus.

Costimulation (Signal 2)

TCR stimulation alone is not sufficient for T cell activation. A second signal delivered by costimulatory receptors is required. A key costimulatory receptor on T cells is CD28, which binds the B7 family costimulatory ligands CD80 and CD86 on mature APCs (Figure 4.2).[20] A fusion protein, CTLA4-Ig (belatacept), that blocks B7-CD28 interaction is a powerful immunosuppressive agent used in clinical transplantation.[21] Sirolimus (rapamycin), inhibits the **mammalian target of rapamycin** (mTOR) protein kinase downstream of CD28, is used in the clinic for the prevention of allograft rejection. Another costimulatory receptor of great interest in transplantation is CD154, also known as CD40 ligand (CD40L) (Figure 4.2).[22-24] CD154 is expressed on activated CD4 T cells, while CD40 is present mainly on B cells, DCs, and macrophages. CD154 was first discovered because of its role in inducing antibody isotype switching in B cells. Isotype switching is the process by which B cells shift from producing immunoglobulin M (IgM) to the more effective IgG antibody isotypes. Therefore, engagement of CD40 by CD154 is an important mechanism by which CD4 T cells provide help to B cells. CD154 is also a key enhancer of T cell stimulation, albeit in an indirect manner. By binding to CD40, it upregulates B7 expression and enhances cytokine production by mature DCs (Figure 4.2). This in turn leads to further costimulation of T cells, especially the CD8 subset.

T cell integrins constitute another group of costimulatory receptors. Integrins extend the interaction between the APC presenting the alloantigen and the alloreactive T cell and by doing so, sustain TCR signaling (signal 1) necessary for full T cell activation (Figure 4.2).[25,26] The integrins LFA-1 and CD2 (LFA-3) on T cells bind to their ligands ICAM-1 and CD58, respectively, on DCs. Blocking LFA-1 or CD2 delays kidney transplant rejection in nonhuman primates and in clinical trials.[27,28] The development and marketing of anti-LFA-1 (efalizumab) and anti-CD2 antibodies (alefacept) for clinical use in autoimmunity and transplantation have been halted due to serious side effects such as progressive multifocal leukoencephalopathy (PML).

Cytokines (Signal 3)

In addition to antigen-recognition (signal 1) and costimulation (signal 2), cytokines play a critical role in T cell activation and proliferation and are often

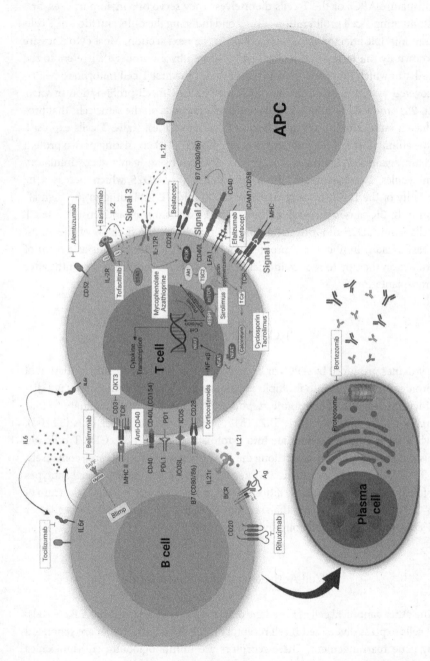

Figure 4.2 Interactions between T cells, B cells, and antigen presenting cells (APCs).

referred to as signal 3 (Figure 4.2).[29] The cytokines involved are proteins secreted by mature APCs or the T cells themselves. They serve two main purposes, first stimulating T cell proliferation and second inducing the differentiation of T cells into multiple effector subsets described in the next section. Most cytokines are known by the term "interleukin" (IL) followed by a number that refers to the order in which they were discovered. IL-2 was the first T cell mitogen to be discovered by virtue of its strong capacity to induce T cell proliferation in vitro. IL-2 is produced by antigen-activated T cells and acts on the same cells that produce it (autocrine) or on neighboring cells (paracrine). Naive T cells express a low affinity form of the interleukin-2 receptor (IL-2R) consisting of two protein chains: gamma (γ) and beta (β). Upon activation by antigen and costimulatory molecules, T cells express a third chain, alpha (α) or CD25, which increases the affinity of the IL-2R by approximately 1,000-fold. IL-2 binding to the high affinity IL-2R causes the proliferation (clonal expansion) of antigen-activated T cells. Anti-CD25 monoclonal antibodies that block the α-chain of the IL-2R (basiliximab) inhibit T cell proliferation and are used in humans as a form of induction therapy to reduce incidence of rejection in the first few months after transplantation.

T Cell Differentiation

Cytokines produced by APCs or by activated T cells direct the differentiation of proliferating T cells into multiple populations or "subtypes" that carry out distinct functions in the immune response.[30,31] CD4 T cells differentiate to four major helper subtypes (Th1, Th2, Th17, and T follicular helper cells [TFHs]), while CD8 T cells differentiate into cytotoxic T cells (CTLs). CD8 T cells can also acquire helper functions along the same lines as CD4 T cells and, conversely, CD4 T cells can be cytotoxic.[32] Moreover, both CD4 and CD8 T cell subtypes often overlap, sharing transcription factors or cytokines, reflecting a spectrum of T cell differentiation rather than separate lineages. Cytokines also assist effector T cells in transitioning to long-lived memory T cells.

B Cell Activation and Differentiation

The other canonical cell of the adaptive immune system is the B cell. Like T cells, B cells express diversified B cell receptors (BCRs) for antigen that are generated by gene rearrangement. These receptors are immunoglobulin (Ig) molecules that, unlike TCR, recognize antigenic epitopes present in whole proteins, independently of MHC molecules (Figure 4.2). The main function of B cells is mediating the humoral immune response. Upon activation by antigen and with the help of CD4 T cells, B cells proliferate and differentiate into antibody (Ab)-producing plasma cells.[33]

B cells also present antigen.[34] Although they are less potent on a per cell basis than DCs or macrophages, their larger numbers following proliferation provide them with the ability to amplify T cell activation and differentiation. B cells also produce effector cytokines such as TNFα, IFNγ, IL-6, IL-12, and IL-17 that are directly injurious to the allograft or provide T cell help, including their differentiation into TFH. Therefore, B cells interact with T cells in a bidirectional manner during the alloimmune response and contribute directly to rejection through Ab or cytokine production (Figure 4.2). The cardinal B cell differentiation pathway is the transformation of B cells into long-lived memory B cells and plasma cells that produce high-affinity, isotype-switched Ab of the IgG, IgA, or IgE class. This transformation occurs in the germinal centers of secondary lymphoid tissues and is guided by T cell help via costimulatory molecules and cytokines (Figure 4.2).[33]

Propagation of the Alloimmune Response

For naive T and B cells, the activation processes described above occur in secondary lymphoid tissues (the spleen and lymph nodes). Once activated, naive T cells differentiate into effector T cells (for example, cytotoxic CD8 T cells) that migrate to the target tissue, the allograft, where the bulk of the antigen resides. Although naive (primary) alloimmune responses are indeed initiated in secondary lymphoid tissues, they are propagated locally in the allograft.[35] First, graft APCs interact with effector T cells in an antigen-specific (cognate) manner to mediate effector T cell transendothelial migration, proliferation, and differentiation.[36] Second, effector T cells differentiate into memory T cells in secondary lymphoid tissues as well as the graft.[37,38] Memory T cells are long-lived, have a low threshold for stimulation, and can be reactivated outside secondary lymphoid tissues, making them a prime player in allograft rejection. Third, chronic inflammation in a transplanted organ gives rise to tertiary lymphoid tissues that then direct naive T cell activation locally.[39] Tertiary lymphoid tissues are often a defining feature of chronic active rejection and in addition to T cell activation, harbor germinal centers that serve as local antibody factories.[40]

The consequence of allorecognition and subsequent initiation and propagation of the alloimmune response manifest as clinical transplant rejection. While the crucial pathways that are targeted by several key immunosuppressive agents were highlighted in this section, the following section will detail the mechanisms of action of individual agents and their associated adverse effects (Table 4.1).

Table 4.1 Mechanism of Action and Adverse Effects of Various Induction Immunosuppressive Agents

Drugs	Mechanism of action	Adverse effects	Comments
Thymoglobulin	Thymoglobulin includes polyclonal antibodies against T-cell markers (CD2, CD3, CD4, CD8, CD11a, CD18, CD25, CD44, CD45), HLA-DR, HLA Class I heavy chains, and β2 microglobulin. Depletes T cells through three different mechanisms: *Apoptosis via activation-induced cell death* *Antibody-dependent cell-mediated cytotoxicity* *Complement-dependent cytotoxicity* Downregulates T cell activation molecules (TCR, CD4, CD8, CD25, HLA I, HLA II & CD45) Binding to selectins and integrin families (CD11a, CD18), thereby preventing T cell help	1. **Serum sickness:** (Arthralgia, myalgias, lymphadenopathy, proteinuria) Can occur 5–15 days after the dose. 2. **Cytokine release syndrome (CRS):** (Caused by cytokine release from activated monocytes and lymphocytes. Reported with rapid infusions) **Five Grades: CRS:** Grade 1—Fever with or without constitutional symptoms Grade 2—Hypotension responding to fluids; hypoxia responding to < 40% FiO2 Grade 3—Hypotension managed with one vasopressor; hypoxia requiring > 40% FiO2 Grade 4—Life-threatening consequences; urgent intervention indicated Grade 5—Death 3. **Hematology:** Leukopenia and thrombocytopenia 4. **Infection and malignancies** including PTLD 5. **Other** adverse reactions: lab abnormalities, abdominal pain, urinary tract infections, anxiety, hypertension, dyspnea, chills, hyperkalemia	**Premedication:** Corticosteroids, acetaminophen, and/or an antihistamine prior to each infusion **Management of CRS:** Supportive measures IL-6R blockade (tocilizumab) for severe cases Anecdotal usage of methylene blue (directly inhibits iNOS and guanyl cyclase)
IL-2R fusion protein (basiliximab)	Basiliximab binds to the α chain of the IL-2R complex (CD25) that is expressed on activated T cells. As a result, T cell activation and proliferation are prevented without cell lysis or depletion.	Basiliximab has no adverse events seen in organ transplantation patients.	

Drug	Description	Adverse effects	Notes
Alemtuzumab (Campath 1H)	Humanized IgG1κ monoclonal antibody that recognizes CD52, expressed on all lymphocytes and causes antibody-dependent cellular cytolysis and complement-mediated lysis of T and B lymphocytes, and also natural killer cells, monocytes, and macrophages.	1. **Common reactions:** upper respiratory and urinary tract infections, lymphopenia, leukopenia, hypothyroidism, tachycardia, skin rashes, pruritus, pyrexia, and fatigue. 2. **Rare but serious effects:** cervicocephalic arterial dissection, stroke, including hemorrhagic and ischemic stroke. 3. **Autoimmune disorders** (Goodpasture's syndrome, Graves' disease, aplastic anemia, ITP, chronic inflammatory demyelinating polyradiculoneuropathy, serum sickness, fatal transfusion associated graft versus host disease, hemophagocytic lymphohistiocytosis) from the emergence of autoreactive B cells) 4. **Anaphylaxis**, first dose reactions—mitigated by subcutaneous administration 5. **Infection/Malignancy:** Reactivation or development of de novo viral (Epstein–Barr virus (EBV) infection, BK, CMV, and progressive multifocal leukoencephalopathy) or fungal infections, malignancy.	Major concern is that of homeostatic repopulation of memory T cells and the risk of late rejection episodes as well as delayed recovery from opportunistic viral infections.
Rituximab	Genetically engineered chimeric murine/human monoclonal antibody directed against the CD20 antigen found on the surface of B lymphocytes (not plasma cells).	1. **Common:** Infusion reactions, leukopenia, thrombocytopenia, abdominal pain (these are not common) 2. **Rare:** cardiac arrythmias 3. **Infection:** occasional reactivation of CMV infection 4. **Other:** significantly increased risk of acute rejection in standard immunological risk renal transplant recipients	Some success in desensitization protocols. Not used as a routine agent for induction.

Immunosuppressive Agents

Immunosuppressive agents principally act through either depleting the lymphocytes, blocking their activation, or diverting their trafficking. The net result of these actions is their therapeutic effect (suppressing rejection). However, undesirable consequences of the resultant immunodeficiency (infections or malignancy) or nonimmune toxicity make therapeutic immunosuppression a double-edged sword. Based on their clinical use, immunosuppressive agents can be divided into those primarily used for induction and those used for maintenance therapy.

Induction Agents
Delayed graft function (DGF) and early acute rejection negatively affect graft survival. Patients with DGF have an increased risk of acute rejection, and the combination is associated with worse graft survival. Induction therapy is specific immunosuppression therapy given at the time of transplantation to lower the incidence of early acute rejection. Induction can be achieved using either monoclonal or polyclonal antibodies that destroy T cells, B cells, or both, or by the use of monoclonal antibodies or fusion proteins that reduce immune responsiveness without lymphodepletion. T cell depletion is often accompanied by cytokine release and the resultant severe systemic symptoms with rabbit antithymocyte globulin (Thymoglobulin, Genzyme). While early rejection risk is mitigated, late rejection that occurs as the lymphocytes reconstitute remains a problem with lymphodepletion. Moreover, the risk of opportunistic infections and lymphoproliferative disorders are the major limitations for the use of lymphodepleting agents. In contrast, nondepleting agents have lower efficacy, but the reduced immunodeficiency and the low nonimmune toxicity given that the target protein expression is limited to the activated immune cells are major advantages. The mechanisms of action of commonly used induction agents and their immune and nonimmune mediated toxicities are detailed in Table 4.1.

Maintenance Immunosuppressive Agents
Uninterrupted access to immunosuppression is paramount to minimize rejection and promote long-term allograft and patient survival. This fundamental principle forms the basis for the use of maintenance immunosuppression in solid organ transplant recipients. Corticosteroids are the oldest immunosuppressive agents to be used in clinical transplantation and continue to be used in the modern era. They exert their effects principally through binding to glucocorticoid receptors (GRs). The ability of GRs to suppress the activity of nuclear transcription factors such as NF-κB and activator protein-1 (AP-1) as well as other key immunomodulatory transcription factors has been a major focus of research.

Since GRs are ubiquitously expressed, glucocorticoids affect virtually all immune cells with precise effects depending on the differentiation and activation state of the cell, making interpretation of in vivo effects in specific cell populations difficult. The metabolic, infectious, and noninfectious complications of the use of corticosteroids are described elsewhere.

Most small molecule immunosuppressive agents used in transplantation are derived from microbial metabolites and target proteins that are highly conserved in evolution. At therapeutic concentrations, these agents typically do not saturate their receptors—the effects are proportional to their blood concentration, making dosing and drug level monitoring crucial in clinical management. The first such small molecule agents, 6 mercaptopurine and its derivative azathioprine, were followed by the CNIs and the inosine monophosphate dehydrogenase inhibitor MMF, and then sirolimus. The mechanisms of action of these small molecule immunosuppressive agents and their immune and nonimmune mediated toxicities are detailed in Table 4.2. The following section details the various induction and maintenance immunosuppressive strategies that form the basis for the medical management of the renal transplant patient.

Immunosuppressive Strategies

Induction

At present, over 80% of KT recipients receive induction therapy with either rabbit antithymocyte globulin (Thymoglobulin, Genzyme), a lymphocyte-depleting polyclonal antibody, or basiliximab (Simulect, Novartis), a non-lymphocyte-depleting monoclonal antibody that targets the IL-2R. Specifically, in patients deemed to be at higher risk for acute rejection (for example, allosensitized recipients with panel reactive antibodies >20%, prior transfusions, black race, higher HLA antigen mismatches), induction with Thymoglobulin was shown to be more protective not only against any acute rejection but also in particular against high-grade rejection episodes, which eventually resulted in approval by the US Food and Drug Administration (FDA) for its usage for induction in patients at high-risk for acute rejection.[41] Basiliximab induction continues to be an alternative in low-risk transplant recipients. Attempts to further mitigate DGF by the addition of agents such as anti-TNF to Thymoglobulin was not shown to be successful, and indeed increased the risk of BK virus infection.[42]

An alternative to Thymoglobulin for depletional induction is alemtuzumab (Campath-1H, Berlex Laboratories), an anti-CD52 T-cell- and B-cell-depleting monoclonal antibody. In corticosteroid sparing immunosuppression strategies, alemtuzumab induction has been shown to reduce the incidence of

Table 4.2 Mechanism of Action and Adverse Effects of Various Maintenance Immunosuppressive Agents

Drugs	Mechanism of action	Adverse effects	Comments
Cyclosporine	11-amino acid cyclic peptide from *Tolypocladium inflatum*. Binds to cyclophilin. The complex inhibits calcineurin phosphatase and thus T cell activation by limiting nuclear translocation of NFAT. Causes specific and reversible inhibition of immunocompetent lymphocytes in the G_0- and G_1- phase of the cell cycle.	**Renal/Vascular:** nephrotoxicity, thrombotic microangiopathy **Endocrine and metabolic:** new-onset diabetes mellitus after transplantation, hirsutism, hyperlipidemia, gynecomastia, hypertrichosis, hypomagnesemia, and hyperuricemia **Electrolytes:** hyperkalemia, Type 4 RTA, edema **Others:** hypertension, hyperkalemia (sometimes with hyperchloremic metabolic acidosis), neurotoxicity (seizures, PRES, anxiety, headache), fever, gum hyperplasia, skin changes, increased infection risk, malignancy.	Cyclosporine is extensively metabolized by CYP 3A isoenzymes, CYP3A4. **Drugs that increase cyclosporine concentration:** CYP3A inhibitors (diltiazem, verapamil, nicardipine, azole antifungals, macrolide antibiotics, methylprednisolone, allopurinol, amiodarone, colchicine, HIV protease inhibitors, grapefruit juice, and nirmatrelvir (Paxlovid) **Drugs that decrease cyclosporine concentration:** CYP3A inducers (rifampicin, carbamazepine, phenytoin, orlistat, octreotide, bosentin, telaprevir, St. John's wort)
Tacrolimus	Macrolide antibiotic from *Streptomyces tsukabaensis*. Binds to FKBP12 The complex inhibits calcineurin phosphatase and thus T cell activation by limiting nuclear translocation of NFAT.	**Renal and Vascular:** nephrotoxicity and thrombotic microangiopathy **Metabolic:** diabetes and IGT **CNS:** neurotoxicity (seizures, PRES, anxiety, headache, tremors, vivid and colorful dreams, nightmares, visual blurring, asthenia) **Electrolytes:** hypomagnesemia, hyperkalemia, Type 4 RTA, edema **Others:** bone pain, leukopenia, alopecia, infection risk, malignancy, myocardial hypertrophy (concentric increases in left ventricular posterior wall and interventricular septum thickness). Rare cases of pure red cell aplasia.	Same as above

Drug	Mechanism	Adverse effects	Notes
Azathioprine	Pro-drug that releases 6-mercaptopurine and thioguanine (6-TGN), by the action of hypoxanthine-guanine phosphoribosyl transferase (HPRT) and thiopurine methyltransferase (TPMT) enzymes. Inhibits purine synthesis (its metabolites are incorporated into the replicating DNA and halt cell division).	Agranulocytosis, dose-dependent leukopenia and thrombocytopenia, macrocytosis and infections Sweet syndrome (acute febrile neutrophilic dermatosis) GI disturbance, hepatotoxicity (a rare, but life-threatening hepatic veno-occlusive disease associated with chronic administration of azathioprine)	Best safety profile in pregnancy Patients with low or absent TPMT activity are at an increased risk of developing severe, life-threatening myelotoxicity if receiving conventional doses of azathioprine (The most common nonfunctional alleles associated with reduced levels of TPMT activity are TPMT*2, TPMT*3A and TPMT*3C)
Sirolimus & Everolimus	Triene macrolide antibiotic from *Streptomyces hygroscopicus* (From Easter Island) Binds to FKBP12. The complex inhibits mTOR and IL-2 driven T cell proliferation.	Hyperlipidemia, hyperglycemia Nephrotoxicity, proteinuria, pedal edema, Lymphocele formation, poor wound healing, wound dehiscence Interstitial lung disease, noninfectious pneumonitis Increases the risk of CNI-induced thrombotic microangiopathy, Infections and malignancy including lymphomas, Angioedema, exfoliative dermatitis Rare: stomatitis, aphthous ulcers, bone necrosis, thromboembolism	Effective in the prevention of NMSC Metabolized by CYP3A4, so similar drug interaction to those of CNI.

(continued)

Table 4.2 Continued

Drugs	Mechanism of action	Adverse effects	Comments
Mycophenolate	Derived from Penicillium molds potent, selective, uncompetitive, and reversible inhibitor of inosine monophosphate dehydrogenase (IMPDH), and therefore inhibits the de novo pathway of guanosine nucleotide synthesis without incorporation into DNA. Inhibits proliferative responses of T- and B-lymphocytes to both mitogenic and allospecific stimulation as well as limits antibody secretion.	Malignancy (including lymphomas) and infection. GI disturbance (diarrhea, dyspepsia, abdominal pain) Progressive multifocal leukoencephalopathy Teratogenic and contraindicated in pregnancy. Neutropenia and pure red cell aplasia	Antimetabolite of choice for renal transplantation Antacids containing magnesium should be spaced from the intake of mycophenolate. Tacrolimus increases blood availability of mycophenolate, while cyclosporine reduces the levels. Concomitant administration with sevelamer would reduce mycophenolate levels.
Belatacept	A selective T-cell (lymphocyte) costimulation blocker, binds to CD80 and CD86 on antigen presenting cells thereby blocking CD28 mediated costimulation of T lymphocytes.	PTLD, especially CNS PTLD and other malignancies Serious infections, including JC virus-associated PML. Rare occurrence of progressive multifocal leukoencephalopathy and Guillain Barré syndrome.	Contraindicated in EBV seronegative patients due to the increased risk of PTLD Reno protective, but Increased risk of acute rejection when compared to tacrolimus.

acute rejection in low-immunological-risk KT recipients when compared to basiliximab induction.[43] Nonetheless, alemtuzumab has never been licensed for use in kidney transplantation, and its use in this setting remains off-label.

Maintenance Immunosuppression

Triple Immunosuppression

While there is no standardized approach to maintenance immunosuppression management in kidney transplantation, a triple immunosuppression regimen comprising of a calcineurin inhibitor, mycophenolate, and corticosteroids represents the most utilized strategy worldwide.[44] Previous studies have established the superiority of mycophenolate over azathioprine for the prevention of acute rejection after transplantation, making mycophenolate the antimetabolite of choice for maintenance immunosuppression.[2] The landmark "Symphony study" in 2007 compared daclizumab (IL-2R antagonist) induction followed by standard dose cyclosporine, MMF, and maintenance corticosteroids to regimes utilizing low-dose cyclosporine, low-dose tacrolimus, or low-dose sirolimus. It established the advantage of the low-dose-tacrolimus-based triple immunosuppression strategy, which has been widely adopted.[5] This tacrolimus-based regimen led to a 2- to 3-fold reduction in the incidence of acute rejection, superior renal function, and better allograft survival compared to the other cyclosporine- and sirolimus-based regimes. There remains an ongoing debate regarding the most appropriate dose of tacrolimus and appropriate mycophenolate exposure for optimal long-term immunosuppression. While the Symphony trial pointed to an optimal tacrolimus trough level of 5–8 ng/mL, uncertainty persists regarding MPA exposure. Furthermore, tacrolimus trough levels lower than 5 ng/mL increase the risk of donor-specific antibody development, thereby heightening the risk for subsequent alloimmune allograft injury.[45] Thus, tacrolimus should generally be dosed to maintain a trough of more than 5 ng/mL.

Corticosteroid-Free Immunosuppression

Chronic corticosteroid usage leads to several well-recognized metabolic and nonmetabolic adverse effects such as glucose intolerance, hyperlipidemia, hypertension, weight gain, premature cataracts, and osteopenia as well as the increase in the risk for infections, thus contributing to increased cardiovascular and infectious mortality and morbidity. Thus, there was an understandable desire to develop steroid-sparing immunosuppressive regimens. Although approximately 30% of all KT recipients in the United States are maintained on a tacrolimus/MPA combination without steroid at 1 year following KT, the true long-term benefits of this approach remain unclear. Earlier attempts at steroid withdrawal with the use of cyclosporine as the CNI led to an unacceptable increase in the incidence of acute rejection. However, corticosteroid withdrawal with the use of tacrolimus and MMF has been shown to be associated with comparable long-term mortality and graft survival when compared to steroid maintenance. Nonetheless concern remains about the greater incidence of acute rejection in a significant minority of patients with steroid avoidance, even with the use of tacrolimus and MMF. While retrospective studies that compared corticosteroid avoidance to historical patient cohorts that remained on maintenance reported a lower incidence of both metabolic and nonmetabolic complications with steroid withdrawal, the true benefits of steroid withdrawal or avoidance are yet to be established in large randomized clinical trials. These factors limit the acceptance of corticosteroid withdrawal as a universal immunosuppression strategy.

CNI Minimization and CNI-Free Immunosuppression

CNIs are nephrotoxic and adversely affect blood pressure, lipid levels, and glucose homeostasis. Thus, a major challenge in the field has been to develop immunosuppressive regimens that limit the incidence of acute rejection like CNIs, but without the adverse renal and cardiovascular side effects. Initial attempts at CNI avoidance utilized the strategy of complete CNI avoidance with daclizumab induction and maintenance immunosuppression with MMF and corticosteroids, but these resulted in unacceptable high rates of acute rejection. When sirolimus, the first mTOR inhibitor (mTORi), was introduced further CNI-avoidance strategies emerged using sirolimus with or without MPA and were investigated in several randomized, controlled trials. Strikingly high acute rejection rates with these approaches led to the abandonment of such strategies.[5,46,47] Furthermore, the need for high mTORi doses (especially for sirolimus) resulted in high rates of complications and withdrawal from studies. Although everolimus in combination with low-dose tacrolimus (target trough tacrolimus levels 1.5 to 3 ng/mL) has been shown to be associated with comparable 1-year acute rejection rates when compared to standard dose CNI with MPA, there was no demonstrable improvement in renal function.[48] Further, the true impact of this regimen on long-term allograft survival and function is not clear.

An alternative approach involves later CNI withdrawal—namely, CNI is withdrawn at some point after transplantation and replaced by an mTORi in combination with MPA and corticosteroids. Two key factors need to be considered for the implementation of this strategy: when to convert to the mTORi and how quickly to discontinue the CNI.

Early conversion is associated with greater improvement in renal function, and late conversion is associated with significant proteinuria. The optimum time for conversion is about 3 months post-transplant. Progressive rather than abrupt discontinuation of the CNI would be preferable given the association of acute rejection with abrupt CNI cessation. However, CNI withdrawal strategies have been marred by a higher incidence of treatment failures, mTORi intolerance, proteinuria, the development of donor-specific antibodies, and higher acute rejection rates.[49-53]

Currently, only one CNI-free regimen, belatacept in combination with mycophenolate and corticosteroids, is FDA approved for use in adult KT recipients (as long as the recipient is seropositive for Epstein–Barr virus [EBV]). Results of the BENEFIT trial have established that belatacept maintenance with mycophenolate and corticosteroids resulted in superior 1-year and 7-year Estimated Glomerular Filtration Rate (eGFR) as well as better patient graft and patient survival at 7 years when compared to a cyclosporine-based maintenance immunosuppression regimen.[54-56] Of note, belatacept usage was associated with a greater incidence of acute rejection episodes, particularly those of high-grade rejection. There was also a greater incidence of post-transplant lymphoproliferative disorder, resulting in the FDA approval being limited to EBV seropositive patients alone.[56] Furthermore, conversion of CNI to belatacept after 6 months post-transplantation in adult renal transplant recipients with stable renal function was again shown to be associated with superior renal function assessed by eGFR.[57] Thus, belatacept-based CNI avoidance or withdrawal regimens could be appropriate in a small proportion of EBV-seropositive patients with no evidence of acute rejection. While the need for in-center infusions limits its widespread clinical applicability, it could also represent an alternative immunosuppressive strategy to improve therapy adherence.

Tacrolimus Monotherapy

Alemtuzumab causes profound depletion of circulating mononuclear cells, with some T cell subsets showing only partial recovery of circulating numbers even beyond the first year post-transplantation. This profound and protracted immune cell depletion gives rise to the tantalizing possibility that induction immunosuppression with alemtuzumab might allow for minimization of maintenance immunosuppression. In line with this notion, several small single-center studies underscored the safety and efficacy of alemtuzumab induction with tacrolimus monotherapy alone in a select group of low-immunological-risk renal transplant recipients.[58-61] In fact, the incidence of early acute rejection was lower with tacrolimus monotherapy when compared to conventional immunosuppression with both tacrolimus and MPA. Data on long-term safety and efficacy of this approach is still lacking, and therefore this strategy has not gained universal acceptance.

Immunosuppression for Special Scenarios

Immunosuppression in the Elderly

Increasing numbers of renal transplants are being performed in transplant recipients aged ≥ 65 years. For example, in the United States, the number of renal transplant recipients >65 years old increased over the past decade from 2,518 in 2008 to 4,427 in 2018.[62] Given that these patients are typically excluded from randomized controlled trials of immunosuppressive agents, insight is largely gained from retrospective studies and registry analyses.

Aging-induced modifications in the immune system are primarily characterized by dysfunctional immune responses and increased systemic inflammation collectively termed "inflamm-aging," and they influence immunosuppression considerations in this population.[63] Inflamm-aging results in chronic, low-grade, systemic inflammation characterized by a shift to the production of pro-inflammatory cytokines including IL-6, IL-1β, TNF-α, and IFN-γ, and reduction of the chemokine receptor expression and expression of several adhesion molecules. This inflammatory status contributes to metabolic dysfunction and insulin resistance and represents a significant risk factor for morbidity and mortality. In addition, the frequency of memory and effector T-cells increases with age. Contrasting these observations, older patients experience thymic involution resulting in reduced number of circulating naive T cells as well as reduced T cell receptor diversity and antibody responses. Clinically, elderly patients have a reduced risk of acute rejection.[64–66] Furthermore, CD4+ T-cell reconstitution after induction with lymphocyte-depleting agents is impaired in older recipients.[67] Alterations in the immune system with aging increase the risk of malignancies.

Aging is also associated with alterations in pharmacokinetics. For example, bioavailability of drugs is usually influenced by decreased intestinal or hepatic first-pass metabolism with aging. In addition, aging is associated with an increase in relative body fat content and a reduction in muscle mass, resulting in a larger volume of distribution of lipophilic drugs such as calcineurin inhibitors and mTORis. Reduction in albumin levels observed with aging results in decreased protein binding of agents such as tacrolimus (typically 99% protein bound), sirolimus (typically 91% protein bound), and MPA (typically 97% protein bound). Protein binding is especially important in the case of MPA, since the free fraction is the active inhibitor of inosine monophosphate dehydrogenase. Hypoalbuminemia could therefore lead to increased pharmacologic exposure to immunosuppressive medications. Finally, aging is also associated with reduced renal and hepatic clearance (reduction in hepatic cytochrome P450).

Table 4.3 Immunosuppression Strategies in the Elderly Kidney Transplant Recipients

Immunological risk	Risk of side effects	Induction immunosuppression	Maintenance immunosuppression
High	Low	Thymoglobulin	Tacrolimus + Mycophenolate + Steroids
High	High	Thymoglobulin	Tacrolimus + Mycophenolate + Steroids or Tailored maintenance regimen per side effects
Low	Low	Basiliximab	CNI minimization ± steroid withdrawal
Low	High	Basiliximab or short course of Thymoglobulin	CNI minimization ± steroid withdrawal

Personalization of immunosuppression management among older transplant recipients may be informed by consideration of recipient factors such as comorbidity burden, measures of biologic age, immunologic risk, measures of immunosenescence, and donor quality. Analysis of data from the United States Renal Data System (USRDS) reveals that older recipients are less likely to receive depletional induction with either Thymoglobulin or alemtuzumab and are more likely to receive induction with basiliximab.[68] While corticosteroid avoidance or withdrawal was not associated with increased risk of acute rejection, maintenance immunosuppression based on mTORi or cyclosporine, or strategies avoiding antimetabolite, were associated with an increase in the incidence of acute rejection.[68] Moreover, studies suggest that the choice of induction and maintenance immunosuppression strategies in older transplant recipients should be based on immunological risk of the recipients as well as the risk of side effects.[69] A summary of potential immunosuppression choices based on these two factors is provided in Table 4.3.

Immunosuppression during Pregnancy

Kidney transplantation restores sexual function and fertility in most patients with end-stage renal disease. Pregnancy in a kidney transplant recipient remains challenging due to side effects of immunosuppression and risk of allograft functional deterioration as well as the risks posed to the mother (e.g., complications such as preeclampsia and hypertension) and the fetus (e.g., complications such as premature birth and small for gestational age). All immunosuppressive drugs commonly used after kidney transplantation cross the placenta to some degree, whereby they pass into the fetal circulation and carry some risk of teratogenic and fetotoxic effects, and some also increase the risk of obstetric complications and maternal disease (Table 4.4). Of the maintenance immunosuppressive agents, mycophenolate stands out with high rates of birth defects and high miscarriage rates.[70] Both corticosteroids and CNIs increase the risk of diabetes and hypertension in pregnancy. Due to paucity of pregnancy outcome data on mTORis and belatacept, they are not considered the drug of choice in women who want to conceive and should be substituted prior to conception. Overall, registry data accumulated over the last six decades suggest that corticosteroids, CNIs, and azathioprine can be used in pregnant transplant recipients with little risk of adverse effects on the fetus or graft and thus remain the maintenance agents of choice in this population.[71] A detailed discussion on this topic is included in Chapter 3, "Wellness after kidney Transplantation."

Immunosuppression in Patients with Cancer

The overall incidence of cancer in renal transplant recipients is 90 per 1,000 patients at 10 years after transplant, which is twice as high as in the general population (c.f. 1.35 times in the dialysis population).[72] The incidence of nonmelanomatous skin cancers is much higher. There is a 50- to 200-fold higher risk for nonmelanoma-skin cancer (NMSC) in transplant recipients, contributing to increased morbidity and sometimes mortality. The excess burden of cancer in KT recipients is largely attributed to long-term immunosuppression; however, the pattern of the increased risk of cancer may differ by the dose and type of immunosuppression.

T-cell-depleting agents, used either for induction therapy or treatment of acute rejection, are associated with an increased risk of early posttransplant lymphoproliferative disorder (PTLD) compared with transplant recipients who received no induction therapy or experienced no acute rejection episodes. In contrast, a 30%–50% lower risk of cancer has been reported in patients treated with mTORis when compared to those receiving a CNI, particularly regarding rates of NMSC. While specific recommendations for immunosuppression management are lacking, the consensus is to reduce immunosuppression dose after cancer diagnosis, given the potential role of immunosuppression in reducing immune surveillance and promoting cancer growth.

Table 4.4 Maintenance Immunosuppressive Agents, Maternal and Fetal Effects

Drugs	In utero exposure	Maternal complications	Fetal complications	Infant exposure via lactation
Corticosteroids	Very low fetal exposure. Pass freely across placenta, 90% inactivated by placental 11-beta-hydroxysteroid dehydrogenase 2	Increased risk of gestational diabetes	**Congenital malformations:** Cleft palate (animal studies). **Other fetal complications:** none	<0.1% in breast milk
CNI (Cyclosporine/Tacrolimus)	Fetal concentration: ~35%–60% of maternal concentration. 70% crossover to fetal circulation	Increased risk of hypertension, dyslipidemia, hyperglycemia, renal dysfunction	**Congenital malformations:** Skeletal retardation (animal studies). None in humans. **Other fetal complications:** Intrauterine growth retardation	Tacrolimus: 0.2% in breast milk. CNIs not absorbed by the infant gut.
Mycophenolate	Readily crosses placenta.	Miscarriage rate of 45%	**Congenital malformations:** High prevalence (26%), Microtia, cleft palate, hypoplastic nails, short 5th finger, corpus callosum agenesis, myelomeningocele, hydronephrosis, ASD, tracheo-esophageal atresia. **Other:** Preterm birth 62%, Low birth weight 31%	Highly protein bound, so very limited excretion, Limited safety data
Azathioprine	Readily crosses placenta. Fetus does not convert AZA from its inactive to the active and possibly teratogenic 6-mercaptopurine.	Safe	**Congenital malformations:** none	Very limited excretion
mTORi	Very limited data	Very limited data	**Congenital malformations:** IUGR, impaired skeletal ossification (animal studies)	Very limited data
Belatacept	Very limited data	Very limited data	Very limited data	Very limited data

Nonmelanoma Skin Cancers

The NMSCs, primarily squamous cell carcinomas (SCCs) and basal cell carcinomas (BCCs), account for 95% of all skin cancers seen in organ transplant recipients. Merkel cell carcinomas and adnexal tumors make up a minority of NMSCs. Risk factors contributing to the development of NMSCs in KT recipients include past medical history of any previous skin cancer, a personal history of significant sun exposure, and a fair skin complexion (phototype) as well as immunosuppressive medication burden. SCCs occur at an earlier age, tend to be aggressive with greater recurrence rates, and infiltrate deeper into the surrounding tissues. As such, the tumors are more likely to involve the adjacent perineural and lymphatic structures and have a higher risk of metastasis in transplant recipients compared to the general population.[73]

Increased immunosuppressive load may lead to a reduction in immune surveillance for these cancers. In addition to impairing immunosurveillance, certain immunosuppressive agents have direct effects on keratinocytes, leading to tumorigenesis and cancer progression. For instance, CNIs induce phenotypic changes in cells and increase tumor invasiveness in nontransformed cells through the activity of transforming growth factor beta (TGF-β).[74,75] Furthermore, cyclosporine induces activating transcription factor 3 production, through inhibition of the CNI/NFAT pathway, which results in the inhibition of p-53-dependent cellular senescence and subsequent uncontrolled tumor growth. Azathioprine, in the presence of UVA light, is associated with producing direct DNA damage through the production of reactive oxygen species.[76]

In addition to cancer-specific therapies, reduction or revision of immunosuppression appears to be the best method to reduce the risk of developing recurrent NMSCs in KT recipients. Mycophenolate was originally developed as an anticancer drug, and acts through blockage of purine biosynthesis, inhibiting inosine monophosphate dehydrogenase. In transplant registry studies mycophenolate-containing regimens have not shown differences in cancer rates compared with mycophenolate-free regimens.[72] The mTORis sirolimus and everolimus have antineoplastic effects attributed to their capacity to restrict uncontrolled cellular growth and to induce apoptosis both by p53-dependent and -independent means and by their ability to inhibit IL-10.[77] In addition, mTORis inhibit the translation of transcription factors resulting in reduced angiogenesis, preventing the multiprotein complexes (mTORC1 and mTORC2) pathway activation, thereby halting cell proliferation, particularly in the setting of cancer development.[78] Indeed, in a retrospective analysis of patients with a history of SCC, sirolimus-switch from a CNI was associated with ~40% reduction in the development of new SCCs. These results were further corroborated in a prospective clinical trial that demonstrated regression of NMSC after sirolimus -switch within 6 months.[79] Taken together, mTORi switch should be considered for

NMSC immunosuppression management. A detailed discussion on this topic is in Chapter 10, "Cancers after Kidney Transplantation."

Opportunistic Infections

As described in the section on immunosuppressive drugs, post-transplant opportunistic infections are a major consequence of the resultant immunodeficiency. Reduction or cessation of immunosuppression remains the mainstay of immunosuppression management in cases of opportunistic infections such as primary EBV disease or PTLD. Furthermore, reduction of immunosuppression, and specifically cessation of antimetabolite agents is shown to be the only effective treatment for BK polyoma virus nephropathy.[80] Antimetabolites are typically withdrawn with the onset of any severe infection with a plan to reintroduce with clinical and microbiological improvement. This is discussed in Chapter 9, "Late Post-Transplant Infections."

Conclusion

In summary, the field of kidney transplantation has come far since the first successful renal transplant in 1954. Major advances in immunosuppression over the last 70 years have played a pivotal role in achieving truly remarkable success. Nonetheless approximately 40% of allografts are still lost by 10 years, and improvement in long-term allograft outcomes remains a major goal. The current "one size fits all" model of immunosuppressive management is a major impediment for further improvement in clinical outcomes given that some patients who are under-immunosuppressed experience alloimmune injury, while others at the opposite end of the spectrum develop infections and cancer. Personalization of immunosuppression informed by risk stratification and possibly immune assays, together with the development of novel targeted therapeutic agents in the future will hopefully deliver further improvements in the health and outcome of patients with renal transplants.

Abbreviations

APC: antigen presenting cell, AZA: azathioprine, BCC: basal cell cancer, BCR: B cell receptor, CNI: calcineurin inhibitor, DC: dendritic cell, DGF: delayed graft function, FDA: Food and Drug Administration, GR: glucocorticoid receptor, HLA: human leukocyte antigen, IFN: interferon, IL: interleukin, KT: kidney transplant, MMF: mycophenolate mofetil,

MPA: mycophenolic acid, mTORi: mammalian target of rapamycin inhibitor, mHAgs: minor histocompatibility antigens, NMSC: nonmelanomatous skin cancer, PML: progressive multifocal leukoencephalopathy, PIR: paired immunoglobulin like-receptor, PTLD: post-transplant lymphoproliferative disorder, TCR: T cell receptor, TFH: T follicular helper cell, TGF-β: transforming growth factor beta, TNF-α: tumor necrosis factor-alpha, USRDS: United States Renal Data System, UVA: ultraviolet A.

References

1. Canadian Multicentre Transplant Study Group. A randomized clinical trial of cyclosporine in cadaveric renal transplantation: analysis at three years. *N Engl J Med.* 1986;314(19):1219–1225.
2. Mathew TH. A blinded, long-term, randomized multicenter study of mycophenolate mofetil in cadaveric renal transplantation: results at three years. Tricontinental Mycophenolate Mofetil Renal Transplantation Study Group. *Transplantation.* 1998;65(11):1450–1454.
3. Nashan B, Moore R, Amlot P, Schmidt AG, Abeywickrama K, Soulillou JP. Randomised trial of basiliximab versus placebo for control of acute cellular rejection in renal allograft recipients. CHIB 201 International Study Group. *Lancet.* 1997;350(9086):1193–1198.
4. Pirsch JD, Miller J, Deierhoi MH, Vincenti F, Filo RS. A comparison of tacrolimus (FK506) and cyclosporine for immunosuppression after cadaveric renal transplantation. FK506 Kidney Transplant Study Group. *Transplantation.* 1997;63(7):977–983.
5. Ekberg H, Tedesco-Silva H, Demirbas A, et al. Reduced exposure to calcineurin inhibitors in renal transplantation. *N Engl J Med.* 2007;357(25):2562–2575.
6. Rostaing L, Bunnapradist S, Grinyo JM, et al. Novel once-daily extended-release tacrolimus versus twice-daily tacrolimus in de novo kidney transplant recipients: two-year results of phase 3, double-blind, randomized trial. *Am J Kidney Dis.* 2016;67(4):648–659.
7. Hariharan S, Israni AK, Danovitch G. Long-term survival after kidney transplantation. *The N Engl J Med.* 2021;385(8):729–743.
8. Lakkis FG, Lechler RI. Origin and biology of the allogeneic response. *Cold Spring Harb Perspect Med.* 2013;3(8):pii: a014993.
9. Klein J, Sato A. The HLA system. *N Engl J Med.* 2000;343(10):702–709.
10. Dierselhuis M, Goulmy E. The relevance of minor histocompatibility antigens in solid organ transplantation. *Curr Opin Organ Transplant.* 2009;14(4):419–425.
11. Alegre ML, Lakkis FG, Morelli AE. Antigen presentation in transplantation. *Trends Immunol.* 2016;37(12):831–843.
12. Larsen CP, Morris PJ, Austyn JM. Migration of dendritic leukocytes from cardiac allografts into host spleens: a novel pathway for initiation of rejection. *J Exp Med.* 1990;171:307–314.
13. Herrera OB, Golshayan D, Tibbott R, et al. A novel pathway of alloantigen presentation by dendritic cells. *J Immunol.* 2004;173(8):4828–4837.
14. Liu Q, Rojas-Canales DM, Divito SJ, et al. Donor dendritic cell-derived exosomes promote allograft-targeting immune response. *J Clin Invest.* 2016;126(8):2805–2820.

15. Marino J, Babiker-Mohamed MH, Crosby-Bertorini P, et al. Donor exosomes rather than passenger leukocytes initiate alloreactive T cell responses after transplantation. *Sci Immunol.* 2016;1(1):aaf8759.
16. Hirayasu K, Arase H. Functional and genetic diversity of leukocyte immunoglobulin-like receptor and implication for disease associations. *J Hum Genet.* 2015;60(11):703–708.
17. Garcia-Sanchez C, Casillas-Abundis MA, Pinelli DF, Tambur AR, Hod-Dvorai R. Impact of SIRPalpha polymorphism on transplant outcomes in HLA-identical living donor kidney transplantation. *Clin Transplant.* 2021 Sep;35(9):e14406. doi: 10.1111/ctr.14406. Epub 2021 Jul 1.
18. Miller JFAP. Effect of neonatal thymectomy on the immunological responsiveness of the mouse. *Proc R Soc Lond B.* 1962;156:415–428.
19. Courtney AH, Lo WL, Weiss A. TCR signaling: mechanisms of initiation and propagation. *Trends Biochem Sci.* 2018;43(2):108–123.
20. Chen L, Flies DB. Molecular mechanisms of T cell co-stimulation and co-inhibition. *Nat Rev Immunol.* 2013;13(4):227–242.
21. Ford ML, Adams AB, Pearson TC. Targeting co-stimulatory pathways: transplantation and autoimmunity. *Nat Rev Nephrol.* 2014;10(1):14–24.
22. Larsen CP, Elwood ET, Alexander DZ, et al. Long-term acceptance of skin and cardiac allografts after blocking CD40 and CD28 pathways. *Nature.* 1996;381(6581):434–438.
23. Elgueta R, Benson MJ, de Vries VC, Wasiuk A, Guo Y, Noelle RJ. Molecular mechanism and function of CD40/CD40L engagement in the immune system. *Immunol Rev.* 2009;229(1):152–172.
24. Kirk AD, Burkly LC, Batty DS, et al. Humanized anti-CD154 monoclonal antibody treatment prevents acute renal allograft rejection in non-human primates. *Nature Med.* 1999;5:686–693.
25. Springer TA, Dustin ML, Kishimoto TK, Marlin SD. The lymphocyte function-associated LFA-1, CD2, and LFA-3 molecules: cell adhesion receptors of the immune system. *Annu Rev Immunol.* 1987;5:223–252.
26. Bockenstedt LK, Goldsmith MA, Dustin M, Olive D, Springer TA, Weiss A. The CD2 ligand LFA-3 activates T cells but depends on the expression and function of the antigen receptor. *J Immunol.* 1988;141(6):1904–1911.
27. Hourmant M, Bedrossian J, Durand D, et al. Multicenter comparative study of an anti-LFA-1 adhesion molecule monoclonal antibody and antithymocyte globulin in prophylaxis of acute rejection in kidney transplantation. *Transplant Proc.* 1995;27(1):864.
28. Weaver TA, Charafeddine AH, Agarwal A, et al. Alefacept promotes co-stimulation blockade based allograft survival in nonhuman primates. *Nat Med.* 2009;15(7):746–749.
29. Curtsinger JM, Mescher MF. Inflammatory cytokines as a third signal for T cell activation. *Curr Opin Immunol.* 2010;22(3):333–340.
30. Dong C. Cytokine regulation and function in T cells. *Annu Rev Immunol.* 2021;39:51–76.
31. Yin X, Chen S, Eisenbarth SC. Dendritic cell regulation of T helper cells. *Annu Rev Immunol.* 2021;39:759–790.
32. Taniuchi I. CD4 helper and CD8 cytotoxic T cell differentiation. *Annu Rev Immunol.* 2018;36:579–601.
33. Cyster JG, Allen CDC. B cell responses: cell interaction dynamics and decisions. *Cell.* 2019;177(3):524–540.

34. Hua Z, Hou B. The role of B cell antigen presentation in the initiation of CD4+ T cell response. *Immunol Rev.* 2020;296(1):24–35.
35. Zhuang Q, Liu Q, Divito SJ, et al. Graft-infiltrating host dendritic cells play a key role in organ transplant rejection. *Nature Communications.* 2016;7:12623.
36. Walch JM, Zeng Q, Li Q, et al. Cognate antigen directs CD8+ T cell migration to vascularized transplants. *J Clin Invest.* 2013;123(6):2663–2671.
37. Chalasani G, Dai Z, Konieczny BT, Baddoura FK, Lakkis FG. Recall and propagation of allospecific memory T cells independent of secondary lymphoid organs. *Proc Natl Acad Sci U S A.* 2002;99(9):6175–6180.
38. Abou-Daya KI, Tieu R, Zhao D, et al. Resident memory T cells form during persistent antigen exposure leading to allograft rejection. *Sci Immunol.* 19th March 2021;6(57):eabc8122. doi10.1126/sciimmunol.abc.8122
39. Nasr IW, Reel M, Oberbarnscheidt MH, et al. Tertiary lymphoid tissues generate effector and memory T cells that lead to allograft rejection. *Am J Transplant.* 2007;7(5):1071–1079.
40. Thaunat O, Field AC, Dai J, et al. Lymphoid neogenesis in chronic rejection: evidence for a local humoral alloimmune response. *Proc Natl Acad Sci U S A.* 2005;102(41):14723–14728.
41. Brennan DC, Daller JA, Lake KD, Cibrik D, Del Castillo D, Thymoglobulin Induction Study Group. Rabbit antithymocyte globulin versus basiliximab in renal transplantation. *N Engl J Med.* 2006;355(19):1967–1977.
42. Hricik DE, Armstrong B, Alhamad T, et al. Infliximab induction lacks efficacy and increases BK virus infection in deceased donor kidney transplant recipients: results of the CTOT-19 trial. *J Am Soc Nephrol.* 2023;34(1):145–159.
43. Hanaway MJ, Woodle ES, Mulgaonkar S, et al. Alemtuzumab induction in renal transplantation. *N Engl J Med.* 2011;364(20):1909–1919.
44. Nelson J, Alvey N, Bowman L, et al. Consensus recommendations for use of maintenance immunosuppression in solid organ transplantation: endorsed by the American College of Clinical Pharmacy, American Society of Transplantation, and the International Society for Heart and Lung Transplantation. *Pharmacotherapy.* 2022;42(8):599–633.
45. Wiebe C, Gibson IW, Blydt-Hansen TD, et al. Rates and determinants of progression to graft failure in kidney allograft recipients with de novo donor-specific antibody. *Am J Transplant.* 2015;15(11):2921–2930.
46. Vincenti F, Ramos E, Brattstrom C, et al. Multicenter trial exploring calcineurin inhibitors avoidance in renal transplantation. *Transplantation.* 2001;71(9):1282–1287.
47. Larson TS, Dean PG, Stegall MD, et al. Complete avoidance of calcineurin inhibitors in renal transplantation: a randomized trial comparing sirolimus and tacrolimus. *Am J Transplant.* 2006;6(3):514–522.
48. Langer RM, Hene R, Vitko S, et al. Everolimus plus early tacrolimus minimization: a phase III, randomized, open-label, multicentre trial in renal transplantation. *Transpl Int.* 2012;25(5):592–602.
49. Guba M, Pratschke J, Hugo C, et al. Early conversion to a sirolimus-based, calcineurin-inhibitor-free immunosuppression in the SMART trial: observational results at 24 and 36months after transplantation. *Transpl Int.* 2012;25(4):416–423.
50. Lebranchu Y, Thierry A, Toupance O, et al. Efficacy on renal function of early conversion from cyclosporine to sirolimus 3 months after renal transplantation: concept study. *Am J Transplant.* 2009;9(5):1115–1123.

51. Schena FP, Pascoe MD, Alberu J, et al. Conversion from calcineurin inhibitors to sirolimus maintenance therapy in renal allograft recipients: 24-month efficacy and safety results from the CONVERT trial. *Transplantation.* 2009;87(2):233–242.
52. Budde K, Becker T, Arns W, et al. Everolimus-based, calcineurin-inhibitor-free regimen in recipients of de-novo kidney transplants: an open-label, randomised, controlled trial. *Lancet.* 2011;377(9768):837–847.
53. Soveri I, Holme I, Holdaas H, Budde K, Jardine AG, Fellstrom B. A cardiovascular risk calculator for renal transplant recipients. *Transplantation.* 2012;94(1):57–62.
54. Vincenti F, Larsen C, Durrbach A, et al. Costimulation blockade with belatacept in renal transplantation. *N Engl J Med.* 2005;353(8):770–781.
55. Vincenti F, Rostaing L, Grinyo J, et al. Belatacept and long-term outcomes in kidney transplantation. *N Engl J Med.* 2016;374(4):333–343.
56. Vincenti F, Charpentier B, Vanrenterghem Y, et al. A phase III study of belatacept-based immunosuppression regimens versus cyclosporine in renal transplant recipients (BENEFIT study). *Am J Transplant.* 2010;10(3):535–546.
57. Budde K, Prashar R, Haller H, et al. Conversion from calcineurin inhibitor- to belatacept-based maintenance immunosuppression in renal transplant recipients: a randomized phase 3b trial. *J Am Soc Nephrol.* 2021;32(12):3252–3264.
58. Tan HP, Donaldson J, Basu A, et al. Two hundred living donor kidney transplantations under alemtuzumab induction and tacrolimus monotherapy: 3-year follow-up. *Am J Transplant.* 2009;9(2):355–366.
59. Margreiter R, Klempnauer J, Neuhaus P, Muehlbacher F, Boesmueller C, Calne RY. Alemtuzumab (Campath-1H) and tacrolimus monotherapy after renal transplantation: results of a prospective randomized trial. *Am J Transplant.* 2008;8(7):1480–1485.
60. Chan K, Taube D, Roufosse C, et al. Kidney transplantation with minimized maintenance: alemtuzumab induction with tacrolimus monotherapy—an open label, randomized trial. *Transplantation.* 2011;92(7):774–780.
61. Welberry Smith MP, Cherukuri A, Newstead CG, et al. Alemtuzumab induction in renal transplantation permits safe steroid avoidance with tacrolimus monotherapy: a randomized controlled trial. *Transplantation.* 2013;96(12):1082–1088.
62. Hart A, Smith JM, Skeans MA, et al. OPTN/SRTR 2018 annual data report: kidney. *Am J Transplant.* 2020;20 Suppl s1:20–130.
63. Fulop T, Larbi A, Dupuis G, et al. Immunosenescence and inflamm-aging as two sides of the same coin: friends or foes? *Front Immunol.* 2017;8:1960.
64. Hirokawa K, Makinodan T. Thymic involution: effect on T cell differentiation. *J Immunol.* 1975;114(6):1659–1664.
65. Frasca D, Diaz A, Romero M, Garcia D, Blomberg BB. B cell immunosenescence. *Annu Rev Cell Dev Biol.* 2020;36:551–574.
66. Schaenman JM, Rossetti M, Sidwell T, et al. Increased T cell immunosenescence and accelerated maturation phenotypes in older kidney transplant recipients. *Hum Immunol.* 2018;79(9):659–667.
67. Longuet H, Sautenet B, Gatault P, et al. Risk factors for impaired CD4+ T-cell reconstitution following rabbit antithymocyte globulin treatment in kidney transplantation. *Transpl Int.* 2014;27(3):271–279.
68. Lentine KL, Cheungpasitporn W, Xiao H, et al. Immunosuppression regimen use and outcomes in older and younger adult kidney transplant recipients: a national registry analysis. *Transplantation.* 2021;105(8):1840–1849.

69. Gill J, Sampaio M, Gill JS, et al. Induction immunosuppressive therapy in the elderly kidney transplant recipient in the United States. *Clin J Am Soc Nephrol.* 2011;6(5):1168–1178.
70. Moritz MJ, Constantinescu S, Coscia LA, Armenti D. Mycophenolate and pregnancy: teratology principles and national transplantation pregnancy registry experience. *Am J Transplant.* 2017;17(2):581–582.
71. McKay DB, Josephson MA, Armenti VT, et al. Reproduction and transplantation: report on the AST Consensus Conference on Reproductive Issues and Transplantation. *Am J Transplant.* 2005;5(7):1592–1599.
72. Chapman JR, Webster AC, Wong G. Cancer in the transplant recipient. *Cold Spring Harb Perspect Med.* 2013 July;3(7):a015677.
73. Lott DG, Manz R, Koch C, Lorenz RR. Aggressive behavior of nonmelanotic skin cancers in solid organ transplant recipients. *Transplantation.* 2010;90(6):683–687.
74. Hojo M, Morimoto T, Maluccio M, et al. Cyclosporine induces cancer progression by a cell-autonomous mechanism. *Nature.* 1999;397(6719):530–534.
75. Wu X, Nguyen BC, Dziunycz P, et al. Opposing roles for calcineurin and ATF3 in squamous skin cancer. *Nature.* 2010;465(7296):368–372.
76. O'Donovan P, Perrett CM, Zhang X, et al. Azathioprine and UVA light generate mutagenic oxidative DNA damage. *Science.* 2005;309(5742):1871–1874.
77. Mungamuri SK, Yang X, Thor AD, Somasundaram K. Survival signaling by Notch1: mammalian target of rapamycin (mTOR)-dependent inhibition of p53. *Cancer Res.* 2006;66(9):4715–4724.
78. Guba M, Graeb C, Jauch KW, Geissler EK. Pro- and anti-cancer effects of immunosuppressive agents used in organ transplantation. *Transplantation.* 2004;77(12):1777–1782.
79. Salgo R, Gossmann J, Schofer H, et al. Switch to a sirolimus-based immunosuppression in long-term renal transplant recipients: reduced rate of (pre-)malignancies and nonmelanoma skin cancer in a prospective, randomized, assessor-blinded, controlled clinical trial. *Am J Transplant.* 2010;10(6):1385–1393.
80. Hariharan S. BK virus nephritis after renal transplantation. *Kidney Int.* 2006;69(4):655–662.

5

Immunological and Nonimmunological Factors Affecting Kidney Transplant Outcomes

Puneet Sood and John Gill

Known knowns and known unknowns influencing kidney transplant survival!

Introduction

A kidney transplant (KT) provides better quality of life and longer survival than treatment with dialysis and is the preferred treatment modality for patients with end-stage kidney disease (ESKD). Over the past few decades, there has been a significant improvement in 1-year graft and patient survival attributable to better immunosuppressant drugs, but with only a modest improvement in long-term outcomes.[1] After the 1st post-transplant year, failure of the allograft—defined as the need for maintenance dialysis or repeat transplantation—and patient death with allograft function are codominant causes of transplant failure.

A failing allograft, defined as estimated glomerular filtration rate (eGFR) less than 20 mL/min with evidence of ongoing GFR loss or macroproteinuria, and allograft failure add significant health and financial burden to the patient and healthcare system. Allograft failure is now the fifth leading cause of dialysis initiation in the United States. Patients who initiate dialysis after transplant failure have high morbidity and mortality. While repeat transplantation is clearly the best treatment, only a minority of patients who suffer allograft failure will undergo repeat transplantation. Repeat transplants account for approximately 10% of kidney transplants (KTs) performed in the United States, compounding the need for organ donation.[2] Repeat transplant recipients have inferior outcomes compared to primary transplant recipients, in part due to higher levels of allosensitization.

Patient death with a functioning allograft is often premature, and only a minority of transplant recipients live a normal life expectancy. The leading causes of death after transplantation include cardiovascular disease (CVD) due to a high prevalence of traditional cardiovascular risk factors that are aggravated by immunosuppressant drugs and suboptimal allograft function. Cancer and infection are the other leading causes of premature death, with cancer deaths exceeding cardiovascular deaths in Australasia.[3–6]

Traditionally factors contributing to allograft failure have been separated from factors contributing to patient death. However, because these factors are often intertwined, this chapter provides a holistic overview of the nonimmunological and immunologic factors contributing to both allograft failure and patient death. The nonimmunological factors impacting patient and allograft survival may be categorized as recipient and donor related.

Nonimmunological Recipient-Related Factors Impacting Patient and Graft Survival

Advanced Recipient Age and Preexisting Cardiovascular Disease

The average age at kidney transplantation is gradually increasing; currently 60% of all KT recipients in the United States are age 50 years and above.[2] Cardiovascular events occur 10–50 times more frequently in KT recipients than in the general population and are more likely to be fatal when they occur.[7,8] Due to this excess mortality, KT recipients achieve only 70%–75% of the life expectancy of age-matched individuals in the general population.[9] Increased CVD in KT patients is the result of a combination of both traditional risk factors and those related to chronic kidney disease (CKD; e.g., advancing age at transplant, a high prevalence of diabetes in ESKD, hypertension, left ventricular hypertrophy, obesity, pre-existing coronary artery disease, smoking, pretransplant dialysis exposure, abnormalities of mineral metabolism leading to vascular calcification, hyperlipidemia, reduced kidney allograft function, and albuminuria), compounded by post-transplant risk factors including immunosuppressant medications, delayed graft function (DGF), chronic inflammation, post-transplant diabetes mellitus (PTDM) and dyslipidemia.[7] Evidence-based therapies to reduce the risk of CVD in the general population have not translated into similar benefits in the transplant population, and there is a need for dedicated studies in KT recipients, as they are excluded from most large CVD trials. As a result, transformative therapies like HMG CoA reductase inhibitors (statins), sodium-glucose cotransporter inhibitors (SGTL2-i), renin-angiotensin-aldosterone system (RAAS) blockade, angiotensin receptor neprolysin inhibitors (ARNIs), and anticoagulants have only low-quality evidence and or uncertain safety to support their use in KT recipients. Consequently, the uptake of these therapies has been slow in KT recipients.[9]

There is an urgent need for high-quality interventional clinical trials specifically designed for this high-risk population.

Post-Transplant Diabetes Mellitus

Post-transplant diabetes mellitus includes pretransplant diabetes and new-onset diabetes after transplant. Diabetes mellitus is common and is the cause of kidney failure in over 30% of transplant recipients in the United States. Patients with ESKD from diabetes have a significantly reduced 5-year patient survival (82% vs. 97%) and graft survival (75% vs. 85%) compared to those with ESKD from cystic kidney disease.[2] The incidence of new-onset diabetes post-transplant has been reported to be 4%–25% and varies with the time since transplant and presence of risk factors.[10] Novel transplant-specific risk factors contributing to PTDM include corticosteroids, calcineurin inhibitor (CNI) therapy, acute rejection, obesity, and hepatitis C positivity. A retrospective analysis of United States Renal Data System (USRDS) data of more than 11,000 KT recipients revealed that PTDM was a strong, independent risk factor for death and death-censored graft loss (DCGL).[11] Novel diabetes therapeutics (e.g., insulin pumps, GLP-1 agonists, SGLT2-i), wearables (e.g., continuous glucose monitors, CGMs) and protocolized management strategies have revolutionized the care of diabetes in the general population, but the utilization and benefits of these therapies in KT recipients are less well understood.

Post-Transplant Malignancy

Malignancy is an important cause of recipient death after KT.[12] The adjusted excess cancer risk is three times higher than in the general population and varies by cancer type (highest with skin cancers), viral etiology (e.g., anogenital cancers, post-transplant lymphoproliferative disorder [PTLD], and Kaposi sarcoma), and overall degree of immune suppression (e.g., PTLD, skin cancers).[13,14] The standardized mortality ratios for all cancers are 1.9 times higher compared to the age- and sex-matched general population with the greatest risk in those with melanoma, urogenital cancers, and non-Hodgkin's lymphoma, where the overall risk of death is 5–10 times greater in KT recipients.[15] The risk of developing malignant melanoma in transplant population is 5–8 times higher than in the general population and has the highest mortality among the post-transplant skin cancers.[16,17] Post-transplant lymphoproliferative disorder warrants special mention: The cumulative incidence of PTLD in adults in the first 10 years after kidney transplantation is 1%–2%.[18] However, the risk of developing PTLD is 10–75 times higher in the EBV-seronegative recipients of seropositive donor organs. An ANZDATA registry analyses revealed survival after PTLD to be around 62%–68% at 1 year, and 41%–48% at 10 years.[19] Post-transplant cancers can be the result of recurrence of a previously treated pretransplant cancer or a de novo malignancy. Careful selection of recipients with prior malignancies, rigorous adherence to age-appropriate cancer screening recommendations, and adoption of novel management protocols for high-risk individuals (e.g., EBV high-risk recipients and dermatology screening) are cornerstones of clinical management. Treatment of cancer is complicated because reductions in immunosuppression as well as the use of immune-based therapies such as checkpoint inhibitors may precipitate allograft rejection.

Post-Transplant Infection

Late post-transplant infections remain an important determinant of adverse graft and patient outcomes.[20,21] Pre-existing exposure or immunity, use of antimicrobial prophylaxis, and the net state of immunosuppression determine susceptibility to and the outcome of post-transplant infection. Infection with BK virus is common in immunocompromised KT recipients, which can lead to BK virus nephropathy (BKVN) and allograft failure.[22] The incidence of BKVN is ~1%–10% in those with viremia, and graft loss occurs in approximately 30% of those cases (range 0–100%).[23] Graft survival rates following a diagnosis of BKVN is worse than either acute rejection or CNI toxicity.[24] In the absence of an effective antiviral agent, the main strategy is to prevent BKN with post-transplant screening, and early reduction of immunosuppressive therapy when there is evidence of viral replication.[22,25] This strategy is not risk free; development of de novo donor-specific antibody (DSA) in 14% and acute rejection in 8%–12% is reported after reduction of immunosuppression for BK viral management.[25-27] BKV specific monoclonal antibodies and adoptive T-cell therapy are novel potential treatments in development for BK virus infection.[28] There is a significant association of BKV infection with CMV reactivation, and combined reactivation is associated with loss of kidney function.[29]

Both CMV and EBV are common in seronegative recipients of seropositive donor KTs. CMV infection is a risk factor for acute rejection and allograft failure.[30-32] Antivirals for primary and secondary prophylaxis as well as for treatment, and evidence-based surveillance protocols have significantly mitigated the overall impact of CMV infection. Patients with primary infection with EBV post-transplant are at increased risk for PTLD (1.7% in EBV seronegative recipients) and have inferior 10-year graft survival (41% vs. 65%)[2,19] EBV infection is also associated with CMV reactivation.[29] Primary EBV infection in the post-transplant period remains an important clinical concern, as there is no effective antiviral treatment. Post-transplant surveillance for EBV viremia followed by reduction in immunosuppression remains the main management strategy.

Recipient Obesity

Obesity (BMI > 30 kg/m^2) is an important problem affecting more than a third of ESKD patients. Obesity is associated with increased surgical complications including delayed wound healing and inferior graft and patient survival. A paired kidney analysis of 44,560 adult recipients of first-time KT from 2001–2016 revealed that BMI > 35 kg/m^2 was associated with increased DGF and DCGL, independent of donor quality. Analyzed as a continuous variable, BMI had an overall hazard ratio (HR) for DCGL of 1.015 (95% confidence interval [CI] 1.010–1.020) per unit increase in BMI (p = 0.001).[33] In a meta-analysis of 17 studies (N = 138,081) comparing obese (BMI > 30 kg/m^2) and nonobese (BMI 18–24.5 kg/m^2) patients, obesity was found to be associated with increased likelihood of DGF (OR 1.68, 95% CI 1.39–2.03) and DCGL (HR 1.06, 95% CI 1.01–1.12) but not mortality.[34] However, obesity was found to modify the effect of KT on the risk of death (66% reduction in BMI < 40 kg/m^2 vs. 48% reduction in those with BMI > 40 kg/m^2).[35] Other studies have confirmed adverse graft and patient outcomes in obese transplant recipients.[34,36–38] Bariatric surgery while on the waitlist, robotic sleeve gastrectomy at the time of KT or minimally invasive robotic-assisted KT are treatment options.[39–42] Weight gain after transplant is common due to a pre-existing sedentary lifestyle, improved appetite post-transplant, steroid use, and higher insulin requirements. There is paucity of data on bariatric surgery after KT, but a single study demonstrated beneficial effects with significant and sustained weight loss, reduction in comorbidities, and improvement in graft function without significant alteration in absorption of immunosuppressive agents.[43] More recently, glucagon-like-peptide (GLP-1) analogues have shown strong promise as a medical therapy for weight loss.[44] A few small retrospective studies of GLP-1 analogue use in solid organ transplant patients primarily for diabetes management have shown that these drugs are effective in promoting weight loss, and do not affect tacrolimus levels.[45] However, the safety and efficacy of GLP-1 inhibitors in the management of obesity in KT recipients needs further study.

Nonimmune Kidney Allograft Injury

Kidney transplant recipients are exposed to a host of nephrotoxic events after transplantation. These include chronic exposure to CNIs, hyperglycemia from uncontrolled diabetes or steroid administration, recurrent infections causing hypotension and sepsis, fluid imbalances and rapid fluid shifts from diuretic use, hospitalizations from unrecognized CHF and diastolic dysfunction, repeated exposure to nephrotoxic antimicrobials, and urological interventions resulting in recurrent Acute Kidney Injuries (AKIs). Repeated AKIs are a strong risk factor for nonrecovery of renal function eventually progressing to graft loss.[46] The progression to graft loss may be accelerated in kidneys with low renal reserve related to donor factors or chronic immune injury. Nonimmune AKI is an important and underemphasized cause of nonimmune graft loss, and multipronged strategies to prevent and minimize the impact of AKI in KT recipients are needed.

Pre-Transplant Dialysis Duration

Dialysis before kidney transplantation is associated with reduced patient and allograft survival. A retrospective cohort study evaluating ~7,000 first kidney recipients in Austrian between 1990 and 2013 found a higher rate of patient death in those with dialysis vintage greater than 1.5 years as compared to preemptive recipients and those with less than 1.5 years of pretransplant dialysis treatment (HR 1.62, 95% CI 1.43–1.83).[47] Similarly, a French transplant registry analyzing 22,345 first kidney-only transplants found preemptive transplantation to be protective against graft loss (HR 0.57, 95% CI 0.51–0.63).[48] A US study found survival of transplant recipients with 10 years or more of pretransplant dialysis treatment to be greater than that of wait-listed candidates with the same dialysis exposure. However, this survival benefit was not observed until two years post-transplantation and was limited to those who underwent transplant using kidneys from donors with favorable characteristics. Whether transplantation of high Kidney Donor Profile Index (KDPI) kidneys is associated with a survival in patients with long dialysis vintage remains unanswered at the current time.[49] Dialysis vintage is also associated with lower allograft survival in living-donor (LD) KT recipients.[50] The association of dialysis exposure with post-transplant outcomes is pertinent, as less than 30% of KTs in the United States are preemptive while 32% have 5 or more years of pretransplant dialysis exposure.[2] The association of pretransplant dialysis exposure varies between countries and even within different regions in the United States and may be related to the quality of dialysis care.[51] To what extent dialysis itself or the characteristics of patients with long dialysis vintage underly the association with post-transplant outcomes is unclear. Irrespective of the mechanism, minimizing dialysis exposure through early referral for transplantation, and LD transplantation is one of the most important modifiable factors limiting allograft and patient survival.

Nonimmunologic Donor-Related Factors Impacting Patient and Graft Survival

The contribution of donor risk factors to post-transplant outcomes should be considered with the understanding that transplantation utilizing kidneys with donor characteristics that portend an increased risk of allograft failure are still associated with significantly better patient survival than continued treatment with dialysis and that recovered deceased donor (DD) kidneys that are utilized successfully for transplantation internationally are frequently underutilized in the United States. Details are discussed below and shown in Table 5.1.

Table 5.1 Nonimmunological Factors Impacting Kidney Transplant Outcome

	Risk factors	Measures	DGF	Acute rejection	Patient loss	Graft loss	Other	Mitigation
							Adverse outcomes	
Recipient	Obesity	BMI>30 kg/m² or >35 kg/m² or >40 kg/m²	50%–60% higher	No impact	No impact	6% higher	Delayed wound healing	Surgical or medical weight loss prior to or after KT
	Primary GN	All GNs combined	No Impact	No impact	Slightly higher	2- to 3-fold higher		Individualized therapy to prevent and treat based on type of recurrent GN
	Diabetes	Pre-transplant diabetes	No impact	No impact	2- to 3-fold higher	No impact	Higher rates of infections	Multipronged diabetes management
	Pretransplant dialysis duration	No dialysis vs. < 1 year on dialysis vs. yearly increment	No impact	No impact	2-fold higher with prolonged dialysis	2-fold higher with prolonged dialysis	Higher rates of CVD and infections	Early referral and listing for transplantation. Encourage **Live Donor** kidney transplantation
	Post-transplant malignancy	Cancer type, organ involved	No impact	Higher with reduction of immunosuppression and certain immunotherapy	Higher based on cancer type	Higher based on cancer type		Reduction of immunosuppression and specific treatment for cancers

(continued)

Table 5.1 Continued

Risk factors	Measures	Adverse outcomes					Mitigation
		DGF	Acute rejection	Patient loss	Graft loss	Other	
Race—African American	2 APLO L1- risk allele	No impact	No impact	No impact	2-fold higher	-	-
Obesity-	BMI >35 kg/m²	30% higher	No impact	No impact	No impact		
Donor—Recipient size mismatch	>30 kg (recipient over donor)	No impact	No impact	No impact	50% higher	-	
Kidney quality [KDPI]	Higher KDPI 1-20% vs 21%–85% and >85%	No impact	No impact	Higher	30%–70% higher	Higher rates of PNF and Lower GFR	High KDPI kidneys are given to older recipients with shorter lifespan
Cold ischemia time (CIT)	Increasing CIT from 6 hours	20%–40% higher	Slight increase	15% higher	10% higher	-	Increased resource utilization through short-term dialysis after transplant
Warm ischemia time (WIT)	Increasing WIT from 20 minutes	No impact	Slight increase	10% higher	10% higher	-	
Kidney histology immediately prior to transplant	Glomerulosclerosis, IFTA	Higher based on severity	No impact	Higher based on severity	Higher based on severity	Lower GFR	
Infections	Infection types: viral and fungal	No impact	Higher based on infection	Higher based on infection	Higher based on infection type	-	Prevention and treatment of infections

Donor

Abbreviations: BMI: body mass index, CIT: cold ischemia time, GFR glomerular filtration rate, KDPI: Kidney Donor Profile Index, LD: living donor, IFTA: interstitial fibrosis and tubular atrophy, WIT: warm ischemia time.

Donor Race

African American (AA) donor race is associated with 20% higher allograft failure among DD transplant recipients. However the basis of this association is unclear and may be confounded by the fact that African American donor kidneys are more likely to be transplanted into African American candidates due to shared ABO blood group and human leukocyte antigens (HLA).[52] A potential genetic basis for this association is the presence of two APLO L1 kidney risk variants. In limited retrospective studies, kidneys with two risk alleles had a twofold increased risk of graft failure compared with kidneys from donors with 1 or 0 APO L1 kidney risk variants.[53] Currently, a National Institutes of Health (NIH)–sponsored study is underway to determine the impact of APO L1 genotype on DD kidney allograft survival.[54]

Donor Obesity

Kidney donor obesity impacts KT outcomes and is in part related to increased warm ischemia time (WIT). A UK transplant registry study from 2003–2015 reported an increased incidence of DGF with donor BMI >35 kg/m^2 compared to BMI 18.5–25 kg/m^2 but no impact on patient and graft survival or 12-month renal function.[55] A large US database analysis of obese LDs and DDs found a graded increase in DCGL with increasing BMI and this association persisted despite adjustment for donor and recipient size mismatch and other donor, recipient, and transplant factors.[56] There remains variation in acceptance of obese DDs. Considerations of LD safety related to obesity are discussed elsewhere.

Donor–Recipient Size and Sex Mismatch

A registry analysis of DD KT between 2000 and 2014 in the United States revealed that a donor-recipient size mismatch of >30 kg (larger recipient) was associated with an increased hazard of graft failure for female recipients of male donors (HR 1.50, 95% CI 1.32–1.70) and for male recipients of female kidney donors (HR 1.35, 95% CI 1.25–1.45).[57] Other studies have found similar adverse outcomes in size-mismatched pairs and that the association is further modified by donor–recipient sex discordance.[58] The association of donor–recipient size mismatch on long-term graft survival is modulated by donor age such that size-mismatched kidneys have excellent graft survival when the donor is of younger age.[59] Recipient height greater than donor height by 5 inches was associated with an increased risk of DCGL and all-cause mortality in both LD and DD transplants.[60] In the absence of consensus recommendations, the impact of these findings on donor acceptance practices is poorly understood and warrants further study.

Donor Kidney Quality

Introduced in 2014, the Kidney Donor Risk Index (KDRI) is a metric used in the United States to measure DD kidney graft quality at the time of organ offer. The KDRI incorporates 10 donor parameters (donor age, height, weight, ethnicity, hypertension, diabetes, stroke as the cause of death, serum creatinine, hepatitis C [HCV] status, and donation after cardiac death). The KDRI is converted into a continuous measure ranging from 1% (high-quality grafts) to 100% (low-quality grafts), named the KDPI (Kidney Donor Profile Index), which estimates the average relative risk of post-transplant graft loss relative to DD kidneys recovered in the previous year.[61] One of the caveats of the KDPI is that there are other factors not currently included in the KDPI calculation (e.g., donor histology, CIT, ex situ machine perfusion, pump parameters, recipient factors) that likely interact with KDPI to influence patient and graft outcomes. Similarly some donor factors included in the KDPI, such as donation after circulatory death and HCV positivity, are no longer considered determinants of allograft survival.[2] In the United States, the allocation system incorporates longevity matching of the kidneys such that low-KDPI organs are preferentially matched to recipients with longest expected post-transplant survival as a strategy to maximize the utility from the available supply of donated kidneys.

Cold Ischemia Time

Cold ischemia time (CIT) is defined as the time from aortic cross-clamp in the donor to reperfusion of the organ. In a registry-based French study, longer CIT was correlated with higher DGF rates: from 22% with a CIT of 6–16 hours to 40% with CIT>24 hours. For each additional hour of CIT, the risk of allograft failure increased by 13% (e.g., increase in CIT from 6 to 12 h resulted in a 8% increase in graft failure) and risk of recipient death increased by a 18% (e.g., an increase in CIT from 6 h to 30 h was associated with a 53% increase in recipient mortality), and this risk was constant regardless of baseline CIT.[62] Other studies have shown a similar detrimental relationship of CIT with poor outcomes.[63] However in a mate kidney analysis of DDs with AKI in the United States, a CIT difference of even up to 15 hours between the mate kidneys did not have an impact on DCGL or patient survival, suggesting that in the setting of a pre-existing donor ischemic insult CIT has little additional impact.[64] A prolonged CIT is also relevant in LDKTs. An ANZDATA registry analysis of 3,717 LDKTs from 1997–2012 found that every hour of increase in CIT was associated with 28% higher odds for DGF. Compared to a CIT of 1–2 hours, a CIT >4–8 hours had an adjusted OR of 1.93 (95% CI 1.21–3.09) for DGF and 1.91 (95% CI 1.05–3.49) for overall survival and DCGL, respectively.[65] Subsequent studies from the National Kidney Registry (NKR) compared shipped kidneys in a kidney paired exchange (KPD) program to unrelated, nonshipped, non-KPD LDKT. In this study, each hour of

CIT was associated with a 5% increase in DGF. However, there was no association with mortality or DCGL (all $p > 0.05$).[66,67] Various strategies including the use of virtual crossmatch techniques are employed to minimize CIT.[68,69]

Warm Ischemia Time

Warm ischemia time (WIT) is defined as the time between when the kidney is taken out of cold storage until perfusion with warm blood and corresponds to the time it takes to anastomose the new graft to the recipient blood vessels. Acceptable WITs have been defined as 20–40 minutes. A prolonged WIT is a consequence of various factors and is associated with poor graft and patient survival. A retrospective adjusted analysis of 131,677 recipients (with 35,901 events) found a graded increase in the composite of graft failure and patient mortality by 23% for every 10 minutes increase in WIT from 20 minutes to >60 minutes when compared with WIT of 10–20 minutes. This association persisted even after stratifying for donor type and DGF.[70] In the Euro-transplant experience of 13,964 DD solitary kidney transplantation, WIT was independently associated with graft loss at 5 years (adjusted HR 1.10 for every 10-minute increase, 95% CI 1.06–1.14, $p < 0.0001$) but it did not influence patient survival. In addition, Donation after Circulatory Death (DCD) kidneys were less tolerant of prolonged WIT than Donation after Brain Death (DBD) kidneys. Other factors associated with a prolonged WIT were multiple vessels, right donor kidney, and donor age but not recipient BMI or retransplantation status.[71] Additional studies have reported association between prolonged WIT higher rates of DGF (OR 3.5, 95% CI 1.6–7.3).[72,73]

Donor Kidney Histology

Donor histology refers to the histopathological state of the allograft immediately prior to transplantation. The role of donor histology in the acceptance of organs for transplantation remains controversial. A 2015 systematic review of empirical evidence from 47 retrospective studies evaluated heterogeneous histopathological criteria and found that no semiquantitative scoring system was conclusively associated with post-transplant outcomes including DGF, graft function, or graft failure.[74] However, a 2022 study using data from 5,997 extended criteria donors and their procurement biopsies from 2008–2012 found glomerulosclerosis (GS) > 5% to be independently associated with an increased all-cause graft failure (HR 1.18, 95% CI 1.06–1.28) and DCGL (HR 1.28, 95% CI 1.08–1.46).[75] Another registry study of 22,006 kidneys from 2005–2014 examined the association of GS on procurement biopsies in KDPI>85 kidneys and found that GS>10% was an independent factor for graft failure (HR 1.27, $p < 0.001$).[76] Challenges with the use of donor histology include the quantity and quality of the biopsy specimen, limited information from frozen sections, and the availability of expert histopathological assessment. At the current time, donor histology is not universally accepted and is neither standardized nor implemented uniformly.

Delayed Graft Function

Delayed graft function is defined as the need for dialysis within the first week of transplantation, irrespective of the indication for dialysis. Because the indications for dialysis are broad and subject to clinical practice variation, reported rates of DGF vary between 5% and 50%.[77] In a registry analysis of 29,528 mate kidney transplants between 1998 and 2011 in which only 1 transplant developed DGF, DGF was associated with graft failure in the first post-transplant year, especially in transplants with concomitant acute rejection (HR 8.22, 95% CI 4.7–14.2).[78] In contrast, the DGF-associated risk of graft failure after the first post-transplant year in patients without acute rejection was far lower (HR 1.15, 95% CI 1.02–1.29). Allograft survival is differentially impacted by duration of DGF and KDPI. A single-center study of 627 patients found that for those with KDPI < 85%, only DGF duration > 14 days impacted 10-year graft survival, while for high KDPI of at least 85%, any duration of DGF was associated with reduced graft survival.[79] The outcomes of LDKT are also impacted by DGF. A UNOS database study analyzing 64,024 LDKTs done between 2000 and 2014 found a DGF rate of 3.4%. Even in recipients of LDKTs, DGF is associated with significantly lower 5-year graft survival when compared with those with no DGF (65% vs. 85%, respectively, $p <$ 0.001). In LD recipients, DGF doubled the risk of subsequent graft failure (HR 2.3, 95% CI 2.1–2.6, $p < 0.001$).[80] A similar registry analysis of ANZDATA for 3,358 adult LDKTs performed between 2004 and 2015 reported a DGF rate of 2.3%. DGF in this analysis was associated with worse patient and graft survival. Risk factors for DGF included right-sided kidney, higher donor BMI, and longer recipient dialysis exposure.[81] The proposed mechanism for DGF causing adverse graft outcomes is increased subclinical inflammation and subclinical T-cell-mediated rejection (TCMR) found on serial protocol and indication biopsies in DGF patients. The TCMR in this group was recurrent and persistent at 12 months and with worse chronicity scores (BANFF IFTA and total i-scores).[82] Systemwide efforts in DD care, ex situ organ preservation, organ allocation, and recipient selection are being undertaken to mitigate factors contributing to DGF. In cases where DGF is anticipated based on KDPI, donor WIT or prolonged CIT, machine perfusion has been shown to decrease DGF and improve overall graft function.[68,83,84]

Immunological Variables Impacting Patient and Graft Survival

Human leukocyte antigen mismatch between the donor and recipient forms the basis for post-transplant de novo DSA development, antibody-mediated graft injury, subsequent recipient sensitization, and an immunological memory response with repeat transplants. In the following section, we will examine the role and intertwined nature of these various factors and how they impact graft survival and repeat transplantations. Details are discussed below and shown in Table 5.2.

Human Leukocyte Antigen Mismatch (DR/A/B)

In one of the earliest reports on the impact of HLA matching on graft outcomes, 7,614 HLA-matched DD transplants were compared with 81,364

Table 5.2 Immunological Factors Impacting Kidney Transplant Outcome

| Factors | Measures | Adverse outcomes | | | | |
		DGF	Acute Rejection	Patient Loss	Graft Loss	Other
HLA match	HLA AB and DR mismatch	No impact	Higher	4% higher	6% higher	Higher rates of sensitization after graft loss
	HLA DR mismatch	No impact	Higher	Slightly higher	12% higher	Higher rates of sensitization alter graft loss
Sensitization	Elevated PRA 0 vs. >80%	Slightly higher	80% higher	1.5-fold higher	2-fold higher	Encourage better matched (molecular level) transplants
	CPRA >98%	Slightly higher	Higher	39% higher	78% higher	Avoid preformed DSA OR repeat mismatches
	Class I and II vs. Class I or Class II	Slightly higher	Higher	Higher	Higher	If the option available, encourage LD paired exchange transplants
Epitope/ eplet mismatches	>14 vs. < 13 eplet mismatches	No impact	5%–12% Higher	Higher	Higher	Higher risk of development of de novo DSA
Post-transplant rejection	TCIAR, AMR, and SCI	No Impact	NA	Higher	Higher	Higher rates of sensitization after graft loss
DGF	Dialysis within 7 days post-transplant	NA	Higher	Higher	Higher	Lower GFR especially among those with higher KDPI

Abbreviations: ABMR: antibody-mediated rejection, CPRA: calculated panel reactive antibody, DGF: delayed graft function, HLA: human leukocyte antigen, GFR glomerular filtration rate, LD: living donor, PRA: panel reactive antibody.

HLA-mismatched transplants. The matched kidneys had a significantly better 10-year graft survival when compared to the mismatched transplants (53% vs. 37%, $p < 0.05$), owing mostly to lesser rejection and fewer immunological graft losses.[85] Later, an analysis of USRDS data reported that compared to 0–1 mismatch (MM), those with higher degrees of MM had a shorter duration of functioning graft. A higher degree of MM was also less likely to receive a second transplant after listing (HR 0.87, 95% CI 0.76–0.98).[86] A subsequent meta-analysis of 23 cohort studies involving 486,608 recipients found that each MM was significantly associate with increased risk of DCGL (HR 1.09, 95% CI 1.06–1.12) and all-cause mortality (HR 1.04, 95% CI 1.02–1.07). The overall graft survival was especially lower with the DR MM (HR 1.12, 95% CI 1.05–1.21).[87] In the United States, ~32% of DDKTs and ~22% of LDKTs have five or more HLA MMs, which presents both a significant challenge and a potential opportunity for intervention.[2] Improved donor–recipient HLA matching using novel technology is discussed later in this section.

Recipient Sensitization

Recipient sensitization is defined as presence of preformed HLA antibodies in prospective recipients and is thought to occur from recipient's lifetime exposure to nonself HLA in the form of prior HLA mismatched tissue/organ transplants, pregnancies, and blood product transfusions. Measured as panel reactive antibody (PRA), determination of a high PRA in earlier years was cell based, which was nonspecific and relatively insensitive in predicting the actual physical cross-match.[88] With the availability of single antigen bead (SAB) assays, PRA was replaced with calculated PRA (CPRA), which in addition to measuring breadth of sensitization also considered donor specificity by listing unacceptable antigens based on presence of DSAs. The literature on association of sensitization with graft outcomes has varied based on how sensitization was measured (PRA vs. CPRA). An ANZDATA registry analysis of 3,171 KT recipients comparing outcomes in those with peak PRA 0% against peak PRA >80% found increased risk of acute rejection, DCGL, and all-cause mortality in the sensitized group independent of HLA MMs and initial immunosuppression.[89] An analysis of 5,315 KT recipients performed between 2000 and 2008 revealed poorer 2-year graft survival of 76.5% in those with both preformed class I/II antibodies as compared with 87.5% for those with none. The survival with class I and class II positive recipients was better if they received a kidney with 0 or 1 mismatch at the ABDR loci.[90] Another analysis of adult-only KTs from 1997 to 2004 comparing PRA≥98% with nonsensitized patients revealed a 10-year actuarial graft survival of 43.9% in highly sensitized versus 52.4% in nonsensitized patients, $p < 0.001$.

The mode of sensitization was important, and those sensitized from a previous transplant had worse graft survival.[91] However, while these studies looked at the breadth of sensitization they failed to consider the donor specificity of the sensitization. In a landmark retrospective observational study of 4,058 zero HLA-A-, B-, DR-, and DQB1-mismtached transplant recipients, a CPRA of 1%–97% when compared to CPRA 0%, was not associated with DCGL (HR 1.07, 95% CI 0.82–1.41). On the other hand, high CPRA, ≥98%, was associated with all-cause graft loss (HR 1.39, 95% CI 1.08--1.79) and DCGL (HR 1.78, 95% CI 1.27–2.49) and the increased graft loss in this group was seen only in those with repeat transplants in the presence of preformed DSA.[92] In summary, sensitization measured as CPRA is indicative of recipient alloreactivity and sensitization is more consequential if its broad, acquired from previous transplants, and donor-specific.

Donor-Specific Antibody

Prior sensitization and donor–recipient HLA MM lead to DSA formation. The presence of preformed DSA at transplant is associated with poor allograft outcome in both DDKT and LDKT recipients. Preformed class II DSA may be more likely to persist post-transplant and to be associated with increased risk of ABMR and graft loss.[93-95] That the effect of DSA on graft outcomes is independent of donor factors has been confirmed in analysis of recipients receiving a kidney from the same donor.[95-98] Similar to preformed DSA, de novo DSA is equally deleterious, with an incidence of subclinical ABMR in up to 53% at 1 year and a higher risk of progression to chronic ABMR and subsequent graft loss.[93,99,100] In general, HLA type and **Mean Fluorescence Index (MFI)** of DSA and its persistence despite treatment provides important prognostication of poor graft outcome and also potential targets to intervene.

Epitope Mismatch

Allograft outcomes are related to degree of recipient–donor HLA disparity. High resolution typing of HLA molecules have led the advance of determining disparity at the level of HLA epitopes. The availability of next-generation sequencing (NGS) has allowed analysis of the three-dimensional structures of HLA molecules allowing the identification of specific regions of the HLA molecule that when disparate between the donor and recipient are immunogenic, called epitopes. Eplets are the configurations of polymorphic amino acid residues on HLA molecules and are the essential part of HLA epitopes recognized by antibodies. Recently published studies supported epitope matching and the resultant eplet MM load as metrics of donor–recipient HLA disparity. A single-center retrospective study of 926 transplant pairs performed between 2004 and 2013 found a significant independent association between antibody-verified eplet MM load and de novo DSA occurrence and graft failure, which they attributed primarily to DQ antibody-verified eplet effects. In this study, the odds for TCMR or ABMR increased by 5% and 12% respectively per antibody-verified DQ MM.[101] Other studies that have included HLA-A, B, DRB, and DRQ eplet MMs have also concluded that a higher burden of class II (DRB + DQB) eplet MMs were more significantly correlated with de novo class II DSA production.[102–104] A nested case-control study of 52 patients with biopsy-proven transplant glomerulopathy found that a higher DR + DQ eplet MM load was almost 4.6 times more likely to be associated with transplant glomerulopathy.[105] Use of eplet mismatching for KT appears very promising. However, further studies are needed to evaluate the long-term effects of eplet MMs at various loci. Studies are also underway to examine if immunosuppression can be safely tailored to the donor–recipient eplet MM load.

Rejection-Related Immunological Graft Injury

Acute allograft rejection is diagnosed when the recipient immune system recognizes the donor HLA as foreign and attacks it, causing TCMR or ABMR. Acute rejection in the 1st year after transplantation is primarily TCMR, with fewer cases of ABMR, whereas after the 1st year, acute rejection is often a combination of ABMR and TCMR.[106] The rejections are graded using the Banff schema, a classification that integrates histological features of immune invasion and injury with serological and molecular diagnostic techniques. The rejection is further classified as subclinical or clinical based on whether the renal function is preserved or not, respectively. The incidence of clinical acute rejection and subclinical rejection during the 1st year after transplantation ranges from 10% to 15% and from 5% to 15%, respectively and are predominantly TCMRs (>90%). Follow-up biopsies of clinical or subclinical TCMR in the same study revealed either a persistent (37%) or a subsequent (26%) TCMR, and both a first or second TCMR event correlated with death-censored and all-cause graft loss when adjusted for baseline covariates and other significant time-dependent covariates such as DGF and ABMR.[107] In addition, subclinical **Borderline Rejection (BL)** or subclinical TCMR within one year are more likely to have a subsequent clinical TCMR (HR 3.8, 95% CI 2.1–7.5) and has a significantly increased risk of DCGL (Adjusted HR 1.99, 95% CI 1.04–3.84).[108] Recent studies have also revealed that even lesser degrees of inflammation that do not meet the Banff schema rejection criteria may impact long-term graft survival. For example, tubulitis alone or with inflammation (but not meeting the TCMR IA threshold) is associated with not only a higher incidence of subsequent TCMR and a higher chronicity score at 1-year but also a higher rate of de novo DSA development compared to those with no inflammation, confirming detrimental effects of even lower degrees of inflammation.[109] In general, immunological graft injury is the result of suboptimal immunosuppressive therapy, particularly in transplant recipients at high immunologic risk; nonadherence to immunosuppressive therapy or a reduction in immunosuppressive medications due to the occurrence of infections; or tumors. In addition, there is a need for identifying patient with subclinical inflammation and rejection with surveillance biopsies for early interventions.[110,111] Studies are ongoing to identify noninvasive biomarkers of early and late immune injury, and to look at what medical interventions would alter the trajectory of long-term outcomes of inflammation and rejection. Both ABMR and TCMR are discussed in detail in other chapters as well. Post-transplant immunological graft injury remains an important clinical event impacting long-term outcome and hence it is prudent to prevent and treat early and late rejections to improve long-term survival further.

Nonrejection Immunological Graft Injury— Primary Glomerulonephritis

As short-term KT allograft survival has improved, nonalloimmune factors like recurrent glomerulonephritis (GN) have emerged as important contributors to medium- and long-term graft outcomes. In the United States, 27% of KT have GN as the cause of kidney failure and the cumulative incidence of glomerular diseases is as high as 42% at 10 years post-transplantation.[112,113] Glomerulonephritis in kidney allograft can present as donor-derived, recurrent, or de novo, and of these, recurrent disease is the most encountered entity post-transplant.[114] Rates of recurrent GN vary according to the type of disease; for example C3GN recurs in more than 90% of recipients, immunoglobulin A nephropathy (IgAN) and membranous nephropathy (MN) in 50%, and focal segmental glomerulosclerosis (FSGS) in 30% of recipients.[113,115-117] For those with IgAN as a cause of ESKD, recurrence of IgAN is the third leading cause of graft loss after chronic allograft nephropathy and death with a functioning graft (DWFG).[118] Recurrence of FSGS predicts poor graft outcomes with 5-year graft survival of 52% as compared to 83% in those with FSGS as cause of ESKD without recurrence.[119] In a largest-to-date ANZDATA registry analysis of 6,597 recipients accumulated over a 30-year period who had a biopsy-proven GN as the primary cause of ESKD, 10% had recurrence over a median of 7.7 years, and of those with recurrence, 44% lost their grafts due to recurrence. The 5-year survival was 30% for recipients with recurrent membranoproliferative GN (MPGN), and 58% for recipients with FSGS, IgAN, and MN. Those with recurrence were twice as likely to lose their allografts compared to those without recurrence.[114] In general, the reported incidence of recurrent GN varies widely depending on the original underlying disease, renal biopsy policies of the referring physicians and transplant programs, and follow-up duration. Biopsy-proven clinical recurrence underestimates the true prevalence of recurrence and its contribution to graft loss. A large collaborative effort by the nephrology, transplant, and pathology communities is required to better understand specific immune predictors, genetic basis, genomic association, and clinical factors associated with recurrence and will give potential targets to intervene to modify the natural history of GN recurrences.[120] As an example, genetic testing of individuals with suspected complement disorders (e.g., C3GN and atypical hemolytic uremic syndrome) can confirm diagnosis, enable an estimated risk of recurrence, and allow possible use of prophylactic terminal complement inhibitors, which have shown to significantly reduce the risk of a hemolytic-uremic syndrome recurrence after transplantation.[121]

Conclusion

Several donor and recipient immune and nonimmune factors impact long-term KT outcomes. Often, several factors operate simultaneously in an individual patient, and their interplay may be more consequential than a single factor. Fortunately, studies have identified several potential targets for intervention to mitigate their impact. A concerted effort by various stakeholders, including the regulatory agencies, transplant centers, professional societies, and patient advocacy groups, is needed to implement effective changes. Thus, beyond identification of various donor and recipient risk factors, it is critical to implement a systematic plan toward mitigating the risk factors, which will improve long-term survival.

References

1. Hariharan S, Israni AK, Danovitch G. Long-term survival after kidney transplantation. *N Engl J Med.* 2021;385(8):729–743.
2. OPTN/SRTR 2021 Annual Data Report: Kidney. *Am J Transplant.* 2023 Feb;23(2):S21–S120. Published online 2023 Feb 27. doi: 10.1016/j.ajt.2023.02.004
3. Yu MY, Kim YC, Lee JP, Lee H, Kim YS. Death with graft function after kidney transplantation: a single-center experience. *Clin Exp Nephrol.* 2018;22(3):710–718.

4. Shimmura H, Tanabe K, Tokumoto T, et al. Analysis of cause of death with a functioning graft: a single-center experience. *Transplant Proc.* 2004;36(7):2026–2029.
5. El-Agroudy AE, Bakr MA, Shehab El-Dein AB, Ghoneim MA. Death with functioning graft in living donor kidney transplantation: analysis of risk factors. *Am J Nephrol.* 2003;23(3):186–193.
6. Ying T, Shi B, Kelly PJ, Pilmore H, Clayton PA, Chadban SJ. Death after kidney transplantation: an analysis by era and time post-transplant. *J Am Soc Nephrol.* 2020;31(12):2887–2899.
7. Stoumpos S, Jardine AG, Mark PB. Cardiovascular morbidity and mortality after kidney transplantation. *Transpl Int.* 2015;28(1):10–21.
8. El-Zoghby ZM, Stegall MD, Lager DJ, et al. Identifying specific causes of kidney allograft loss. *Am J Transplant.* 2009;9(3):527–535.
9. Vinson AJ, Singh S, Chadban S, et al. Premature death in kidney transplant recipients: the time for trials is now. *J Am Soc Nephrol.* 2022;33(4):665–673.
10. Davidson J, Wilkinson A, Dantal J, et al. New-onset diabetes after transplantation: 2003 international consensus guidelines. Proceedings of an international expert panel meeting. Barcelona, Spain, February 19, 2003. *Transplantation.* 2003;75(10 Suppl):SS3–24.
11. Kasiske BL, Snyder JJ, Gilbertson D, Matas AJ. Diabetes mellitus after kidney transplantation in the United States. *Am J Transplant.* 2003;3(2):178–185.
12. Krynitz B, Edgren G, Lindelof B, et al. Risk of skin cancer and other malignancies in kidney, liver, heart and lung transplant recipients 1970 to 2008—a Swedish population-based study. *Int J Cancer.* 2013;132(6):1429–1438.
13. Webster AC, Craig JC, Simpson JM, Jones MP, Chapman JR. Identifying high risk groups and quantifying absolute risk of cancer after kidney transplantation: a cohort study of 15,183 recipients. *Am J Transplant.* 2007;7(9):2140–2151.
14. Webster AC, Wong G, Craig JC, Chapman JR. Managing cancer risk and decision making after kidney transplantation. *Am J Transplant.* 2008;8(11):2185–2191.
15. Au EH, Chapman JR, Craig JC, et al. Overall and site-specific cancer mortality in patients on dialysis and after kidney transplant. *J Am Soc Nephrol.* 2019;30(3):471–480.
16. Mittal A, Colegio OR. Skin cancers in organ transplant recipients. *Am J Transplant.* 2017;17(10):2509–2530.
17. Robbins HA, Clarke CA, Arron ST, et al. Melanoma risk and survival among organ transplant recipients. *J Invest Dermatol.* 2015;135(11):2657–2665.
18. Francis A, Johnson DW, Teixeira-Pinto A, Craig JC, Wong G. Incidence and predictors of post-transplant lymphoproliferative disease after kidney transplantation during adulthood and childhood: a registry study. *Nephrol Dial Transplant.* 2018;33(5):881–889.
19. Francis A, Johnson DW, Craig J, Teixeira-Pinto A, Wong G. Post-transplant lymphoproliferative disease may be an adverse risk factor for patient survival but not graft loss in kidney transplant recipients. *Kidney Int.* 2018;94(4):809–817.
20. Fishman JA. Infection in organ transplantation. *Am J Transplant.* 2017;17(4):856–879.
21. van Delden C, Stampf S, Hirsch HH, et al. Burden and timeline of infectious diseases in the first year after solid organ transplantation in the Swiss Transplant Cohort Study. *Clin Infect Dis.* 2020;71(7):e159–e169.
22. Sood P, Senanayake S, Sujeet K, et al. Management and outcome of BK viremia in renal transplant recipients: a prospective single-center study. *Transplantation.* 2012;94(8):814–821.

23. Hirsch HH, Brennan DC, Drachenberg CB, et al. Polyomavirus-associated nephropathy in renal transplantation: interdisciplinary analyses and recommendations. *Transplantation.* 2005;79(10):1277–1286.
24. Trofe J, Hirsch HH, Ramos E. Polyomavirus-associated nephropathy: update of clinical management in kidney transplant patients. *Transpl Infect Dis.* 2006;8(2):76–85.
25. Schaub S, Hirsch HH, Dickenmann M, et al. Reducing immunosuppression preserves allograft function in presumptive and definitive polyomavirus-associated nephropathy. *Am J Transplant.* 2010;10(12):2615–2623.
26. Hardinger KL, Koch MJ, Bohl DJ, Storch GA, Brennan DC. BK-virus and the impact of pre-emptive immunosuppression reduction: 5-year results. *Am J Transplant.* 2010;10(2):407–415.
27. Cheungpasitporn W, Kremers WK, Lorenz E, et al. De novo donor-specific antibody following BK nephropathy: the incidence and association with antibody-mediated rejection. *Clin Transplant.* 2018;32(3):e13194.
28. Jahan S, Scuderi C, Francis L, et al. T-cell adoptive immunotherapy for BK nephropathy in renal transplantation. *Transpl Infect Dis.* 2020;22(6):e13399.
29. Blazquez-Navarro A, Dang-Heine C, Wittenbrink N, et al. BKV, CMV, and EBV interactions and their effect on graft function one year post-renal transplantation: results from a large multi-centre study. *EBioMedicine.* 2018;34:113–121.
30. Opelz G, Dohler B, Ruhenstroth A. Cytomegalovirus prophylaxis and graft outcome in solid organ transplantation: a collaborative transplant study report. *Am J Transplant.* 2004;4(6):928–936.
31. Kotton CN, Kumar D, Caliendo AM, et al. International consensus guidelines on the management of cytomegalovirus in solid organ transplantation. *Transplantation.* 2010;89(7):779–795.
32. Kotton CN, Kumar D, Caliendo AM, et al. The Third International Consensus Guidelines on the management of cytomegalovirus in solid-organ transplantation. *Transplantation.* 2018;102(6):900–931.
33. Sureshkumar KK, Chopra B, Josephson MA, Shah PB, McGill RL. Recipient obesity and kidney transplant outcomes: a mate-kidney analysis. *Am J Kidney Dis.* 2021;78(4):501–510 e501.
34. Hill CJ, Courtney AE, Cardwell CR, et al. Recipient obesity and outcomes after kidney transplantation: a systematic review and meta-analysis. *Nephrol Dial Transplant.* 2015;30(8):1403–1411.
35. Gill JS, Lan J, Dong J, et al. The survival benefit of kidney transplantation in obese patients. *Am J Transplant.* 2013;13(8):2083–2090.
36. Aziz F, Ramadorai A, Parajuli S, et al. Obesity: an independent predictor of morbidity and graft loss after kidney transplantation. *Am J Nephrol.* 2020;51(8):615–623.
37. Kwan JM, Hajjiri Z, Metwally A, Finn PW, Perkins DL. Effect of the obesity epidemic on kidney transplantation: obesity is independent of diabetes as a risk factor for adverse renal transplant outcomes. *PLoS ONE.* 2016;11(11):e0165712.
38. Erturk T, Berber I, Cakir U. Effect of obesity on clinical outcomes of kidney transplant patients. *Transplant Proc.* 2019;51(4):1093–1095.
39. Sheetz KH, Gerhardinger L, Dimick JB, Waits SA. Bariatric surgery and long-term survival in patients with obesity and end-stage kidney disease. *JAMA Surg.* 2020;155(7):581–588.

40. Oberholzer J, Giulianotti P, Danielson KK, et al. Minimally invasive robotic kidney transplantation for obese patients previously denied access to transplantation. *Am J Transplant*. 2013;13(3):721–728.

41. Tzvetanov IG, Spaggiari M, Tulla KA, et al. Robotic kidney transplantation in the obese patient: 10-year experience from a single center. *Am J Transplant*. 2020;20(2):430–440.

42. Spaggiari M, Di Cocco P, Tulla K, et al. Simultaneous robotic kidney transplantation and bariatric surgery for morbidly obese patients with end-stage renal failure. *Am J Transplant*. 2021;21(4):1525–1534.

43. Yemini R, Nesher E, Winkler J, et al. Bariatric surgery in solid organ transplant patients: long-term follow-up results of outcome, safety, and effect on immunosuppression. *Am J Transplant*. 2018;18(11):2772–2780.

44. Wilding JPH, Batterham RL, Calanna S, et al. Once-weekly semaglutide in adults with overweight or obesity. *N Engl J Med*. 2021;384(11):989–1002.

45. Thangavelu T, Lyden E, Shivaswamy V. A retrospective study of glucagon-like peptide 1 receptor agonists for the management of diabetes after transplantation. *Diabetes Ther*. 2020;11(4):987–994.

46. Chawla LS, Eggers PW, Star RA, Kimmel PL. Acute kidney injury and chronic kidney disease as interconnected syndromes. *N Engl J Med*. 2014;371(1):58–66.

47. Haller MC, Kainz A, Baer H, Oberbauer R. Dialysis vintage and outcomes after kidney transplantation: a retrospective cohort study. *Clin J Am Soc Nephrol*. 2017;12(1):122–130.

48. Prezelin-Reydit M, Combe C, Harambat J, et al. Prolonged dialysis duration is associated with graft failure and mortality after kidney transplantation: results from the French transplant database. *Nephrol Dial Transplant*. 2019;34(3):538–545.

49. Rose C, Gill J, Gill JS. Association of kidney transplantation with survival in patients with long dialysis exposure. *Clin J Am Soc Nephrol*. 2017;12(12):2024–2031.

50. Gill JS, Rose C, Joffres Y, Landsberg D, Gill J. Variation in dialysis exposure prior to nonpreemptive living donor kidney transplantation in the United States and its association with allograft outcomes. *Am J Kidney Dis*. 2018;71(5):636–647.

51. Gill JS, Clark S, Kadatz M, Gill J. The association of pretransplant dialysis exposure with transplant failure is dependent on the state-specific rate of dialysis mortality. *Am J Transplant*. 2020;20(9):2481–2490.

52. Gill JS, Kelly B, Tonelli M. Time to abolish metrics that sustain systemic racism in kidney allocation. *JAMA*. 2023;329(11):879–880.

53. Freedman BI, Pastan SO, Israni AK, et al. APOL1 genotype and kidney transplantation outcomes from deceased African American donors. *Transplantation*. 2016;100(1):194–202.

54. Freedman BI, Moxey-Mims MM, Alexander AA, et al. APOL1 long-term kidney transplantation outcomes network (APOLLO): design and rationale. *Kidney Int Rep*. 2020;5(3):278–288.

55. Arshad A, Hodson J, Chappelow I, et al. The impact of donor body mass index on outcomes after deceased kidney transplantation—a national population-cohort study. *Transpl Int*. 2018;31(10):1099–1109.

56. Naik AS, Zhong Y, Parasuraman R, et al. The temporal and long-term impact of donor body mass index on recipient outcomes after kidney transplantation—a retrospective study. *Transpl Int*. 2020;33(1):59–67.

57. Miller AJ, Kiberd BA, Alwayn IP, Odutayo A, Tennankore KK. Donor–recipient weight and sex mismatch and the risk of graft loss in renal transplantation. *Clin J Am Soc Nephrol.* 2017;12(4):669–676.

58. Tillmann FP, Quack I, Woznowski M, Rump LC. Effect of recipient–donor sex and weight mismatch on graft survival after deceased donor renal transplantation. *PLoS ONE.* 2019;14(3):e0214048.

59. Lepeytre F, Delmas-Frenette C, Zhang X, et al. Donor age, donor–recipient size mismatch, and kidney graft survival. *Clin J Am Soc Nephrol.* 2020;15(10):1455–1463.

60. Tandukar S, Wu C, Hariharan S, Puttarajappa C. Impact of size matching based on donor-recipient height on kidney transplant outcomes. *Transpl Int.* 2022;35:10253.

61. Rao PS, Schaubel DE, Guidinger MK, et al. A comprehensive risk quantification score for deceased donor kidneys: the Kidney Donor Risk Index. *Transplantation.* 2009;88(2):231–236.

62. Debout A, Foucher Y, Trebern-Launay K, et al. Each additional hour of cold ischemia time significantly increases the risk of graft failure and mortality following renal transplantation. *Kidney Int.* 2015;87(2):343–349.

63. Hansson J, Mjornstedt L, Lindner P. The risk of graft loss 5 years after kidney transplantation is increased if cold ischemia time exceeds 14 hours. *Clin Transplant.* 2018;32(9):e13377.

64. Xia Y, Friedmann P, Cortes CM, Lubetzky ML, Kayler LK. Influence of cold ischemia time in combination with donor acute kidney injury on kidney transplantation outcomes. *J Am Coll Surg.* 2015;221(2):532–538.

65. Krishnan AR, Wong G, Chapman JR, et al. Prolonged ischemic time, delayed graft function, and graft and patient outcomes in live donor kidney transplant recipients. *Am J Transplant.* 2016;16(9):2714–2723.

66. Treat E, Chow EKH, Peipert JD, et al. Shipping living donor kidneys and transplant recipient outcomes. *Am J Transplant.* 2018;18(3):632–641.

67. Nassiri N, Kwan L, Bolagani A, et al. The "oldest and coldest" shipped living donor kidneys transplanted through kidney paired donation. *Am J Transplant.* 2020;20(1):137–144.

68. Wey A, Foutz J, Gustafson SK, et al. The Collaborative Innovation and Improvement Network (COIIN): effect on donor yield, waitlist mortality, transplant rates, and offer acceptance. *Am J Transplant.* 2020;20(4):1076–1086.

69. Puttarajappa CM, Jorgensen D, Yabes JG, et al. Trends and impact on cold ischemia time and clinical outcomes using virtual crossmatch for deceased donor kidney transplantation in the United States. *Kidney Int.* 2021;100(3):660–671.

70. Tennankore KK, Kim SJ, Alwayn IP, Kiberd BA. Prolonged warm ischemia time is associated with graft failure and mortality after kidney transplantation. *Kidney Int.* 2016;89(3):648–658.

71. Heylen L, Pirenne J, Samuel U, et al. The impact of anastomosis time during kidney transplantation on graft loss: a Eurotransplant cohort study. *Am J Transplant.* 2017;17(3):724–732.

72. Marzouk K, Lawen J, Alwayn I, Kiberd BA. The impact of vascular anastomosis time on early kidney transplant outcomes. *Transplant Res.* 2013;2(1):8.

73. Ferede AA, Walsh AL, Davis NF, et al. Warm ischemia time at vascular anastomosis is an independent predictor for delayed graft function in kidney transplant recipients. *Exp Clin Transplant.* 2020;18(1):13–18.

74. Wang CJ, Wetmore JB, Crary GS, Kasiske BL. The donor kidney biopsy and its implications in predicting graft outcomes: a systematic review. *Am J Transplant.* 2015;15(7):1903–1914.
75. Stewart DE, Foutz J, Kamal L, et al. The independent effects of procurement biopsy findings on 10-year outcomes of extended criteria donor kidney transplants. *Kidney Int Rep.* 2022;7(8):1850–1865.
76. Cheungpasitporn W, Thongprayoon C, Vaitla PK, et al. Degree of glomerulosclerosis in procurement kidney biopsies from marginal donor kidneys and their implications in predicting graft outcomes. *J Clin Med.* 2020;9(5):1469. https://doi.org/10.3390/jcm 9051469
77. Zens TJ, Danobeitia JS, Leverson G, et al. The impact of kidney donor profile index on delayed graft function and transplant outcomes: a single-center analysis. *Clin Transplant.* 2018;32(3):e13190.
78. Gill J, Dong J, Rose C, Gill JS. The risk of allograft failure and the survival benefit of kidney transplantation are complicated by delayed graft function. *Kidney Int.* 2016;89(6):1331–1336.
79. Schrezenmeier E, Muller M, Friedersdorff F, et al. Evaluation of severity of delayed graft function in kidney transplant recipients. *Nephrol Dial Transplant.* 2022;37(5):973–981.
80. Redfield RR, Scalea JR, Zens TJ, et al. Predictors and outcomes of delayed graft function after living-donor kidney transplantation. *Transpl Int.* 2016;29(1):81–87.
81. Mogulla MR, Bhattacharjya S, Clayton PA. Risk factors for and outcomes of delayed graft function in live donor kidney transplantation—a retrospective study. *Transpl Int.* 2019;32(11):1151–1160.
82. Cherukuri A, Mehta R, Sood P, Harihuran S. Early allograft inflammation and scarring associate with graft dysfunction and poor outcomes in renal transplant recipients with delayed graft function: a prospective single center cohort study. *Transpl Int.* 2018;31(12):1369–1379.
83. Moers C, Smits JM, Maathuis MH, et al. Machine perfusion or cold storage in deceased-donor kidney transplantation. *N Engl J Med.* 2009;360(1):7–19.
84. O'Callaghan JM, Morgan RD, Knight SR, Morris PJ. Systematic review and meta-analysis of hypothermic machine perfusion versus static cold storage of kidney allografts on transplant outcomes. *Br J Surg.* 2013;100(8):991–1001.
85. Takemoto SK, Terasaki PI, Gjertson DW, Cecka JM. Twelve years' experience with national sharing of HLA-matched cadaveric kidneys for transplantation. *N Engl J Med.* 2000;343(15):1078–1084.
86. Foster BJ, Dahhou M, Zhang X, Platt RW, Smith JM, Hanley JA. Impact of HLA mismatch at first kidney transplant on lifetime with graft function in young recipients. *Am J Transplant.* 2014;14(4):876–885.
87. Shi X, Lv J, Han W, et al. What is the impact of human leukocyte antigen mismatching on graft survival and mortality in renal transplantation? A meta-analysis of 23 cohort studies involving 486,608 recipients. *BMC Nephrol.* 2018;19(1):116.
88. Gebel HM, Bray RA, Nickerson P. Pre-transplant assessment of donor-reactive, HLA-specific antibodies in renal transplantation: contraindication vs. risk. *Am J Transplant.* 2003;3(12):1488–1500.
89. Lim WH, Chapman JR, Wong G. Peak panel reactive antibody, cancer, graft, and patient outcomes in kidney transplant recipients. *Transplantation.* 2015;99(5):1043–1050.

90. Susal C, Dohler B, Opelz G. Presensitized kidney graft recipients with HLA class I and II antibodies are at increased risk for graft failure: a Collaborative Transplant Study report. *Hum Immunol.* 2009;70(8):569–573.

91. Redfield RR, Scalea JR, Zens TJ, et al. The mode of sensitization and its influence on allograft outcomes in highly sensitized kidney transplant recipients. *Nephrol Dial Transplant.* 2016;31(10):1746–1753.

92. Lan JH, Kadatz M, Chang DT, Gill J, Gebel HM, Gill JS. Pretransplant calculated panel reactive antibody in the absence of donor-specific antibody and kidney allograft survival. *Clin J Am Soc Nephrol.* 2021;16(2):275–283.

93. Senev A, Lerut E, Van Sandt V, et al. Specificity, strength, and evolution of pretransplant donor-specific HLA antibodies determine outcome after kidney transplantation. *Am J Transplant.* 2019;19(11):3100–3113.

94. Redondo-Pachon D, Perez-Saez MJ, Mir M, et al. Impact of persistent and cleared preformed HLA DSA on kidney transplant outcomes. *Hum Immunol.* 2018;79(6):424–431.

95. Morrison AH, Gupta M, Lloyd K, et al. Class and kinetics of weakly reactive pretransplant donor-specific HLA antibodies predict rejection in kidney transplant recipients. *Transplant Direct.* 2019;5(8):e478.

96. Michielsen LA, Wisse BW, Kamburova EG, et al. A paired kidney analysis on the impact of pre-transplant anti-HLA antibodies on graft survival. *Nephrol Dial Transplant.* 2019;34(6):1056–1063.

97. Kamburova EG, Wisse BW, Joosten I, et al. Differential effects of donor-specific HLA antibodies in living versus deceased donor transplant. *Am J Transplant.* 2018;18(9):2274–2284.

98. Ziemann M, Altermann W, Angert K, et al. Preformed donor-specific HLA antibodies in living and deceased donor transplantation: a multicenter study. *Clin J Am Soc Nephrol.* 2019;14(7):1056–1066.

99. Haas M, Mirocha J, Reinsmoen NL, et al. Differences in pathologic features and graft outcomes in antibody-mediated rejection of renal allografts due to persistent/recurrent versus de novo donor-specific antibodies. *Kidney Int.* 2017;91(3):729–737.

100. Aubert O, Loupy A, Hidalgo L, et al. Antibody-mediated rejection due to preexisting versus de novo donor-specific antibodies in kidney allograft recipients. *J Am Soc Nephrol.* 2017;28(6):1912–1923.

101. Senev A, Coemans M, Lerut E, et al. Eplet mismatch load and de novo occurrence of donor-specific anti-HLA antibodies, rejection, and graft failure after kidney transplantation: an observational cohort study. *J Am Soc Nephrol.* 2020;31(9):2193–2204.

102. Sakamoto S, Iwasaki K, Tomosugi T, et al. Analysis of T and B cell epitopes to predict the risk of de novo donor-specific antibody (DSA) production after kidney transplantation: a two-center retrospective cohort study. *Front Immunol.* 2020;11:2000.

103. Kishikawa H, Kinoshita T, Hashimoto M, et al. Class II HLA eplet mismatch is a risk factor for de novo donor-specific antibody development and antibody-mediated rejection in kidney transplantation recipients. *Transplant Proc.* 2018;50(8):2388–2391.

104. Lachmann N, Niemann M, Reinke P, et al. Donor-recipient matching based on predicted indirectly recognizable HLA epitopes independently predicts the incidence of de novo donor-specific HLA antibodies following renal transplantation. *Am J Transplant.* 2017;17(12):3076–3086.

105. Sapir-Pichhadze R, Tinckam K, Quach K, et al. HLA-DR and -DQ eplet mismatches and transplant glomerulopathy: a nested case-control study. *Am J Transplant.* 2015;15(1):137–148.
106. Nickerson PW. What have we learned about how to prevent and treat antibody-mediated rejection in kidney transplantation? *Am J Transplant.* 2020;20(Suppl 4):12–22.
107. Rampersad C, Balshaw R, Gibson IW, et al. The negative impact of T cell-mediated rejection on renal allograft survival in the modern era. *Am J Transplant.* 2022;22(3):761–771.
108. Mehta RB, Melgarejo I, Viswanathan V, et al. Long-term immunological outcomes of early subclinical inflammation on surveillance kidney allograft biopsies. *Kidney Int.* 2022;102(6):1371–1381.
109. Mehta RB, Tandukar S, Jorgensen D, et al. Early subclinical tubulitis and interstitial inflammation in kidney transplantation have adverse clinical implications. *Kidney Int.* 2020;98(2):436–447.
110. Sharma A, Cherukuri A, Mehta RB, Sood P, Hariharan S. High calcineurin inhibitor intrapatient variability is associated with renal allograft inflammation, chronicity, and graft loss. *Transplant Direct.* 2019;5(2):e424.
111. Dierickx D, Habermann TM. Post-transplantation lymphoproliferative disorders in adults. *N Engl J Med.* 2018;378(6):549–562.
112. Saran R, Robinson B, Abbott KC, et al. US Renal Data System 2019 annual data report: epidemiology of kidney disease in the United States. *Am J Kidney Dis.* 2020;75(1 Suppl 1):A6–A7.
113. Cosio FG, Cattran DC. Recent advances in our understanding of recurrent primary glomerulonephritis after kidney transplantation. *Kidney Int.* 2017;91(2):304–314.
114. Allen PJ, Chadban SJ, Craig JC, et al. Recurrent glomerulonephritis after kidney transplantation: risk factors and allograft outcomes. *Kidney Int.* 2017;92(2):461–469.
115. Regunathan-Shenk R, Avasare RS, Ahn W, et al. Kidney transplantation in C3 glomerulopathy: a case series. *Am J Kidney Dis.* 2019;73(3):316–323.
116. Grupper A, Cornell LD, Fervenza FC, Beck LH, Jr., Lorenz E, Cosio FG. Recurrent membranous nephropathy after kidney transplantation: treatment and long-term implications. *Transplantation.* 2016;100(12):2710–2716.
117. Uffing A, Perez-Saez MJ, Mazzali M, et al. Recurrence of FSGS after kidney transplantation in adults. *Clin J Am Soc Nephrol.* 2020;15(2):247–256.
118. Moroni G, Belingheri M, Frontini G, Tamborini F, Messa P. Immunoglobulin A nephropathy: recurrence after renal transplantation. *Front Immunol.* 2019;10:1332.
119. Francis A, Trnka P, McTaggart SJ. Long-term outcome of kidney transplantation in recipients with focal segmental glomerulosclerosis. *Clin J Am Soc Nephrol.* 2016;11(11):2041–2046.
120. Zanoni F, Khairallah P, Kiryluk K, Batal I. Glomerular diseases of the kidney allograft: toward a precision medicine approach. *Semin Nephrol.* 2022;42(1):29–43.
121. Zuber J, Frimat M, Caillard S, et al. Use of highly individualized complement blockade has revolutionized clinical outcomes after kidney transplantation and renal epidemiology of atypical hemolytic uremic syndrome. *J Am Soc Nephrol.* 2019;30(12):2449–2463.

6

Short-Term and Late
T-Cell-Mediated Rejection after
Kidney Transplantation

Rajil B. Mehta and Maarten Naesens

T-cell Rejection—an expected, but unwanted event after kidney transplantation!

Introduction: The Definition of T-Cell-Mediated Rejection

Alloimmune T cell responses are central in the pathogenesis of rejection. T cells are activated by exposure to alloantigens followed by expansion of T cell clones, differentiation into effector cells, and migration into the graft, leading to tissue destruction. From the early days of kidney transplantation, this immune infiltration into the graft was recognized as rejection, even prior to the development of a classification system of rejection. Over the years, this understanding has evolved as has the recognition of the prognostic implications of varying severity of rejection. This chapter provides details of T-cell-medicated rejection (TCMR) including historical perspective, classification, clinical features, current management and its shortcomings, as well as future directions.

History and Banff Classification

Histological classification of acute rejection was necessary to establish consensus on the characteristics of inflammation for the definition of rejection. The Banff Classification, initiated in 1991, has been adopted and revised periodically, and is currently used for diagnosis of rejection.[1] During the initial Banff meetings, it was recognized that tubulitis and intimal arteritis are key histological lesions in acute rejection. Further it was felt that a certain threshold of tubulitis was necessary to be called a rejection, while interstitial inflammation was considered of relevance only when accompanied by tubulitis. Cases not reaching the thresholds for diagnosis of acute rejection but with only mild/moderate interstitial inflammation and mild tubulitis were considered "very mild acute rejection" (coined "border-line changes"). Over the past three decades, the definitions established in Banff '91 for diagnosis of "acute rejection" (later renamed "cell-mediated rejection" and "T-cell-mediated rejection" [TCMR], to make the distinction from antibody-mediated rejection phenotypes) have remained relatively unchanged. TCMR is further subclassified in grades I, II, and III, based on the presence and extent of tubulitis as well as intimal arteritis.

In addition to acute forms of cellular rejection, chronic rejection has been recognized since the early days of the Banff classification, but its definition has evolved over time. After the recognition in Banff '05 that the definition of "chronic/sclerosing allograft nephropathy" was not specific for alloimmune in-volvement, more detailed definitions of chronic rejection were proposed. The definition of "chronic active TCMR" introduced with Banff '05 was restricted to inflammatory arteriopathy, but since Banff '17 expanded to include inflamma-tion is atrophic and sclerotic areas.[2]

The Banff classification is used today by pathologists and clinicians all over the world and has been instrumental in creating a common language for the defini-tion and classification of different types of kidney rejection. Banff classification required modifications, as ambiguities are uncovered along with the introduction of newer technologies and unraveling of innovative pathobiological pathways.

Clinical Presentation of TCMR

The clinical features of TCMR can vary. In the pioneering days of clinical kidney transplantation, severe rejection manifested as fever, allograft pain and ten-derness, and worsening renal function. In the modern era of potent immuno-suppression, TCMR is usually asymptomatic and manifests only as an increase in serum creatinine. This is generally referred to as "clinical rejection," when accompanied by worsening renal function and diagnosed in a "clinically indi-cated" biopsy (indication/for-cause biopsy).

Since the late 1980s, it was noted that cell-mediated rejections can also be observed with little or no change in the serum creatinine values, coined "sub-clinical rejection." These histological changes can only be picked up on protocol or surveillance biopsies as there are no associated symptoms and no rise in creatinine noted. These surveillance biopsies are performed at predetermined time points as ascertained by the institution. The most common time points for performance of a surveillance biopsies are 3 months and 1 year. Only about 17% of transplant centers in the United States perform surveillance biopsies for all patients, and another 20% or so perform surveillance biopsies in select recipients.[3] These subclinical rejections may be associated with worse kidney transplant function although their long-term impact has not been clearly elucidated. However, detection of TCMR at time of graft dysfunction clearly has worse prognosis compared to TCMR or borderline changes detected in surveillance biopsies. The relevance of different grades of TCMR with regard to graft longevity is less clear. The performance of surveillance biopsies for the detection of subclinical TCMR remains a debated topic and is the subject of ongoing studies. In addition to creatinine monitoring and evaluation of proteinuria, other noninvasive tests have been proposed for diagnosis of rejection and thus offer novel indications to perform a biopsy or measures to avoid a biopsy.

Mixed Rejection

Antibody-mediated rejection (AMR, discussed in Chapter 7) was described in the mid-1990s and introduced in Banff '97. AMR represents a different pathway for destruction of the renal parenchyma, mediated by antibodies (primarily targeting mismatched donor human leukocyte antigen [HLA] molecules). However, AMR cannot be dissociated from alloimmune T cell responses, as T cell help is required for B cell activation. Furthermore, biopsies that not only fulfill the definition of TCMR but also simultaneously fulfill the AMR criteria of the Banff classification (see Figure 6.1), are termed "mixed rejection," given the combination of histopathological features of both types of rejection. Mixed rejections tend to be more severe and refractory to treatment and are commonly seen in the

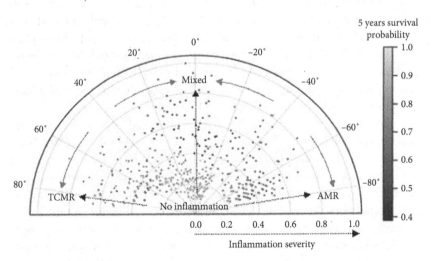

Figure 6.1 Prognostic implications of varying types and severity of rejection.
Adapted from Vaulet et al.; JASN 2022.

setting of nonadherence with immunosuppressive therapy. Schematic representation of rejection is shown in Figure 6.1.

Early versus Late TCMR

Acute TCMR and borderline changes are typically observed in the first few weeks and months after transplantation; protocol biopsy studies have demonstrated that later episodes of TCMR are less common. Nevertheless, cases of severe TCMR after nonadherence illustrate the importance of long-term maintenance immunosuppressive therapy, and show that the alloimmune responses do not completely wane over time. The development of chronic active TMCR has also been related to underimmunosuppression, a further indication of persistent immune responses against the graft.

Pros and Cons of the Banff Classification

The Banff classification, which has been extensively used to grade the types and severity of rejections has been instrumental in unifying the definitions and concepts of rejection in solid organ transplantation. It has been extremely useful in furthering the understanding of the different types of rejection and currently remains the most widely used system for the diagnosis and classification of rejection. The Banff classification system gets modified every 2 years based on technological advances and other developments with clinical findings of newer studies. A recent version is shown in Table 6.1.

Despite these merits of the Banff classification, there are limitations. Probably the biggest limitation is the lack of reproducibility across different institutions and the subjectivity involved in the scoring of the primary lesions used for the diagnostic classification. Additionally, sampling error is an inherent error in any histology-based study, as the inflammatory processes may be patchy. Gene expression profiling in kidney transplant biopsies has been proposed and holds promise for more objective evaluation of kidney transplant rejection. However, they are not yet considered standard of care; at the current time, histopathology remains the gold standard for the diagnosis of rejection. A more conceptual issue with the Banff classification is that it dichotomizes continuous disease processes and severity spectra into presence/absence of disease (subtypes). Shortcomings of the Banff classification are shown in Table 6.2. Cases that are clinically and histologically very similar but fall just below or above the iteratively defined Banff thresholds are classified differently and receive different treatment. Also, cases with high inflammatory lesion scores can fall into the same category as

Table 6.1 Adapted from "The Banff 2019 Kidney Meeting Report"; AJT 2020

Category 3: Borderline (Suspicious) for acute TCMR

Foci of tubulitis (t1, t2, or t3) with mild interstitial inflammation (ii), or mild (t1) tubulitis with moderate-severe interstitial inflammation (i2 or 13)

No intimal or transmural arteritis (v = 0)

Category 4: TCMR

Acute TCMR

Grade IA: Interstitial inflammation involving >25% of nonsclerotic cortical parenchyma (i2 or 13) with moderate tubulitis (t2) involving 1 or more tubules, not including tubules that are severely atrophic

Grade IB: Interstitial inflammation involving >25% of nonsclerotic cortical parenchyma (i2 or i3) with severe tubulitis (t3) involving 1 or more tubules, not including tubules that are severely atrophic

Grade IIA: Mild to moderate intimal arteritis (v1), with or without interstitial inflammation and/or tubulitis

Grade IIB: Severe intimal arteritis (v2), with or without interstitial inflammation and/or tubulitis

Grade III: Transmural arteritis and/or arterial fibrinoid necrosis involving medial smooth muscle with accompanying mononuclear cell intimal arteritis (v3), with or without interstitial inflammation and/or tubulitis

Chronic active TCMR

Grade IA: Interstitial inflammation involving >25% of sclerotic cortical parenchyma (i-IFTA2 or i-IFTA3) AND > 25% of total cortical parenchyma (ti2 or ti3) with moderate tubulitis (t2 or t-IFTA2) involving 1 or more tubules, not including severely atrophic tubules; other known causes of i-IFTA should be ruled out

Grade IB: Interstitial inflammation involving >25% of sclerotic cortical parenchyma (i-IFTA2 or i-IFTA3) AND > 25% of total cortical parenchyma (ti2 or ti3) with severe tubulitis (t3 or t-IFTA3) involving 1 or more tubules, not including severely atrophic tubules; other known causes of i-IFTA should be ruled out

Grade II: Chronic allograft arteriopathy (arterial intimal fibrosis with mononuclear cell inflammation in fibrosis and formation of neointima). This may also be a manifestation of chronic active or chronic ABMR or mixed ABMR/TCMR

---

lower inflammatory scores, as there is no granular evaluation of disease severity apart from the three Banff TCMR grades (I, II, III) based on the presence/absence of intimal arteritis. The place of "borderline changes" is even more cumbersome, and it often remains unclear whether the lower grade inflammation of cases with borderline changes represents rejection or not. The true implication of borderline changes remains unclear at this time, although several studies have noted negative prognostic features of this detection, be it clinical or subclinical. Centers tend to treat cases of borderline changes in indication biopsies, but not in protocol biopsies, although clinical practice is heterogeneous. This dilemma has arisen as many of these cases also seem to resolve on their own, despite the

Table 6.2 Shortcomings of Current Methods in Diagnosis and Treatment of TCMR

Shortcomings of current diagnostic methods	Potential solutions
Invasive	Testing through noninvasive means
Subjectivity in pathology reading	Computerized or automated readings
Inflammation may be patchy and hence could be missed	Use of a biomarker that correlates with extent of inflammation
Severity of inflammation does not always correlate with changes in renal function	Use of a biomarker that correlates with extent and severity of inflammation
Shortcomings of current treatment methodology	Potential solutions
Return of creatinine to baseline after treatment may not always correlate with resolution of inflammation	Follow-up biopsies or use of noninvasive testing that indicates resolution of inflammation
No standard method to follow up treatment of subclinical TCMR	Follow-up biopsies or use of noninvasive testing that indicates resolution of inflammation

progression of certain others. Identifying beforehand which cases will progress and which will resolve remains a challenge.

Treatment of TCMRFrom the days before the definition of AMR, treatment of acute TCMR consisted primarily of steroids (see Table 6.3). Higher grades of rejection have been treated either with steroid boluses or with antithymocyte globulin (T-cell-depleting antibodies) as severe rejections can be resistant to steroids, especially in instances where intimal arteritis is noted. Many acute cases of TCMR encountered in clinical practice, whether clinical or subclinical, are of grade Banff IA. These have been traditionally treated with steroid boluses following by addition or continuation of oral steroids. In general, the responsiveness of TCMR to steroids seems very good.

Despite the successful treatment of acute TCMR, studies have found that persistent and recurrent TCMR are seen in a sizable proportion of patients. Given the lack of studies that demonstrated full resolution of inflammation with a follow-up biopsy, the proportion of patients with persistent TCMR remains unclear. In cases of clinical acute TCMR, one could assume that the inflammation resolved if the renal function improved back to the baseline after treatment. However, this becomes challenging in the case of subclinical acute TCMR, where graft function (per definition stable) is not a readout for treatment effect. Persistent or recurrent acute TCMR associates with increased risk of graft

Table 6.3 Commonly Used Treatment Regimens and Variations in Approach for Treatment of Different Grades of TCMR Noted on Surveillance

TCMR histological diagnosis	Treatment options
Normal Biopsy or biopsy with minor interstitial inflammation in the absence of tubulitis	No intervention
Borderline Change Suspicious for TCMR (Banff 2019)—tubulitis with interstitial inflammation	Observation Optimize immunosuppression (MPA and TAC dose) One to three doses of solumedrol doses ranging from 250 to 500 mg intravenously depending on the clinical context
Banff IA TCMR	Three doses of solumedrol 250–500 mg intravenously with continuation of low dose prednisone in steroid free regimens Optimize immunosuppression (MPA and TAC dose)
Banff IB TCMR or higher	Three doses of solumedrol 250–500 mg intravenously with continuation of low dose prednisone. Antithymocyte globulin 3–6 mg/kg intravenously depending on the clinical context Optimize immunosuppression (MPA and TAC dose)

failure, as illustrated recently.[4] Follow-up biopsies may be useful, however, this not been adopted as standard of care.

While there are very limited controlled studies on the best treatment of acute TCMR over the past two decades, even less is known about the treatment options for chronic active TCMR. In the initial studies contributing to the definition of this more recently defined phenotype there was an association between i-IFTA, a determining lesion of the phenotype, and lower immunosuppression. This may indicate that underimmunosuppression is a risk factor for chronic active TCMR, and that prevention and perhaps treatment could consist of optimizing immunosuppressive doses and regimens. Whether treatment of chronic active TCMR with steroids and/or thymoglobulin is beneficial needs to be further explored.[5]

Noninvasive Biomarkers for TCMR

Several biomarkers are being explored with the aim of developing a noninvasive test to diagnose acute clinical and subclinical rejection and for follow-up of resolution after rejection treatment. This is a rapidly evolving area. The use of biomarkers such as donor-derived cell-free DNA as well as peripheral blood gene expression profiling are being investigated and also used clinically at the current time, at least in the United States. Urinary chemokines CXCL9 and CXCL10 also hold promise as noninvasive markers for ongoing rejection. None of these tests seems to be specific for TCMR. The clinical utility of noninvasive biomarkers for rejection will likely become apparent with time. Noninvasive testing for the diagnosis of rejection is an attractive tool given the ease of testing for the patient. However, the specific information conveyed by these tests and its utility in the clinical setting is yet to be defined. Additionally, the frequency of performance of the testing, cost-effectiveness, and so forth, need to be further elucidated.[6,7]

Moving Forward

Relation between Histological Phenotype of TCMR and Infiltrating Cell Patterns

Currently, the definition of acute and chronic active TCMR and borderline changes suspicious of acute TCMR is based on the histological pattern of tubulointerstitial monocytic inflammation and intimal arteritis. The suggestion in its name that this phenotype of rejection is mediated by infiltrating T cells stems from extensive research in early decades of clinical transplantation about the role of T cells in transplant rejection. However, in practice, the infiltrate in TCMR does not solely consist of T cells and is often very monocyte-rich.[8] In addition, not all T cells are cytotoxic, and part of the T cell infiltration is regulatory in nature. Currently, it is not well charted how the cell-subtype distribution relates to the histological pattern of inflammation in TCMR, and it is largely unclear how the infiltrating cell distribution relates to treatment response and outcome. Further research is necessary to elucidate this.

Relation to the Underlying Cause of Inflammation

Tubulointerstitial inflammation, the hallmark of acute and chronic active TCMR and borderline changes suspicious for TCMR, is not specific for alloimmune responses. This inflammatory pattern is also observed in viral nephropathy (e.g., BK virus nephropathy [BKVN] and adenovirus infections), drug-induced tubulointerstitial nephritis, and crystal nephropathy. It remains essential to distinguish the alloimmune-mediated inflammation (rejection) from these other processes. BKVN can be diagnosed by attention to viral cytopathic changes in light microscopy, specific stains (SV40 or BKV stain for BKVN), and blood PCR. For drug-induced tubulointerstitial nephritis, no specific markers exist. It is unclear whether viral or drug-induced inflammatory processes could instigate secondary alloimmune activation.

The role of primary T cell alloimmune responses, as convincingly evidenced in the first decades of clinical kidney transplantation by extensive preclinical models, remains up to the present time, despite the use of combinations of strong immunosuppressants. This is indicated by the significant associations between donor–recipient HLA gene mismatches and the risk for acute TCMR and graft failure.[9,10] However, more recent preclinical models indicated not only that T cell allorecognition plays a role but also that innate immune allorecognition could contribute to the phenotypes observed in clinical practice. More specifically, a potential role of the CD47-sirpalpha pathway in allorecognition by monocytes was demonstrated in preclinical models,[11] and first clinical studies may suggest that this new type of allorecognition could indeed contribute to the tubulointerstitial inflammation observed in clinical practice.[12] Given the lack of statistical power in this clinical study, further research is needed before conclusions can be made on the potential role of innate allorecognition in the clinical phenotype of tubulointerstitial inflammation.

Mixed Rejection

As noted above, mixed rejection is defined as the co-occurrence of AMR and TCMR. This combined phenotype has been studied only scarcely, and it is not clear whether this combination of tubulointerstitial inflammation and microvascular inflammation in the same biopsy is the hallmark of two independent processes. It is more likely that this combined phenotypic presentation is the reflection of a single underlying immune process. For instance, TCMR and borderline changes are often observed in the context of AMR, with intimal arteritis a lesion largely contributing to this mixed phenotype. Similarly, peritubular capillaritis is a hallmark of AMR, but in the context of TCMR or borderline changes it is considered less informative for the definition of AMR, and cases of potential mixed rejection may be underrecognized by this current Banff rule. Whether such mixed types of rejection have different pathophysiology and outcome than isolated TCMR or AMR, and require different treatments, has not been studied.

Biopsy-Based Transcript Analysis for Diagnosis of TCMR

In the current Banff classification, TCMR and borderline changes are defined exclusively by histological criteria. Over the past two decades, several research groups have detailed the transcriptomic profile of TCMR in kidney transplant biopsies, first by using genome-wide microarrays[13] but more recently also more targeted gene transcript expression analyses.[14] For AMR, the option to use a gene expression classifier is included since Banff '13, but not for TCMR or borderline changes. Whether the biopsy-based transcript analyses are sufficiently validated for diagnosis of TCMR in clinical routine remains an ongoing debate. It remains unclear which classifiers and thresholds can be proposed for the diagnosis of TCMR. Furthermore, the standardization and clinical availability of biopsy-based transcript analysis is another obstacle that will need to be overcome, if biopsy-based transcript analysis is to be widely used clinically.

Machine Learning and Artificial Intelligence for TCMR

Given the complexity of the Banff classification and the difficulty of correctly applying the Banff rules based on lesion scores, attempts are under way to automate the interpretation of Banff lesion scores in diagnostic categories. A recent study points to the great potential of such an approach using machine-learning classifiers.[15] Another approach points to the potential of mathematical reclassification of biopsies based on Banff lesion scores and indicates that data-driven reclassification could simplify the system by eliminating the clinically difficult category "borderline."[16] However, the clinical feasibility and validity of this reclustering have yet to be demonstrated. Perhaps even more promising is the calculation of activity and chronicity indices based on individual Banff lesion scores, on top of the diagnostic classification[16] (Figure 6.1). Activity and chronicity indices are independently related to graft failure rates and can potentially provide an indication of the reversibility of (active) disease versus futility of treatment of (chronic) disease phenotypes. The added value of such approaches for clinical decision-making has not yet been demonstrated.

Machine learning and artificial intelligence are promising on the basis of not only individual Banff lesion scores, which are notoriously observer-dependent, but also rapid advances in the availability of digital scans, which enable deep learning on entire slides. Although not yet ready for routine clinical application, initial reports indicate the great potential of such approaches for automated biopsy segmentation and structural annotation[17] as well as the diagnosis of rejection.[18] More sophisticated algorithms that distinguish between TCMR and AMR, and between different subtypes of TCMR (acute vs. chronically active), are not yet defined, but several research teams are working on such algorithms with the ultimate goal of bringing these innovations to clinical practice.

Conclusion

TCMR is not an uncommon finding on allograft biopsies, both indication as well as surveillance. Although the gold standard for diagnosis has been histology, there is a potential for use of supplementary tools that could perhaps be used to overcome the shortcomings of histology. Additionally, there is a clinical need for tools that would help identify resolution of inflammation following treatment. The overarching goal in such an endeavor would be to ultimately help improve long-term kidney allograft survival.

References

1. Solez K, Axelsen RA, Benediktsson H, et al. International standardization of criteria for the histologic diagnosis of renal allograft rejection: the Banff working classification of kidney transplant pathology. *Kidney Int.* 1993;44(2):411–422.
2. Haas M, Loupy A, Lefaucheur C, et al. The Banff 2017 Kidney Meeting report: revised diagnostic criteria for chronic active T cell-mediated rejection, antibody-mediated rejection, and prospects for integrative endpoints for next-generation clinical trials. *Am J Transplant.* 2018;18(2):293–307.
3. Mehta R, Cherikh W, Sood P, Hariharan S. Kidney allograft surveillance biopsy practices across US transplant centers: a UNOS survey. *Clin Transplant.* 2017;31(5):e12945.
4. Rampersad C, Balshaw R, Gibson IW, et al. The negative impact of T cell-mediated rejection on renal allograft survival in the modern era. *Am J Transplant.* 2022;22(3):761–771.
5. Kung VL, Sandhu R, Haas M, Huang E. Chronic active T cell-mediated rejection is variably responsive to immunosuppressive therapy. *Kidney Int.* 2021;100(2):391–400.
6. Huang E, Mengel M, Clahsen-van Groningen MC, Jackson AM. Diagnostic potential of minimally invasive biomarkers: a biopsy-centered viewpoint from the Banff Minimally Invasive Diagnostics Working Group. *Transplantation.* 2023;107(1):45–52.
7. Puttarajappa CM, Mehta RB, Roberts MS, Smith KJ, Hariharan S. Economic analysis of screening for subclinical rejection in kidney transplantation using protocol biopsies and noninvasive biomarkers. *Am J Transplant.* 2021;21(1):186–197.
8. Calvani J, Terada M, Lesaffre C, et al. In situ multiplex immunofluorescence analysis of the inflammatory burden in kidney allograft rejection: a new tool to characterize the alloimmune response. *Am J Transplant.* 2020;20(4):942–953.
9. Senev A, Coemans M, Lerut E, et al. Eplet mismatch load and de novo occurrence of donor-specific anti-HLA antibodies, rejection, and graft failure after kidney transplantation: an observational cohort study. *J Am Soc Nephrol.* 2020;31(9):2193–2204.
10. Wiebe C, Kosmoliaptsis V, Pochinco D, et al. HLA-DR/DQ molecular mismatch: a prognostic biomarker for primary alloimmunity. *Am J Transplant.* 2019;19(6):1708–1719.
11. Dai H, Friday AJ, Abou-Daya KI, et al. Donor SIRPalpha polymorphism modulates the innate immune response to allogeneic grafts. *Sci Immunol.* 2017;2(12):eaam6202.

12. Garcia-Sanchez C, Casillas-Abundis MA, Pinelli DF, Tambur AR, Hod-Dvorai R. Impact of SIRPalpha polymorphism on transplant outcomes in HLA-identical living donor kidney transplantation. *Clin Transplant*. 2021;35(9):e14406.

13. Halloran PF, Einecke G. Microarrays and transcriptome analysis in renal transplantation. *Nat Clin Pract Nephrol*. 2006;2(1):2–3.

14. Mengel M, Loupy A, Haas M, et al. Banff 2019 Meeting report: molecular diagnostics in solid organ transplantation—consensus for the Banff Human Organ Transplant (B-HOT) gene panel and open source multicenter validation. *Am J Transplant*. 2020;20(9):2305–2317.

15. Labriffe M, Woillard JB, Gwinner W, et al. Machine learning-supported interpretation of kidney graft elementary lesions in combination with clinical data. *Am J Transplant*. 2022;22(12):2821–2833.

16. Vaulet T, Divard G, Thaunat O, et al. Data-driven chronic allograft phenotypes: a novel and validated complement for histologic assessment of kidney transplant biopsies. *J Am Soc Nephrol*. 2022;33(11):2026–2039.

17. Farris AB, Moghe I, Wu S, et al. Banff Digital Pathology Working Group: going digital in transplant pathology. *Am J Transplant*. 2020;20(9):2392–2399.

18. Kers J, Bulow RD, Klinkhammer BM, et al. Deep learning-based classification of kidney transplant pathology: a retrospective, multicentre, proof-of-concept study. *Lancet Digit Health*. 2022;4(1):e18–e26.

7

Short-Term and Late Antibody-Mediated Rejection after Kidney Transplantation

Carrie Schinstock and Marta Crespo

Antibody Mediated Rejection—determined by history, memory and underimmunosuppression!

Introduction

Antibody-mediated rejection (ABMR) remains an important cause of renal allograft loss in the current era. A large multicenter observational study of over 5,000 kidney transplant recipients since 2006 showed that 30% of all death-censored allograft losses were associated with ABMR.[1] Our understanding of ABMR has expanded in concert with advances in human leukocyte antigen (HLA) antibody detection techniques and standardization of renal allograft histology interpretation with the Banff classification, yet our treatment approach for late active and chronic ABMR remains limited. This chapter discusses various aspects of ABMR including the clinical presentations of ABMR, the mechanisms of ABMR, and treatment strategies. In addition, we also discuss the importance of microvascular inflammation and the histologic features suggestive of ABMR without detectable HLA donor-specific antibody (DSA).

Mechanism of Antibody-Mediated Production and Allograft Injury

Alloantibodies directed toward HLA and blood ABO antigens are the most relevant in kidney transplantation. This chapter will mainly focus on alloantibody directed toward HLA because these antibodies (DSAs) are the most studied and deleterious to the allograft.

Generation of Alloantibody

The bone marrow continuously generates a vast assortment of diverse naive B cells expressing unique cell surface immunoglobulin (B cell receptors). The naive B cell's immunoglobulin can interact with an enormous variety of antigens, including the diverse class I and class II HLA molecules that are relevant in kidney transplant. These CD19 and CD20 positive mature, but naive, B cells remain in a dormant state until they encounter antigen in secondary lymphoid tissue. Upon antigen exposure and subsequent activation by T cells that have encountered the same antigen, the B cell antigen-specific population rapidly proliferates and differentiates into memory B cells and CD38 positive plasma cells (either short-lived or long-lived). Plasma cells become terminally differentiated and constitutively secrete enormous quantities amounts of antibody. Numerous cytokines are also involved in promoting the development and maturation of B cells to plasma cells (see Figure 7.1).

Alloantibody Injury to Allograft

Direct binding of DSA to the endothelium and subsequent activation combined with complement activation and the recruitment of an inflammatory cells infiltrating the allograft are the key general mechanisms of ABMR. Accumulating evidence also suggests that natural killer (NK) cells play a key role in antibody-mediated allograft injury[2] as increased NK cell transcripts are associated with ABMR. Complement activation and its downstream effects also leads to allograft injury in ABMR. Several clinical studies have shown that C4d staining of the microvasculature (e.g., peritubular and glomerular capillaries) is associated with ABMR, graft dysfunction, and failure (see Figure 7.2).

Histological Features of ABMR with HLA DSA

The Banff classification was devised to standardize kidney allograft pathological findings and definitions. For the histologic diagnosis of active ABMR, three key criteria must be met:

   i. Histologic evidence of tissue injury,
   ii. Evidence of antibody interaction with the endothelium, and
   iii. Serologic evidence of DSA.

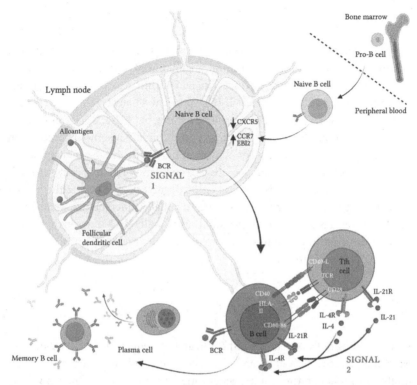

Figure 7.1 Generation of alloantibody. B cells are activated by two signals. The first is the antigen recognition through their B cell receptor (BCR), which triggers the downregulation of CXCR5 and the upregulation of CCR7 and EBI2. The second is a consequence of the interaction between B cells and T follicular helper cells (Tfh), mediated by costimulatory molecules such as CD28 and CD40L on T cells and CD80/86 and CD40 on B cells, together with the secretion of IL-4 and IL-21 by Tfh. The B cell antigen specific population rapidly proliferates and differentiates into memory B cells and CD38 positive plasma cells.
Figures created by D. Linas & M Crespo. CCR7: C-C motif chemokine receptor 7, CXCR5: C-X-C motif chemokine receptor type 5, IL-4: interleukin 4, IL-21: interleukin 21, IL-4R: interleukin 4 receptor, IL-21R: interleukin 21 receptor, TCR: T cell receptor

Histologic evidence of tissue injury (criteria i) is usually manifested by microvascular inflammation in peritubular and glomerular capillaries (e.g., peritubular capillaritis = Banff "ptc" score and glomerulitis = Banff "g" score). Together these scores must be $\geq$ to 2. Thrombotic microangiopathy or unexplained acute tubular necrosis can also fulfill the criteria for tissue injury. Antibody-mediated injury to the endothelium (criteria ii) can be fulfilled with microvascular inflammation

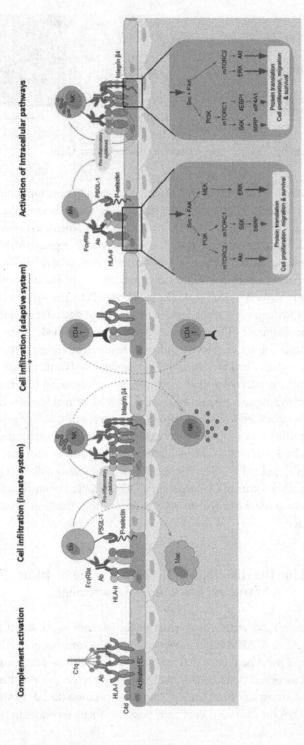

Figure 7.2 Mechanisms of alloantibody injury to the allograft.

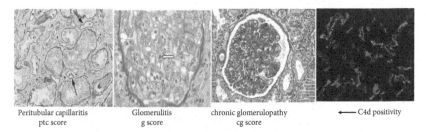

| Peritubular capillaritis | Glomerulitis | chronic glomerulopathy | C4d positivity |
| ptc score | g score | cg score | |

Figure 7.3 Histological features of active and chronic active AMR.

or C4d positivity. Importantly, having microvascular inflammation fulfills both the histologic evidence of tissue injury (criteria i) and antibody interaction with the endothelium (criteria ii). C4d positivity is *not* a requirement to make a diagnosis of ABMR,[3] and patients with both C4d-positive and -negative ABMR have inferior allograft survival compared to patients without ABMR.[4] Additionally, C4d-positive cases can become C4d-negative and can be present later with acute active or chronic active ABMR. Serological evidence of circulating DSA (criteria iii) is necessary to diagnose ABMR derived from HLA antigens (see Figure 7.3).

A histologic diagnosis of chronic active ABMR can be made if the biopsy meets the criteria for active ABMR and with features of allograft chronicity. These chronic features include chronic glomerulopathy (Banff cg score > 0), severe peritubular capillary basement membrane multilayering (requires electronic microscopy), or unexplained new-onset arterial intimal fibrosis. Chronic active ABMR is associated with a poor prognosis. In one study, 60% of grafts with chronic active ABMR on a 1-year biopsy either failed or lost > 50% of their allograft function by 5 years after transplantation.[5] Many patients with chronic active ABMR have minimal or no interstitial fibrosis, suggesting a distinct process separate from other forms of chronic injury. Occasionally, the chronic features are present in the absence of microvascular inflammation. This is termed chronic inactive ABMR.

Taking the Histological Diagnosis to the Bedside: A Framework to Guide Management

The Banff classification system has been a major advance in standardizing the histologic diagnosis of ABMR, but it oversimplifies the complexity in ABMR in practice. First, it must be recognized that ABMR is a chronic progressive disease. The DSA associated with ABMR may have been present prior to transplant or develop post-transplant from underimmunosuppression (i.e., de novo DSA). The source of DSA can also vary. Very early post-transplant increases in DSA can be driven by memory B cell responses, while persistently elevated DSA may be the result of constant secretion of alloantibody by plasma cells. These factors are important to consider for clinical trial design and treatment strategies.

A consensus conference sponsored by the Transplantation Society considered the limitations of using histology alone for the diagnosis of ABMR and a framework of the clinical phenotypes of ABMR was constructed.[6] The purpose of this framework was to aid ABMR clinical trial design and guide patient management.

Clinical phenotypes of ABMR are shown in Table 7.1.

Hyperacute Rejection

Hyperacute rejection occurs minutes to hours post-transplant leading to almost immediate allograft loss. The incidence is related to the level of DSA at the time of transplantation. The exact level of DSA that leads to this complication is unknown, but patients who go to transplant with a positive complement-dependent cytotoxicity (CDC) crossmatch are at substantial risk (20%–50%) for this event. For this reason, kidney transplant should not be performed if the CDC crossmatch is positive.

Early Acute Active ABMR (<30 Days Post-Transplant)

Even if hyperacute rejection is avoided, patients with DSA at transplant still have a high incidence of early acute active ABMR within the first 2 weeks after transplantation, typically during a memory B cell response. The incidence of early ABMR depends on the level of DSA at baseline but may be as high as 40%–50% in the context of positive crossmatch transplantation with desensitization.[7,8] Uncommonly, early active ABMR occurs among patients with a prior sensitizing history (blood transfusions, pregnancy, and prior transplant). In these cases, DSA was not apparent pretransplant, but rapidly increases in the first 2 weeks post-transplant.

From a histologic perspective, patients with early acute active ABMR (< 30 days post-transplant) meet the criteria for ABMR based on the Banff criteria.[9] However, evidence of C4d deposition in the peritubular capillaries is almost universally present and the degree of microvascular inflammation (peritubular and/ or glomerular capillaritis) varies. Depending on the severity of the rejection, thrombotic microangiopathy and evidence of acute tubular injury may also be present.[3]

Because of the high incidence of early acute active ABMR among patients with preformed DSA, we recommend close monitoring of DSA for the first

Table 7.1 Clinical Phenotypes of Antibody-Mediated Rejection

Timing	Donor-specific antibody	Histology	Clinical presentation	Standard of care	Consider adjunctive therapies
Hyperacute rejection (hours post-transplant)	Preexisting	Diffuse inflammation, necrosis, and thrombotic microangiopathy	Abrupt graft loss	Graft cannot usually be salvaged.	NA
Early active (< 30 days post-transplant)	Preexisting or patient is nonimmunologically naive with history of sensitizing events (pregnancy, transplant, or blood transfusions)	Banff active ABMR C4d positivity and thrombotic microangiopathy usually present. Banff cg = 0.	Abrupt allograft dysfunction correlating with increased DSA quantity usually 7–10 days post-transplant.	Plasmapheresis (daily or alternate day x 6 based on DSA titer) (1C) IVIG 100 mg/kg after each plasmapheresis treatment or 2 g/kg at the end of plasmapheresis treatments (1C) Corticosteroids (EO)	Complement inhibitors (2B) Rituximab 375 mg/m² (2B) Splenectomy (3C)
Late (> 30 days post-transplant)	Preexisting	Banff active or Chronic active ABMR (continuum) +/- C4d positivity	+/- allograft dysfunction and proteinuria	Plasmapheresis (daily or alternate day x 6 based on DSA titer) (1C) IVIG 100 mg/kg after each plasmapheresis treatment or 2 g/kg at the end of plasmapheresis treatments (1C) Corticosteroids (EO)	Rituximab 375 mg/m² (2B)
	De novo (MOST COMMON)	Banff active or Chronic active ABMR (continuum) +/- C4d positivity. Concomitant TCMR often present with de novo DSA.	+/- allograft dysfunction and proteinuria	Optimize baseline immunosuppression. Treatment of concomitant T-cell-mediated rejection (corticosteroids or depleting antibody) Evaluate and management nonadherence	IVIG (3C)

Source: Adapted from Table 2 Schinstock et al. Recommended Treatment for Antibody-mediated Rejection after kidney transplantation: The 2019 Expert Consensus from the Transplantation Society Working Group. *Transplantation* 2020;104(5):911–922.[6]

2 weeks in this group (i.e., postoperative days 7, 10, and 14) and as needed if there is allograft dysfunction. Increases in DSA during this time warrants consideration for urgent kidney biopsy and probable treatment.

With aggressive treatment, early acute ABMR can be managed. In some cases, the ABMR can completely resolve with concomitant reduction or even resolution of circulating DSA. In other cases, DSA can persist chronically, leading to chronic active ABMR, as discussed in the next section.

Treatment of early acute ABMR generally consists of a course of plasmapheresis and intravenous immunoglobulin (IVIG) to remove DSA that has rapidly increased resulting from the amnestic response. Recommendations from the expert consensus conference suggest that the plasmapheresis and IVIG treatment course be limited to a maximum of six sessions given the potential for complications and lack of benefit from an extended course. Adjunctive therapies such as eculizumab and rituximab can also be used if available, but the evidence supporting these adjunctive therapies is mainly based on small single-center studies.[10]

Late ABMR: Active and Chronic Active ABMR

Advances in DSA detection techniques have made it easier to avoid pretransplant DSA. Thus, the risk and incidence of early active ABMR within the first 30 days post-transplant is now very low unless transplant is performed with known DSA. Most cases of ABMR in current practice are now detected *late* (>30 days post-transplant) and are associated with inferior allograft survival.[11,12] These cases can occur when DSA was present at the time of transplant or if de novo DSA forms after transplant.

Late ABMR in a patient with known *pretransplant DSA* can represent ongoing inflammation/injury after an early acute ABMR episode or can appear later. The onset can be insidious, subclinical, and unrecognized without histologic surveillance. Therefore, the histologic features found on the biopsy may be more reflective of the timing of the biopsy rather than the mechanisms of disease. For example, if the biopsy is done very early in the course of disease, chronic histologic features of ABMR (cg score >0 or transplant glomerulopathy) may not have had time to develop.

Late ABMR now usually develops in the context of de novo DSA from underimmunosuppression.[13] This underimmunosuppression could result from administration of lower doses of immunosuppressive medications mandated by a physician due to concurrent complications (infection or tumors) or due to medication nonadherence. Because these rejections are associated with underimmunosuppression, they are often "mixed" and include histologic features of T-cell-mediated rejection (TCMR). Unfortunately, concomitant features of TCMR are associated with an inferior prognosis.[14] Like late ABMR associated with preexisting DSA, whether the histology is active or chronic active ABMR depends on the timing of the diagnosis and biopsy. A histologic diagnosis of chronic active ABMR also does not account for the spectrum of activity and chronicity. Cases of chronic active ABMR cases include those with moderate to severe microvascular inflammation with mild chronicity or cases with mild microvascular inflammation with severe chronicity.

Unfortunately, ABMR that is detected beyond the first month post-transplant is more difficult to treat. The data supporting plasmapheresis, IVIG, or rituximab is mixed and largely based on evidence from nonrandomized observational trials in heterogeneous populations. Expert opinion suggests considering a limited trial of plasmapheresis, IVIG, or rituximab for patients who do NOT have moderate to severe chronic features of ABMR on their biopsy and had evidence of DSA prior to transplant. Complement inhibitors are not currently recommended for ABMR that is found > 30 days post-transplant, based on a small single-center study that showed that eculizumab does not prevent chronic active ABMR or improve long-term allograft survival among patients who received a positive crossmatch kidney transplant.[15]

Most ABMR that is currently encountered in practice today is the result of de novo DSA. Expert consensus suggests that the approach to treatment should be management of any TCMR if present and optimizing the maintenance immunosuppression. In general, aggressive treatments with plasmapheresis, and so forth, are NOT recommended in the context of de novo DSA because they do not target the source of the antibody.

Clinical trials to date in ABMR have been limited by small sample sizes and heterogeneous patient populations.[16] With improved understanding of ABMR and multiple novel therapeutics on the horizon (IgG endopeptidases, anti-CD38, anti-IL-6, neonatal Fc Receptor (FcRn) antagonists, etc.), we are hopeful that that the landscape for ABMR treatment will change. It is increasingly recognized that ABMR is largely a chronic disease that will likely require long-term treatment with combination therapy.

Adjuvant Tests for ABMR Diagnosis

While histology remains the gold standard for ABMR diagnosis in the current era, new tools are available for ABMR diagnosis. Gene expression studies have shown that ABMR is associated with increased NK cell and endothelial cell transcripts,[2] therefore increased expression of validated gene transcripts in the biopsy tissue indicative of ABMR can be used to indicate antibody injury to the endothelium (criteria ii) even if microvascular inflammation or C4d is absent. This is uncommonly done in clinical practice, however.[17] Routinely incorporating gene expression to clinical care is complicated by the fact that discrepancies between the gene expression studies and histology can occur in up to 40% of cases,[18] gene expression tests are costly, and some require testing fresh kidney allograft biopsy tissue. Advances in technology are leading to broader implementation and use of formalin-fixed, paraffin-embedded samples for reduced cost.[19]

Noninvasive peripheral blood testing for rejection with donor-derived cell free DNA is also being utilized for screening purposes.[20] If the donor-derived cell free DNA percentage increases beyond a prespecified threshold, rejection (ABMR or TCMR) remains a possibility. However, kidney biopsy is recommended for confirmation. Immunosuppression should not be altered based on abnormal donor-derived cell free DNA alone. Currently, noninvasive tests are not part of the Banff ABMR classification system.

ABMR without Detectable HLA Antibody

It remains unclear how to best classify patients who have histologic features suggestive of ABMR without detectable circulating HLA antibody. Patients in this category have been reclassified with the various Banff classification systems.[21] Studies have suggested that microvascular inflammation independent of DSA status is relevant,[22] and reports of aggressive features of ABMR have been identified even after transplantation from an HLA-identical donor.[23] Historically, these studies were difficult to interpret because of the insensitivity of HLA DSA testing, but HLA DSA testing methods have improved substantially, and unexplained microvascular inflammation is increasingly recognized.[24] Among a cohort of 935 kidney transplant recipients who received surveillance biopsy, 9% had histologic features of ABMR without detectable DSA, and 13% had ABMR with detectable DSA. In this study, patients with histologic features of ABMR without DSA had superior allograft survival compared to those individuals with ABMR associated with detectable DSA.[25] In contrast, a multicenter study of allograft biopsies obtained mainly for indication purposes showed similar allograft survival whether DSA was present or undetectable if histologic features of ABMR were present. The study found similar transcript expression among DSA negative and DSA positive cases.[26] The proposed mechanisms of ABMR without detectable DSA include:

   i) Non-HLA-antibody-mediated injury,[27]
   ii) Intragraft antibody adsorption,

iii) Antibodies against self-epitopes, and

iv) Missing self- and NK-cell-driven allorecognition.[28]

The main non-HLA antibodies investigated include anti-major-histocompatibility complex class I–related chain A, anti-Laminin G, anticollagen, antiendothelin-1 type A receptor, and antibodies toward the angiotensin 2 receptor (anti-AT1R).[29] Unfortunately, most studies in this area have major limitations including the lack of consistency in testing methods, and concurrent comprehensive testing for HLA DSA has not always been reported.[30] For these reasons, routine testing for non-HLA with broad panels is not currently recommended and the limitations of the testing methods must be considered when interpreting the results.[30]

Prevention of Rejection

Given the adverse outcomes associated with rejection even when treated, it is important to avoid rejection if possible. The growth of kidney paired donation programs and sensitive DSA testing have made it possible to avoid DSA pretransplant in most circumstances, but the development of de novo DSA remains a problem. Studies have repeatedly shown the importance of maintaining therapeutic drug levels[31] and medication adherence[32,33] to prevent both TCMR and de novo DSA. Improved HLA matching of donor–recipient pairs has also been increasingly recognized to prevent both TCMR and ABMR.

HLA matching has been traditionally done at the whole antigen level considering only HLA A, B, and DR antigens because of the strong DR-DQ linkage disequilibrium. However, recent studies have shown that up to 15% of patients completely matched at DR have 1 or 2 DQ mismatches.[34] This is important because DQ mismatches have been repeatedly shown to be associated with de novo DQ DSA and ABMR.[35] Recent studies have shown that the number of DR/DQ eplet-mismatches also has prognostic significance,[36] but the optimal way to incorporate eplet matching (matching at amino-acid level) into clinical practice remains to be determined. Stratifying patients into low-, intermediate-, and high-risk groups based on the eplet load alone may be overly simplistic due to the linear association between eplet load and de novo DSA[36] and the fact that certain eplet mismatches and epitopes may be more immunogenic.[37] While it remains unclear how to integrate HLA matching in practice and allocation, data strongly supports HLA matching (especially Class-2) if possible to avoid de novo DSA, rejection, and premature allograft failure at least in younger recipients who may be become a candidate for retransplantation in future.

Conclusion

ABMR remains an important cause of late allograft dysfunction leading to failure, and it results from preexisting or de novo DSA. Microvascular inflammation with peritubular and glomerular capillaritis are the main histologic features of active ABMR with or without evidence of complement activation with C4d positivity. It is often a chronic progressive disease with the eventual development of chronic glomerulopathy with ongoing inflammation leading to chronicity. Management of ABMR can be challenging given the paucity of randomized controlled clinical trials and heterogeneous patient populations. Combining the histologic features of ABMR with the timing of ABMR and DSA information can be used to inform treatment decisions. Given the current lack of effective treatment options, it is best to avoid ABMR with appropriate support and means to prevent medication nonadherence and a focus toward better HLA-matching strategies. In the future there is a need for clinical trials of novel agents, an improved understanding of the pathophysiology and significance of histologic features of ABMR without DSA, and how to better allocate kidneys considering the importance of HLA matching at least for younger recipients.

References

1. Merzkani MA, Bentall AJ, Smith BH, et al. Death with function and graft failure after kidney transplantation: risk factors at baseline suggest new approaches to management. *Transplant Direct.* 2022;8(2):e1273.
2. Hidalgo LG, Sis B, Sellares J, et al. NK cell transcripts and NK cells in kidney biopsies from patients with donor-specific antibodies: evidence for NK cell involvement in antibody-mediated rejection. *Am J Transplant.* 2010;10(8):1812–1822.
3. Haas M, Sis B, Racusen LC, et al. Banff 2013 meeting report: inclusion of C4d-negative antibody-mediated rejection and antibody-associated arterial lesions. *Am J Transplant.* 2014;14(2):272–283.
4. Orandi BJ, Alachkar N, Kraus ES, et al. Presentation and outcomes of C4d-negative antibody-mediated rejection after kidney transplantation. *Am J Transplant.* 2016;16(1):213–220.
5. Cosio FG, Grande JP, Wadei H, Larson TS, Griffin MD, Stegall MD. Predicting subsequent decline in kidney allograft function from early surveillance biopsies. *Am J Transplant.* 2005;5(10):2464–2472.
6. Schinstock CA, Mannon RB, Budde K, et al. Recommended treatment for antibody-mediated rejection after kidney transplantation: the 2019 expert consensus from the Transplantation Society Working Group. *Transplantation.* 2020;104(5):911–922.
7. Vo AA, Peng A, Toyoda M, et al. Use of intravenous immune globulin and rituximab for desensitization of highly HLA-sensitized patients awaiting kidney transplantation. *Transplantation.* 2010;89(9):1095–1102.

8. Stegall MD, Diwan T, Raghavaiah S, et al. Terminal complement inhibition decreases antibody-mediated rejection in sensitized renal transplant recipients. *Am J Transplant*. 2011;11(11):2405–2413.
9. Loupy A, Haas M, Roufosse C, et al. The Banff 2019 kidney meeting report (I): updates on and clarification of criteria for T cell- and antibody-mediated rejection. *Am J Transplant*. 2020;20(9):2318–2331.
10. Tan EK, Bentall A, Dean PG, Shaheen MF, Stegall MD, Schinstock CA. Use of eculizumab for active antibody-mediated rejection that occurs early post-kidney transplantation: a consecutive series of 15 cases. *Transplantation*. 2019;103(11):2397–2404.
11. Loupy A, Suberbielle-Boissel C, Hill GS, et al. Outcome of subclinical antibody-mediated rejection in kidney transplant recipients with preformed donor-specific antibodies. *Am J Transplant*. 2009;9(11):2561–2570.
12. Bentall A, Cornell LD, Gloor JM, et al. Five-year outcomes in living donor kidney transplants with a positive crossmatch. *Am J Transplant*. 2013;13(1):76–85.
13. Schinstock CA, Cosio F, Cheungpasitporn W, et al. The value of protocol biopsies to identify patients with de novo donor-specific antibody at high risk for allograft loss. *Am J Transplant*. 2017;17(6):1574–1584.
14. Wiebe C, Gibson IW, Blydt-Hansen TD, et al. Rates and determinants of progression to graft failure in kidney allograft recipients with de novo donor-specific antibody. *Am J Transplant*. 2015;15(11):2921–2930.
15. Schinstock CA, Bentall AJ, Smith BH, et al. Long-term outcomes of eculizumab-treated positive crossmatch recipients: allograft survival, histologic findings, and natural history of the donor-specific antibodies. *Am J Transplant*. 2019;19(6):1671–1683.
16. Wan SS, Ying TD, Wyburn K, Roberts DM, Wyld M, Chadban SJ. The treatment of antibody-mediated rejection in kidney transplantation: an updated systematic review and meta-analysis. *Transplantation*. 2018;102(4):557–568.
17. Schinstock CA, Askar M, Bagnasco SM, et al. A 2020 Banff Antibody-Mediated Injury Working Group examination of international practices for diagnosing antibody-mediated rejection in kidney transplantation—a cohort study. *Transpl Int*. 2021;34(3):488–498.
18. Madill-Thomsen K, Perkowska-Ptasinska A, Bohmig GA, et al. Discrepancy analysis comparing molecular and histology diagnoses in kidney transplant biopsies. *Am J Transplant*. 2020;20(5):1341–1350.
19. Mengel M, Loupy A, Haas M, et al. Banff 2019 Meeting Report: Molecular diagnostics in solid organ transplantation-Consensus for the Banff Human Organ Transplant (B-HOT) gene panel and open source multicenter validation. *Am J Transplant*. 2020;20(9):2305–2317.
20. Jordan SC, Bunnapradist S, Bromberg JS, et al. Donor-derived cell-free DNA identifies antibody-mediated rejection in donor specific antibody positive kidney transplant recipients. *Transplant Direct*. 2018;4(9):e379.
21. Callemeyn J, Ameye H, Lerut E, et al. Revisiting the changes in the Banff classification for antibody-mediated rejection after kidney transplantation. *Am J Transplant*. 2021;21(7):2413–2423.
22. Gupta A, Broin PO, Bao Y, et al. Clinical and molecular significance of microvascular inflammation in transplant kidney biopsies. *Kidney Int*. 2016;89(1):217–225.
23. Grafft CA, Cornell LD, Gloor JM, et al. Antibody-mediated rejection following transplantation from an HLA-identical sibling. *Nephrol Dial Transplant*. 2010;25(1):307–310.

24. Parajuli S, Redfield RR, Garg N, et al. Clinical significance of microvascular inflammation in the absence of anti-HLA DSA in kidney transplantation. *Transplantation*. 2019;103(7):1468–1476.

25. Senev A, Coemans M, Lerut E, et al. Histological picture of antibody-mediated rejection without donor-specific anti-HLA antibodies: clinical presentation and implications for outcome. *Am J Transplant*. 2019;19(3):763–780.

26. Halloran PF, Madill-Thomsen KS, Pon S, et al. Molecular diagnosis of ABMR with or without donor-specific antibody in kidney transplant biopsies: differences in timing and intensity but similar mechanisms and outcomes. *Am J Transplant*. 2022;22(8):1976–1991.

27. Lefaucheur C, Louis K, Philippe A, Loupy A, Coates PT. The emerging field of non-human leukocyte antigen antibodies in transplant medicine and beyond. *Kidney Int*. October 2021;(4):787–798.

28. Callemeyn J, Senev A, Coemans M, et al. Missing self-induced microvascular rejection of kidney allografts: a population-based study. *J Am Soc Nephrol*. 2021;32(8):2070–2082.

29. Lefaucheur C, Viglietti D, Bouatou Y, et al. Non-HLA agonistic anti-angiotensin II type 1 receptor antibodies induce a distinctive phenotype of antibody-mediated rejection in kidney transplant recipients. *Kidney Int*. 2019;96(1):189–201.

30. Tambur A, Bestard, Campbell P, et al. Sensitization in transplantation: Assessment of Risk 2022 Working Group meeting report. *Am J Transplant*. 2023;23(1):133–149.

31. Davis S, Gralla J, Klem P, Stites E, Wiseman A, Cooper JE. Tacrolimus intrapatient variability, time in therapeutic range, and risk of de novo donor-specific antibodies. *Transplantation*. 2020;104(4):881–887.

32. Schinstock CA, Dadhania DM, Everly MJ, et al. Factors at de novo donor-specific antibody initial detection associated with allograft loss: a multicenter study. *Transpl Int*. 2019;32(5):502–515.

33. Nevins TE, Nickerson PW, Dew MA. Understanding medication nonadherence after kidney transplant. *J Am Soc Nephrol*. 2017;28(8):2290–2301.

34. Lim WH, Chapman JR, Coates PT, et al. HLA-DQ mismatches and rejection in kidney transplant recipients. *Clin J Am Soc Nephrol*. 2016;11(5):875–883.

35. DeVos JM, Gaber AO, Knight RJ, et al. Donor-specific HLA-DQ antibodies may contribute to poor graft outcome after renal transplantation. *Kidney Int*. 2012;82(5):598–604.

36. Senev A, Coemans M, Lerut E, et al. Eplet mismatch load and de novo occurrence of donor-specific anti-HLA antibodies, rejection, and graft failure after kidney transplantation: an observational cohort study. *J Am Soc Nephrol*. 2020;31(9):2193–2204.

37. Kramer C, Heidt S, Claas FHJ. Towards the identification of the relative immunogenicity of individual HLA antibody epitopes. *Hum Immunol*. 2019;80(4):218–220.

8

Cardiovascular Disease and Metabolic Complications after Kidney Transplantation

Chien-Jung Lin, Krista L. Lentine, and Adnan Sharif

Cardiac Disease—a dominant clinical event impacting kidney transplant recipients!

Introduction

Cardiovascular disease (CVD) remains the leading cause of death for people with chronic kidney disease with or without kidney transplant and accounts for 30% of post-transplant hospitalizations and one-third of deaths in kidney transplant recipients.[1-3] Among all renal replacement therapy options, kidney transplantation is the best option to reduce long-term cardiovascular risk in comparison to remaining on dialysis. For example, using registry data from the United States, Meier-Kriesche and colleagues demonstrated successful kidney transplantation halts progression of CVD risk in kidney transplant recipients compared to patients wait-listed but remaining on dialysis, albeit with an early 3-month period of heightened cardiovascular risk immediately postoperatively.[4] However, death with a functioning graft is the leading cause of late allograft loss and CVD remains one of the leading causes of death post-transplantation.[5] This may relate to progression of pretransplantation CVD or development of de novo disease post-transplantation, influenced by the milieu of immunosuppression contributing to cardiometabolic risk burden. To improve long-term outcomes further after kidney transplantation, reducing the morbidity and/or mortality associated with CVD is a priority for transplant professionals. In this chapter, we review the range of metabolic complications and CVD observed for kidney transplant candidates and recipients.

Incidence, Prevalence, and Risk Factors for CVD in Kidney Transplant Patients

In the latest 2020 report from the United States Renal Data System (USRDS), CVD of any type was present in 75.8% of patients receiving hemodialysis, 65.4% of patients receiving peritoneal dialysis, and 52.0% of patients with a kidney transplant.[6] Older kidney failure patients were more likely to have CVD than younger ones, regardless of kidney replacement therapy modality, while patterns by sex and race/ethnicity were more heterogeneous. While transplantation reduces CVD burden compared to dialysis, the incidence of CVD post-transplantation is still increased comparable to the general population.[7]

Both traditional and nontraditional cardiovascular risk factors contribute to CVD risk in this population (Figure 8.1). Kidney transplant patients have high prevalence of traditional CVD risk factors including hypertension,[8] preexisting or post-transplantation diabetes,[9] dyslipidemia,[10] and smoking.[11] Some of these metabolic risk factors are preexisting or develop de novo secondary to the adverse metabolic effects of immunosuppression. Other nontraditional CVD risk factors for kidney transplant patients include post-transplant anemia, hyperhomocysteinemia, chronic inflammation, proteinuria, and suboptimal allograft function.[7]

Impact of CVD on Transplant Outcomes

Cardiovascular disease is associated with risk for major adverse cardiovascular events (MACE). In a UK study of a large kidney transplant cohort (N = 30,325), MACE occurred in 2.6% (n = 781) of all kidney transplant recipients within the 1st year post-transplant.[12] Of these 781 events, 201 occurred during the index admission for kidney transplantation surgery (25.7% of all 1st-year MACE and 0.7% of all kidney transplant procedures). In an adjusted Cox proportional hazard model, nonfatal MACE within the 1st year post-transplant was associated with significant long-term mortality risk (hazard ratio [HR] 2.59; 95% confidence interval [CI] 2.34–2.88).[12] The multicenter SCORe study prospectively collected data on MACE rates after kidney transplantation between 2003 and 2008 in Ontario, Canada.[13] After a mean follow-up of 4.5 years with 1,301 kidney transplant recipients, 7% of individuals experienced MACE episodes.[13] Current estimates from North America tend to report higher incidence of MACE, ranging from 3.0% to 8.7% within the 1st year after kidney transplant surgery.[14,15]

While the full spectrum of CVD post-transplantation is broad and encompasses many diseases (e.g., coronary artery disease [CAD], heart failure, valvopathy, cerebrovascular disease, pulmonary hypertension, and cardiac

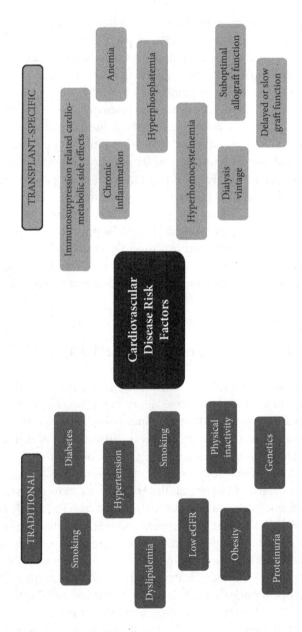

Figure 8.1 Traditional and transplant-specific CVD risk factors.

arrhythmias), the focus for the rest of this chapter will be on CAD. Atherosclerotic CAD comprises clinical entities that include asymptomatic subclinical atherosclerosis and its clinical complications such as angina pectoris, myocardial infarction (MI), and sudden cardiac death. With regard to MIs, cumulative incidence ranges from 9% to 17% by 3 years after transplant listing, and from 5% to 11% after kidney transplantation, with post-transplant MI strongly associated with risk for death-censored graft failure and death.[16] Therefore, strategies to reduce CAD morbidity and mortality after kidney transplantation is an important part of improving long-term outcomes.

Role of Screening for CAD after Kidney Transplant

Routine clinical care of kidney transplant recipients should include surveillance of cardiometabolic risk factors and timely intervention to modify risk. Various CVD risk calculators are utilized among the general population, but few have been robustly validated for use in kidney transplant patients. Heleniak et al. retrospectively analyzed various CVD risk prediction scores in kidney transplant patients and found QRISK2 and Pol-SCORE scales to be more predictive in assessing CVD risk compared to PROCAM and Framingham.[17] Using data from the Assessment of Lescol in Renal Transplantation (ALERT) trial cohort, a formula for 7-year CAD risk calculation among prevalent kidney transplant patients was developed that demonstrates areas under the receiver operating characteristic curve of 0.74 in both assessment and test samples.[18] However, this has not been validated in any external kidney transplant cohorts and at present the best screening for CAD among kidney transplant recipients is through monitoring of traditional and nontraditional risk factors.

Prevention of CAD in Kidney Transplant Recipients

Measures to prevent CVD in kidney transplant recipients are shown in Table 8.1.

Lifestyle Measures

Although transplant-specific evidence to support nonpharmacological interventions is limited, encouraging patients to live active, healthy lifestyles after kidney transplantation is recommended to reduce CAD risk.[19] While more definitive studies are warranted, there are suggestions of positive impact on post-transplant cardiometabolic parameters with lifestyle intervention. For example,

Table 8.1 Prevention and Management of CVD in Kidney Transplant Recipients

	Measures	Key points
Prevention of CAD in kidney transplant recipients		
Lifestyle modifications	Diet and exercise, achieve/maintain acceptable BMI, and abstain from tobacco use	First-line approach
Daily ASA	Questionable benefit in patients without CAD	CVD risk reduction offset by increased bleeding risk
BP management	Goal—130/80 mm/Hg—preferably with calcium blocker or ACEi.	Self-monitoring BP at home Caution: ACEi and ARB can decrease GFR and increase blood serum K level
Diabetes management	Optimal diabetes control with oral medications or insulin—consider using GLP-1 agonist or SGLT-2 inhibitor	Aim for HBA1C around 7.0%
Lipidemia	Statin use to control lipidemia	To decrease CVD risk
Preservation of renal function	Preserving GFR by avoiding acute rejection and CNI nephrotoxicity	
Management of established CAD in kidney transplant recipients		
Lifestyle modifications	Diet and exercise, achieve/maintain acceptable BMI, and abstain from tobacco use. Periodic evaluation by a cardiologist	First line of treatment
Daily ASA	Used to prevent coronary events	CVD risk reduction supersedes bleeding risk
BP management	130/80 mm/Hg—preferably with beta blocker, calcium blocker, ACEi, or ARB.	Cautions: diltiazem, verapamil, and nicardipine can increase CNI level. ACEi and ARB can decrease GFR and increase blood K level
Diabetes management	Optimal diabetes control with oral medications and insulin—consider using GLP-1 agonist or SGLT-2 inhibitor	Aim for HBA1C around 7.0%
Lipidemia	Statin use to control lipidemia followed by ezetimibe as a second agent. Emerging role of PCSK9 inhibitors.	To decrease CVD risk
Cardiac intervention	PCI with drug eluting stent placement; CABG when indicated	Minimize contrast exposure for those with low GFR.

Kuningas et al. conducted a randomized controlled trial among nondiabetic kidney transplant recipients to receive active lifestyle intervention (support from a dietician trained with behavior change methodology) versus standard of care in the CAVIAR (Comparing glycemic benefits of Active Versus passive lifestyle Intervention in kidney Allograft Recipients) study.[20] Short-term intervention of 6 months' duration had impressive benefits including weight loss, fat mass reduction, and reduced risk for new-onset diabetes. However, behavior change intervention must be long-term and a continuous process. Cessation of the 6-month active intervention at CAVIAR study closure subsequently led to regression of any attained benefits, with no difference observed between study participants 3 years after study recruitment.[21] Further work should study long-term benefits of lifestyle intervention, with behavior change methodology firmly embedded. Behavior change approaches after kidney transplantation would also benefit lifestyle measures to attenuate unhealthy practices such as smoking.[22]

Aspirin Prophylaxis

Aspirin is commonly used for primary or secondary prevention of cardiovascular events in the general population. However, the evidence base for use of aspirin as prophylaxis for prevention of CAD in a kidney transplant population is unclear. In a systematic review and meta-analysis of observational cohort studies, the pooled risk ratio of MACE or mortality in kidney transplant recipients who received aspirin was 0.86 (95% CI 0.52–1.43) with significant heterogeneity (I^2 = 64%).[23] However, if the meta-analysis was limited to studies with adjusted analyses to minimize confounding, then the pooled risk ratio of MACE or mortality was 0.72 (95% CI 0.59–0.88) with less heterogeneity (I^2 = 0%).[23] While aspirin prophylaxis may yield additional allograft-specific benefits (e.g., reduced risk of allograft thrombosis or attrition) that indirectly will attenuate CVD risk, data with regard to side effects such as minor or major bleeding are limited.

Blood Pressure Management

Hypertension is the most prevalent CAD risk factor among kidney transplant patients, with reported rates up to 90%.[24] Currently recommended blood pressure targets for kidney transplant patients from both the 2012 Kidney Disease Improving Global Outcomes (KDIGO) Hypertension guidelines and 2017 American College of Cardiology/American Heart Association Hypertension Guidelines is less than 130/80 mmHg.[24] In addition to traditional risk factors (e.g., age, sex, obesity, pretransplant history), transplant-specific risk factors include donor-derived factors (e.g., increased donor age), allograft function, immunosuppression, transplant renal artery stenosis, and the presence of angiotensin II type 1-receptor activating antibodies.

Treatment of post-transplant hypertension should include lifestyle intervention and pharmacological intervention when that alone is insufficient. While achieving the target blood pressure is more important than choice of antihypertensive, some evidence exists for hierarchy of choice. In a systematic review and meta-analysis of 71 randomized controlled trials, Pisano and colleagues compared the efficacy of several antihypertensive agents.[25] Calcium channel blockers reduced the risk of graft loss estimated as Relative Risk (RR 0.58, 95% CI 0.38–0.89) and increased glomerular filtration rate (GFR) when compared with either placebo/no treatment (mean difference 3.08 mL/min, 95% CI 0.38–5.78) or angiotensin-converting enzyme inhibitors (ACEi)/angiotensin receptor blockers (ARB) therapy (mean difference 11.07, 95% CI 6.04–16.09). However, ACEi treatment also reduced the risk of graft loss (RR 0.62, 95% CI 0.40–0.96) but was associated with slightly decreased GFR and increased hyperkalemia risk. In contrast, ARBs did not lower the risk of graft loss, while also increased the risk of hyperkalemia. Most included studies suffer from lack of hard outcomes (e.g., CVD risk reduction, survival), short duration, and lack of contemporary pharmacotherapies. Clinical phenotype, underlying risk factors, and timing post-transplant should dictate choice of antihypertensive agents with the aim to achieve target blood pressure control.

Diabetes Management

Despite diabetes being one of the leading causes of kidney failure, and post-transplantation diabetes being a major complication associated with kidney transplantation, the safety and efficacy of glucose-lowering agents as treatment is unclear according to a Cochrane review of published studies.[26] Evidence from existing studies examining the effect of intensive insulin therapy, dipeptidyl peptidase-4 (DPP-4) inhibitors, sodium glucose cotransporter (SGLT)-2 inhibitors, and glitazones are rated low to very low certainty. There are no studies examining the effects of biguanides, glinides, glucagon-like peptide (GLP)-1 agonists, or sulfonylureas. Overall, most studies have an unclear to high risk of bias.

Any form of diabetes is a CAD risk factor for kidney transplant recipients. Post-transplantation diabetes, which is time-dependent and accrues with time, can contribute to MACE risk that is higher than in nondiabetic recipients,[27] but event rates are lower compared to kidney transplant recipients with pretransplantation diabetes. The impressive cardiorenal benefits observed with new antidiabetic agents like GLP-1 agonists or SGLT-2 inhibitors in the general population have great potential to translate to kidney transplant recipients[28] but long-term efficacy data in a post-transplant setting is lacking.

Dyslipidemia Management

Dyslipidemia is common after kidney transplantation, but the evidence base for lipid-lowering therapy improving CAD outcomes is mixed. In the original ALERT study, there was a significant (35%) reduction in the incidence of MI and cardiac death among fluvastatin-treated patients, although the 13% reduction in the primary efficacy endpoint (occurrence of MACE) did not achieve statistical significance.[29] In a planned extension study where all study participants were offered fluvastatin therapy, significant reductions in MACE (21%) and cardiac death or nonfatal MI (29%) were observed.[30] In a meta-analysis of published studies including chronic kidney disease (CKD), dialysis, and transplant patients, the investigators report strong evidence base for statin use with CKD stages 1–3, weak evidence for statin use in both CKD stage 4 and after kidney transplantation, and no evidence base for statin use in CKD stage 5/dialysis.[31] Therefore, statins are encouraged to reduce CAD risk after kidney transplantation but efficacy may vary by level of kidney allograft function.

Allograft-Specific Risk Prevention Measures

Low eGFR and proteinuria are independent risk factors in the general population.[32] Translating this to kidney transplant patients, optimizing allograft function should reduce long-term CVD risk and strategies to attenuate long-term allograft attrition are discussed in other chapters.

Transplant Patients with Prior CAD

The 2012 American College of Cardiology (ACC)/American Heart Association (AHA) guidelines on stable ischemic heart disease, 2021 guideline for coronary artery revascularization, 2019 European Society of Cardiology (ESC) guidelines, and 2022 AHA guidelines for coronary heart disease for transplant candidates, on chronic coronary syndromes provide a framework on the management of preexisting CAD, although some adjustments specific for the kidney transplant recipient are warranted.[33–36] Management of renal transplant patients with CVD is illustrated in Table 8.1.

Patients with existing CAD should be evaluated at least annually by a cardio-vascular practitioner, including assessment of overall clinical status, medication compliance, and risk profile. Laboratory tests should be performed at least every other year, including lipid profile, renal function, complete blood count, and possibly cardiac biomarkers.[37] A 12-lead ECG should be obtained as needed to define heart rate and heart rhythm, as well as to detect silent ischemia/infarction, given angina is less common and silent ischemia more common in kidney transplant.[38] Echocardiogram assesses ventricular function, chamber dimension, and valvular abnormalities; it may be beneficial to obtain every 3–5 years.[37]

The role of routine CAD surveillance after kidney transplant remains poorly defined. It has been demonstrated that noninvasive stress testing shows reduced accuracy in patients with CKD.[39] A retrospective study suggested nuclear stress test in the post-transplant population predicted risk of cardiovascular hospitalization and death.[40] By contrast, the recent randomized POST-PCI trial cast doubt on the utility of routine surveillance stress testing in patients with high-risk features after PCI. However, this trial included only 5% of patients with CKD and 3% on dialysis.[41] Coronary computed tomography angiography (CTA) should not be used for follow-up of patient with established CAD given the lack of functional information on ischemia and the prevalence of coronary calcium in transplant patients, which diminishes the utility of coronary CTA.

Continued risk factor modification is of utmost importance in managing patients with known CAD. KDIGO guidelines suggest managing cardiovascular disease "at least as intensively in kidney transplant recipients as in the general population." Unfortunately, studies have shown inadequate control of these risk factors in kidney transplant recipients.

Hypertension is prevalent in kidney transplant recipients. The optimal agent or combinations for hypertension in this population have not been defined. ACE inhibitors and ARBs are recommended to reduce ischemic events in patients with CAD and concurrent heart failure, hypertension, or diabetes, comorbidities many kidney transplant recipients have. Widespread use of ACEi or ARB in this population is limited by the inherent hemodynamic effect leading to lowering GFR, although these agents also slow down the progress loss of renal function. Calcium channel blockers (CCBs) such as amlodipine can be used as antianginal and antihypertensive agents. Some evidence suggests nifedipine may be superior to lisinopril in renal function and blood pressure control.[42] Caution is advised with use of this class of agents in transplant recipients, as diltiazem, verapamil, and nicardipine can increase blood levels of calcineurin inhibitors.

Dyslipidemia should be managed according to guidelines. The ALERT trial demonstrated no difference in combined cardiovascular end point but a favorable reduction in the separate outcomes of cardiac death and nonfatal MI with fluvastatin.[29] Subsequent meta-analyses suggested a likely benefit for statin use in reducing the outcome of major vascular event, coronary revascularization or stroke, and mortality. Overall, given the likely benefit and little harm, initiation and continuation of statin therapy in patients with functioning kidney transplants are recommended.[43] The concurrent use of statins and CNIs should be approached with caution given their potential drug–drug interactions.[44] Ezetimibe is a second-line agent when additional lipid control is needed. Emerging evidence suggests PCSK9 inhibitors are a safe and promising approach to dyslipidemia in kidney transplant recipients.

Management of CAD after Transplant

Acute coronary syndrome is not uncommon in kidney transplant recipients. While renal transplant reduces CVD risk for those with CKD, data from USRDS indicated a cumulative MI incidence of 11% at 3 years after transplant, with a mortality of 28% 1 year after the infarction.[16,45] Therefore, acute coronary syndrome remains an important post-transplant comorbidity to improve transplant outcomes.

Timely revascularization and medical therapy are the cornerstone of acute coronary syndrome management, as have been described in American and European guidelines.[34,46–48] While these guidelines were built on an evidence base where kidney transplant recipients were largely excluded or underrepresented in randomized controlled trials, they serve as foundations of management strategies that may be tailored for kidney transplant recipients.

Coronary angiography and percutaneous coronary intervention (PCI) present unique challenges to graft function. The antiplatelet agents used for acute coronary syndrome (ACS), including aspirin, and P2Y12 inhibitors (clopidogrel, ticagrelor, prasugrel) do not require dose adjustment to renal function. Ticagrelor and prasugrel are more potent than clopidogrel and are associated with reduced ischemic events and increased bleeding. The choice of dual antiplatelet therapy (DAPT) and its duration should be tailored to the patient characteristics. Most anticoagulants and glycoprotein 2b3a antagonists used in the cardiac catheterization lab require dose adjustment in CKD, except unfractionated heparin and abciximab.[16]

With regard to procedural considerations, iodinated contrast during angiography may cause contrast-induced nephropathy. Radial artery access is recommended as first-line choice in the guidelines, femoral vascular access ipsilateral to transplant renal artery should be performed with caution. Best practices have been suggested in the cardiac catheterization laboratory to minimize contrast-induced nephropathy in patients with CKD.[34] There is understandable reluctance to coronary angiography and revascularization in this population, despite observational data suggesting revascularization with PCI or CABG poses little risk for graft loss.[37] Studies with real-life registries revealed that renal transplant patients with STEMI are more likely to receive reperfusion therapies compared to CKD patients, but less likely than non-CKD patients. Risk-adjusted in-hospital mortality among the renal transplant group with STEMI was markedly lower compared with the stage 5D CKD group but similar compared with the non-CKD group.[49]

The modality of revascularization should be individualized. Observational data suggested that coronary artery bypass surgery (CABG) and PCI had similar rates of graft failure. CABG was associated with a higher adjusted risk of death within 3 months but lower mortality beyond 6 months.[50] As indicated in cardiology guidelines, a heart team approach should be used to determine the optimal modality and extent of revascularization in an individualized fashion.

Medical therapy is the other pillar in the long-term management of ACS. While ACEi/ARB and mineralocorticoid receptor antagonist use should be cautious in patients with renal dysfunction, beta-blocker and lipid-lowering agent use are generally not limited by renal function. However, use of medical therapy in the real world has been suboptimal. Use of Organ Procurement and Transplantation Network (OPTN) registry and linked pharmacy billing claims data demonstrated the prescription for beta blockers, antiplatelet agents, ACE inhibitors/ARBs, and statins were submitted in only 40%–80% of patients within 60 days after acute MI in kidney transplant recipients.[51] Together, these real-world data indicate opportunities for quality improvement in caring for CAD in kidney transplant recipients.

Pulmonary HTN Secondary to CAD

Pulmonary hypertension (PH) is defined as mean pulmonary artery pressure of >20 mmHg. The World Health Organization (WHO) classification categorizes PH into 5 groups:

1. Group 1: pulmonary arterial hypertension,
2. Group 2: PH due to left heart disease,
3. Group 3: PH due to respiratory system disease,
4. Group 4: PH due to chronic thromboembolism and thromboembolic, and
5. Group 5: PH due to multifactorial causes.

The most common type of PH in CKD patients, Group 2 PH is due to elevated left atrial filling pressure from heart failure with preserved or reduced ejection fraction. PH related to CAD and ischemic cardiomyopathy can cause heart failure with reduced ejection fraction in CKD patients. Conversely, chronic hypertension, diabetes, and uremia, conditions common in CKD patients, can cause diastolic dysfunction, which in turn lead to heart failure with preserved ejection fraction. Contributing causes of PH often coexist in kidney transplant recipients.[52] A study of national sample of Medicare-insured US kidney transplant recipients found that PH is diagnosed in 1 in 10 patients within 3 years after kidney transplant, and is associated with an increased risk of death and graft failure.[53]

While right heart catheterization remains the gold standard, echocardiography is a noninvasive, less expensive, and more widely available test to diagnose PH. Echocardiographic measures of diastolic dysfunction are associated with adverse cardiovascular outcomes in both the pre- and post-transplant periods, despite normal left ventricle (LV) systolic function.[54] Hence, when evaluating the prognostic impact of PH in group 2 patients, consideration must be given to the presence and severity of underlying CAD, LV and right ventricle (RV) systolic function, LV diastolic function, presence and severity of LV hypertrophy, and symptom severity.

Future Directions

The ACC/AHA and ESC guidelines were established on studies in which kidney transplant recipients were underrepresented or excluded. Observational data suggest suboptimal penetration of guideline use in caring for CAD in kidney transplant recipients, an opportunity for quality improvement. Future registry-based or multicenter studies are needed to confirm the adaptability of these guidelines in kidney transplant recipients.

Conclusions

Despite progress made in the past decades, CAD remains a major comorbidity and adverse risk factor for kidney transplant recipients. Guidelines from major cardiovascular societies have established a standard of care in patients with existing CAD and ACS. Although the evidence base is largely from non-kidney-transplant recipients, these guidelines provide a basis to be adapted in this patient population. The management of stable CAD and ACS requires a multidisciplinary approach in consideration of the attributes of kidney transplant recipients. Future research is needed to fill the knowledge gaps in the management of CAD in this unique patient population.

Acknowledgments

We thank Saint Louis University Public Health student Kennan Maher for assistance with manuscript preparation.

References

1. Mathur AK, Chang YH, Steidley DE, et al. Patterns of care and outcomes in cardiovascular disease after kidney transplantation in the United States. *Transplant Direct.* 2017;3:e126.
2. Hart A, Smith JM, Skeans MA, et al. OPTN/SRTR 2017 annual data report: kidney. *Am J Transplant.* 2019;19(Suppl 2):19–123.
3. Jankowski J, Floege J, Fliser D, Bohm M, Marx N. Cardiovascular disease in chronic kidney disease: pathophysiological insights and therapeutic options. *Circulation.* 2021;143:1157–1172.
4. Meier-Kriesche HU, Schold JD, Srinivas TR, Reed A, Kaplan B. Kidney transplantation halts cardiovascular disease progression in patients with end-stage renal disease. *Am J Transplant.* 2004;4:1662–1668.
5. Ojo AO, Hanson JA, Wolfe RA, Leichtman AB, Agodoa LY, Port FK. Long-term survival in renal transplant recipients with graft function. *Kidney Int.* 2000;57:307–313.
6. USRDS. *2022 Annual data report.* https://usrds-adr.niddk.nih.gov/2022. Accessed February 7, 2023.
7. Stoumpos S, Jardine AG, Mark PB. Cardiovascular morbidity and mortality after kidney transplantation. *Transpl Int.* 2015;28:10–21.
8. Tantisattamo E, Molnar MZ, Ho BT, et al. Approach and management of hypertension after kidney transplantation. *Front Med (Lausanne).* 2020;7:229.
9. Sharif A, Cohney S. Post-transplantation diabetes—state of the art. *Lancet Diabetes Endocrinol.* 2016;4:337–349.
10. Badiou S, Cristol JP, Mourad G. Dyslipidemia following kidney transplantation: diagnosis and treatment. *Curr Diab Rep.* 2009;9:305–311.
11. Hurst FP, Altieri M, Patel PP, et al. Effect of smoking on kidney transplant outcomes: analysis of the United States Renal Data System. *Transplantation.* 2011;92:1101–1117.
12. Anderson B, Qasim M, Evison F, et al. A population cohort analysis of English transplant centers indicates major adverse cardiovascular events after kidney transplantation. *Kidney Int.* October 2022;102(4):876–884.
13. Ribic CM, Holland D, Howell J, et al. Study of cardiovascular outcomes in renal transplantation: a prospective, multicenter study to determine the incidence of cardiovascular events in renal transplant recipients in Ontario, Canada. *Can J Kidney Health Dis.* 2017;4:2054358117713729.
14. Kasiske BL, Israni AK, Snyder JJ, Camarena A, Investigators C. Design considerations and feasibility for a clinical trial to examine coronary screening before kidney transplantation (COST). *Am J Kidney Dis.* 2011;57:908–916.
15. Ying T, Gill J, Webster A, et al. Canadian-Australasian randomised trial of screening kidney transplant candidates for coronary artery disease—a trial protocol for the CARSK study. *Am Heart J.* 2019;214:175–183.

16. Lentine KL, Brennan DC, Schnitzler MA. Incidence and predictors of myocardial infarction after kidney transplantation. *J Am Soc Nephrol*. 2005;16:496–506.
17. Heleniak Z, Komorowska-Jagielska K, Debska-Slizien A. Assessment of cardiovascular risk in renal transplant recipients: preliminary results. *Transplant Proc*. 2018;50:1813–1817.
18. Soveri I, Holme I, Holdaas H, Budde K, Jardine AG, Fellstrom B. A cardiovascular risk calculator for renal transplant recipients. *Transplantation*. 2012;94:57–62.
19. Baker LA, March DS, Wilkinson TJ, et al. Clinical practice guideline exercise and lifestyle in chronic kidney disease. *BMC Nephrol*. 2022;23:75.
20. Kuningas K, Driscoll J, Mair R, et al. Comparing glycaemic benefits of active versus passive lifestyle intervention in kidney allograft recipients: a randomized controlled trial. *Transplantation*. 2020;104:1491–1499.
21. Kuningas K, Driscoll J, Mair R, Day E, Sharif A. Short-term healthy lifestyle intervention and long-term behavior change after kidney transplantation: findings from the CAVIAR study. *Am J Kidney Dis*. 2023;81:249–252.
22. Devresse A, Gohy S, Robert A, Kanaan N. How to manage cigarette smoking in kidney transplant candidates and recipients? *Clin Kidney J*. 2021;14:2295–2303.
23. Cheungpasitporn W, Thongprayoon C, Mitema DG, et al. The effect of aspirin on kidney allograft outcomes: a short review to current studies. *J Nephropathol*. 2017;6:110–117.
24. Loutradis C, Sarafidis P, Marinaki S, et al. Role of hypertension in kidney transplant recipients. *J Hum Hypertens*. 2021;35:958–969.
25. Pisano A, Bolignano D, Mallamaci F, et al. Comparative effectiveness of different antihypertensive agents in kidney transplantation: a systematic review and meta-analysis. *Nephrol Dial Transplant*. 2020;35:878–887.
26. Lo C, Toyama T, Oshima M, et al. Glucose-lowering agents for treating pre-existing and new-onset diabetes in kidney transplant recipients. *Cochrane Database Syst Rev*. 2020;8:CD009966.
27. Lim WH, Lok CE, Kim SJ, et al. Impact of pretransplant and new-onset diabetes after transplantation on the risk of major adverse cardiovascular events in kidney transplant recipients: a population-based cohort study. *Transplantation*. 2021;105(11):2470–2481.
28. Yeggalam A, Liebich JA, Yu K, et al. Safety and efficacy of sodium-glucose cotransporter-2 inhibitors in patients with kidney transplantation and diabetes mellitus. *Diabetes Obes Metab*. 2023;25:1777–1780.
29. Holdaas H, Fellstrom B, Jardine AG, et al. Effect of fluvastatin on cardiac outcomes in renal transplant recipients: a multicentre, randomised, placebo-controlled trial. *Lancet*. 2003;361:2024–2031.
30. Holdaas H, Fellstrom B, Cole E, et al. Long-term cardiac outcomes in renal transplant recipients receiving fluvastatin: the ALERT extension study. *Am J Transplant*. 2005;5:2929–2936.
31. Messow CM, Isles C. Meta-analysis of statins in chronic kidney disease: who benefits? *QJM*. 2017;110:493–500.
32. Matsushita K, Coresh J, Sang Y, et al. Estimated glomerular filtration rate and albuminuria for prediction of cardiovascular outcomes: a collaborative meta-analysis of individual participant data. *Lancet Diabetes Endocrinol*. 2015;3:514–525.
33. Fihn SD, Gardin JM, Abrams J, et al. 2012 ACCF/AHA/ACP/AATS/PCNA/SCAI/STS guideline for the diagnosis and management of patients with stable ischemic

heart disease: executive summary: a report of the American College of Cardiology Foundation/American Heart Association task force on practice guidelines, and the American College of Physicians, American Association for Thoracic Surgery, Preventive Cardiovascular Nurses Association, Society for Cardiovascular Angiography and Interventions, and Society of Thoracic Surgeons. *Circulation.* 2012;126:3097–3137.

34. Lawton JS, Tamis-Holland JE, Bangalore S, et al. 2021 ACC/AHA/SCAI guideline for coronary artery revascularization: executive summary: a report of the American College of Cardiology/American Heart Association Joint Committee on Clinical Practice Guidelines. *Circulation.* 2022;145:e4–e17.

35. Knuuti J, Wijns W, Saraste A, et al. 2019 ESC guidelines for the diagnosis and management of chronic coronary syndromes. *Eur Heart J.* 2020;41:407–477.

36. Cheng XS, VanWagner LB, Costa SP, et al. Emerging evidence on coronary heart disease screening in kidney and liver transplantation candidates: a scientific statement from the American Heart Association: endorsed by the American Society of Transplantation. *Circulation.* 2022;146:e299–e324.

37. Ferguson ER, Hudson SL, Diethelm AG, Pacifico AD, Dean LS, Holman WL. Outcome after myocardial revascularization and renal transplantation: a 25-year single-institution experience. *Ann Surg.* 1999;230:232–241.

38. Schmidt A, Stefenelli T, Schuster E, Mayer G. Informational contribution of noninvasive screening tests for coronary artery disease in patients on chronic renal replacement therapy. *Am J Kidney Dis.* 2001;37:56–63.

39. Bangalore S. Stress testing in patients with chronic kidney disease: the need for ancillary markers for effective risk stratification and prognosis. *J Nucl Cardiol.* 2016;23:570–574.

40. Abuzeid W, Iwanochko RM, Wang X, Kim SJ, Husain M, Lee DS. Prognostic impact of SPECT-MPI after renal transplantation. *J Nucl Cardiol.* 2017;24:295–303.

41. Park DW, Kang DY, Ahn JM, et al. Routine functional testing or standard care in high-risk patients after PCI. *N Engl J Med.* 2022;387:905–915.

42. Midtvedt K, Hartmann A, Foss A, et al. Sustained improvement of renal graft function for two years in hypertensive renal transplant recipients treated with nifedipine as compared to lisinopril. *Transplantation.* 2001;72:1787–1792.

43. Cholesterol Treatment Trialists Collaboration, Herrington WG, Emberson J, et al. Impact of renal function on the effects of LDL cholesterol lowering with statin-based regimens: a meta-analysis of individual participant data from 28 randomised trials. *Lancet Diabetes Endocrinol.* 2016;4:829–839.

44. Wiggins BS, Saseen JJ, Pagell RL, et al. Recommendations for management of clinically significant drug-drug interactions with statins and select agents used in patients with cardiovascular disease: a scientific statement from the American Heart Association. *Circulation.* 2016;134:e468–e95.

45. Kasiske BL, Maclean JR, Snyder JJ. Acute myocardial infarction and kidney transplantation. *J Am Soc Nephrol.* 2006;17:900–7.

46. O'Gara PT, Kushner FG, Ascheim DD, et al. 2013 ACCF/AHA guideline for the management of ST-elevation myocardial infarction: a report of the American College of Cardiology Foundation/American Heart Association Task Force on Practice Guidelines. *Circulation.* 2013;127:e362–e425.

47. Amsterdam EA, Wenger NK, Brindis RG, et al. 2014 AHA/ACC Guideline for the management of patients with non-ST-elevation acute coronary syndromes: a report

of the American College of Cardiology/American Heart Association Task Force on Practice Guidelines. *J Am Coll Cardiol.* 2014;64:e139–e228.

48. Collet JP, Thiele H, Barbato E, et al. 2020 ESC guidelines for the management of acute coronary syndromes in patients presenting without persistent ST-segment elevation. *Eur Heart J.* 2021;42:1289–367.

49. Gupta T, Kolte D, Khera S, et al. Management and outcomes of ST-segment elevation myocardial infarction in US renal transplant recipients. *JAMA Cardiol.* 2017;2:250–258.

50. Charytan DM, Li S, Liu J, Qiu Y, Herzog CA. Risks of death and graft failure after surgical versus percutaneous coronary revascularization in renal transplant patients. *J Am Heart Assoc.* 2013;2:e003558.

51. Lentine KL, Villines TC, Xiao H, et al. Cardioprotective medication use after acute myocardial infarction in kidney transplant recipients. *Transplantation.* 2011;91:1120–1126.

52. Lentine KL, Villines TC, Axelrod D, Kaviratne S, Weir MR, Costa SP. Evaluation and management of pulmonary hypertension in kidney transplant candidates and recipients: concepts and controversies. *Transplantation.* 2017;101:166–181.

53. Lentine KL, Lam NN, Caliskan Y, et al. Incidence, clinical correlates, and outcomes of pulmonary hypertension after kidney transplantation: analysis of linked US registry and medicare billing claims. *Transplantation.* 2022;106:666–675.

54. McGregor E, Jardine AG, Murray LS, et al. Pre-operative echocardiographic abnormalities and adverse outcome following renal transplantation. *Nephrol Dial Transplant.* 1998;13:1499–1505.

9

Late Post-Transplant Infections

George T. John and Rajiv Khanna

*Interaction between immunosuppression, immunity
and infections post-transplant!*

Introduction

"Immunosuppression without side-effects—A dream" is an apt statement for the
topic "infection after kidney transplantation." Transplant recipients with kidney
disease, especially those who have diabetes and liver disease, have lower immunity and are at a higher risk for post-transplant infections while receiving maintenance immunosuppression. Cancer, infections, and cardiovascular diseases
are known to negatively impact kidney transplant (KT) outcomes. However,
due to marked improvements in medical management and preventive strategies,
there has been a decline in mortality from infectious complications after transplantation. Infectious complications account for 19% of deaths in KT recipients
(KTRs), with a standardized incidence ratio of 7.8, compared with matched general population in Australia and New Zealand. Risk factors of infections include
T-cell-depleting therapy, deceased donor transplantation, older age, diabetes,
female sex, and marginalized individual. However, death related to infection
accounts to over 50% of deaths among KTRs in the developing world. In this
chapter we discuss various infections with viral, fungal, and mycobacterial
organisms in KTRs. Details of specific infections are illustrated in Table 9.1.

CMV Infection

Cytomegalovirus (CMV) is a DNA virus and is the most common infective
agent seen after transplantation.[1] High-risk CMV mismatch, characterized by
donor CMV IgG+ and recipient CMV IgG- status (D+R-) is the most important risk factor for CMV infection.[2] In addition, use of depleting antibodies
and antimetabolites such as mycophenolate (MMF) and rejection treatment increase the risk of CMV infection. Registry studies have shown inferior patient

Table 9.1 Select Late Post-Transplant Infections with Risk Factors, Key Clinical Features, Treatment Options, and Potential Preventive Strategies

	Risk factors	Clinical features	Diagnosis	Treatment	Prevention
CMV-DNA virus	High-risk recipients (D+R-), depleting antibody, antimetabolites	Viral syndrome, pneumonitis gastritis, enteritis, hepatitis	CMV—NAAT/QPCR testing, BAL or biopsy of affected organ	decrease immunosuppression; IV or oral ganciclovir. Recurrent and resistant infection treated with cidofovir, foscarnet, and or mirabavir	Valganciclovir prophylaxis for 90–200 days, Use of paired exchange KT to avoid high-risk transplants
BKV-DNA virus	Depleting antibody and antimetabolites	None, elevated serum creatinine	Routine screening (blood and urine), Renal biopsy	Decrease immunosuppression—taper and discontinue antimetabolites; IVIG, cidofovir	Early detection through aggressive screening for BKV DNA in blood and urine during first 2 years post-transplant
EBV-DNA virus	High-risk recipients (D+R-), depleting antibody, antimetabolites	Viral syndrome, Lymphadenopathy, organ involvement	EBV—NAAT, biopsy of lymph node or affected organ	Decrease immunosuppression—decrease and discontinue Antimetabolites. Rituximab and RCHOP for PTLD when indicated	Early detection using NAAT testing and use of paired exchange KT to avoid high-risk transplants
Tuberculosis (TB)	Older age, diabetes, Hep C, liver disease depleting antibody	Pulmonary (cough, fever, and hemoptysis) and extra pulmonary (lymph nodes, skin, soft tissue, and CNS)	BAL, lung biopsy, biopsy of lymph node or affected organ	Combination therapy with rifampicin, INH or rifabutin and quinolone	INH prophylaxis?

(continued)

Table 9.1 Continued

	Risk factors	Clinical features	Diagnosis	Treatment	Prevention
Aspergillosis—Filamentous fungus	COPD, diabetes, DGF, acute rejection, CMV infection	Pulmonary symptoms (cough, fever, and shortness of breath) or CNS symptoms	BAL or lung biopsy or biopsy of the affected organ or tissues (CNS)	Voriconazole or liposomal amphotericin B Second-line agents: posaconazole and caspofungin	None
Cryptococcal—fungal	Diabetes, liver disease, and depleting antibody. Exposure to pigeon droppings	Lung and CNS involvement; occasionally joint and soft tissue	BAL, CSF examination or biopsy of the affected organ	Liposomal amphotericin B and flucytosine, followed by fluconazole for 8 weeks and then a maintenance course for 6–12 months	None
Pneumocystis jirovecii Pneumonia (PJP)	Older age, depleting antibody, use of mTORi, prior rejection, CMV infection	Respiratory—fever, cough, and shortness of breath	BAL, lung biopsy	Oral or IV—Trimethoprim-sulfamethoxazole (TMP/SMX). Secondary agents: pentamidine, atovaquone, dapsone with trimethoprim or primaquine	Oral trimethoprim-sulfamethoxazole (TMP/SMX) for 6–12 months. Alternatives are atovaquone, dapsone, or monthly pentamidine inhalation.
Nocardia (gram-positive filamentous rod)	Diabetes, older recipients and use of depleting antibody	Skin, joint and CNS involvement	Aspiration or biopsy of the affected organ	Trimethoprim-sulfamethoxazole (TMP/SMX), 3rd generation cephalosporins, carbapenems and amikacin	Prophylaxis with trimethoprim-sulfamethoxazole (TMP/SMX) used for PJP prevention may benefit nocardia prevention

Organism	Population	Clinical presentation	Diagnosis	Treatment	Prophylaxis
Histoplasmosis (Fungus—*Histoplasma capsulatum*)	Transplant recipients residing around Ohio and Mississippi river valleys	Fever, cough, and shortness of breath	BAL, lung biopsy, urine Histo antigen	Oral itraconazole and IV amphotericin in severe cases	None
Blastomycosis dermatitidis—fungal	Transplant recipients residing in Wisconsin and Minnesota	Fever and cough with pulmonary involvement. Can present with skin and soft tissue lesions	BAL, lung biopsy, or biopsy of the affected organ	Itraconazole or lipid formulation amphotericin followed by itraconazole. Secondary agents—voriconazole, posaconazole or fluconazole	None
Coccidiodomycosis immitis—fungal	Transplant recipients residing in southwestern part of United States and Mexico	Fever and cough with pulmonary involvement. Can present with lymphadenopathy	BAL, lung, or lymph-node biopsy	oral azoles (itraconazole, ketoconazole) or amphotericin	None

and allograft survival among KTRs with high-risk CMV status.[1] CMV infection is seen usually within 1 year post-transplantation. However, late infections, including recurrent and resistant infection are increasingly common and are seen beyond 1 year post-transplantation.[3]

CMV can be transmitted through the transplanted kidney and can replicate after transplantation with immunosuppression. Virus can also remain dormant in the recipient at the time of transplant and can get reactivated post-transplant with immunosuppression. Currently T cell responses, specific B cell responses, and antibody-dependent cellular cytotoxicity are deemed important components of the immune response mediating protection from CMV. Absence of humoral immunity or CMV-specific T cell response at the time of transplantation and inability to mount immune responses to the virus upon exposure, due to concurrent immunosuppression, remains a critical step toward post-transplant CMV infection.[4,5]

A CMV infection can manifest as mild viral syndrome to severe invasive disease including pneumonitis, enteritis, hepatitis, and bone marrow suppression. CMV infection is diagnosed by the presence of CMV viremia using a nucleic acid amplification test (NAAT) or quantitative polymerase chain reaction (Q PCR) testing, or documentation of viral particles and viral cytopathic effect in the affected organ.

A CMV infection can be prevented by administration of valganciclovir prophylaxis for 90 days post-transplant. Prophylaxis for 200 days is recommended for high-risk (D+R-) recipients.[1] The dose of ganciclovir must be adjusted for renal function. Subtherapeutic prophylactic dose is associated with breakthrough infection. CMV infection is frequent after valganciclovir prophylaxis among high-risk patients. Late, recurrent infections and resistant CMV infections can occur in high-risk patients as well among those who were given subtherapeutic doses or long duration of prophylaxis with valganciclovir.

Symptomatic CMV infections and those with significant viremia should be treated with reduction of immunosuppression, usually reduction or discontinuation of antimetabolites such as MMF with concomitant antiviral therapy with valganciclovir or IV ganciclovir for few weeks. Resolution of CMV viremia should be documented before discontinuation of ganciclovir. Administration of ganciclovir is commonly associated with neutropenia. Resistant CMV infections can be confirmed through mutations in UL97 (kinase) and UL54 (DNA polymerase). Based on resistance pattern, alternative antiviral agents such as foscarnet, cidofovir, and maribavir can be administered to treat the infection. Leflunomide is an effective slow-acting drug that inhibits viral capsid assembly.[6] Letermovir is another antiviral agent but is associated with rapid development of resistance. Preliminary studies show promising results with adoptive T cell therapy.

BKV Infection

BK virus is a polyoma virus, and infection was first described in a patient in 1971. It is a common infection manifesting as viruria in approximately 30%, viremia in 10%, and BKV nephritis in less than 3% after kidney transplantation. Infection remains dormant and asymptomatic in renal tubular, ureteric, and bladder epithelial cells. It persists in the kidney, leuckocytes, and brain.[7]

Ischemia-reperfusion injury may influence BK virus replication along with tacrolimus administration via FK-binding protein. An adequate BKV-specific cellular response controls its latency and suppresses BK viremia. BKPyV-specific CD4[+] T cells play a direct role in controlling BKV infection by mediating the expression of proinflammatory cytokines, including interferon γ (IFNγ), tumor necrosis factor (TNF), and lysozyme B.[8] The degree of T cell suppression correlates with replication and BKV-nephropathy (BKVN). BKV-specific immunoglobulin G (IgG) antibodies found in 70%–90% of healthy individuals do not totally prevent BK viral reactivation.[9] However, if recipient antibodies are genotype specific, it could be protective. Immunosuppression plays a major role in the development of BKV infection. T-cell-depleting agents with administration of MMF and tacrolimus along with high dose of steroids are known to increase the chance of BKV replication and infection. However, sirolimus and cyclosporine appear to reduce viral replication.

Asymptomatic BK viruria and viremia can progress to BKVN, which can manifest as renal allograft dysfunction. Ureteral stenosis and hemorrhagic cystitis can occur rarely after KT, however are more commonly seen after hematopoietic stem cell transplantation. In those with unbridled replication, BK viruria precedes viremia by a median of 1 month and viremia precedes BKVN by 2 months. Viremia ($>1 \times 10^4$ copies/mL) has the best sensitivity (100%), specificity (88%–96%), and positive predictive value (50%–82%) of BKVN, which occurs most often within 2 years of transplantation. However, late BKV infection including BKVN can occur and is often associated with poor outcome due to delay in the diagnosis as aggressive surveillance wanes beyond 2 years post-transplantation.

Polymerase chain reaction (PCR) or NAATs are the common diagnostic tools. Higher donor-derived cell-free DNA (dd-cfDNA) levels were associated with higher BK viral loads and BKVN and may serve as a noninvasive prognostic injury marker.[10]

A histopathological diagnosis, BKVN is characterized by the presence of basophilic virus inclusion bodies in the nucleus of epithelial cells, tubulitis with interstitial infiltrates, and SV40/BKV IgG immunostaining or intratubular inclusion bodies indicating virus particles. BKVN in early stages is focal with a false negative rate of up to 30%.[11] Later stages show moderate to severe fibrosis and tubular atrophy. The interstitial inflammation and tubulitis often resemble acute cellular rejection. The Banff working group scoring system based on these characteristics is simple and useful in prognostication.[12]

Reduction of immunosuppression is the mainstay of treatment. The most common approach is to reduce or discontinue antimetabolites first, followed by reduction in tacrolimus dose. Anecdotally, switching from tacrolimus to cyclosporine has been effective. Cidofovir inhibits BK virus DNA polymerase in human proximal tubules and appears to be effective. However, therapeutic dose of cidofovir has been associated with significant nephrotoxicity. A lipid conjugate of cidofovir, brincidofovir has minimal nephrotoxicity, but oral administration has been associated with higher GI toxicity and is not available for clinical use. Leflunomide and its newer formulation FK778 have not been proven to be effective in clinical trials. IV immunoglobulin (IVIG) contains neutralizing antibodies against all BKV genotypes, is well tolerated, and, in retrospective studies, has shown to have some transient efficacy in viral clearance.[13] However, IVIG does not have good intracellular penetration and has a short half-life to have efficacious antiviral effects. Preliminary results with novel monoclonal antibodies against BKV and adoptive T cell therapy appear promising.

EBV Infection

Epstein-Barr virus (EBV), also called human herpes virus 4, has a seroprevalence of 90% in many parts of the world and remains latent after primary infection in B lymphocytes. In renal transplant recipients it can lead to an array of manifestations both with reactivation and with a new, acute infection. Those include asymptomatic states, infectious mononucleosis syndrome and posttransplant lymphoproliferative disorder (PTLD). PTLD usually presents with extra-nodal masses in the gastrointestinal tract (15%–30%), liver and skin (5%–10%), lungs, central nervous system (20%–25%), and in the allograft (20%–25%) with or without type B symptoms of weight loss, night sweats, or fever.[14] Please see Chapter 10 on cancer and transplantation for more details about EBV and PTLD.

Tuberculosis

In areas with low tuberculosis (TB) endemicity, the prevalence among KTs is 0.5%–6.4%, rising to 12%–20% in highly endemic areas.[15] Factors affecting TB incidence after transplant include T-cell-depleting therapies, treatment of graft rejection, renal insufficiency, chronic liver disease, diabetes mellitus, hepatitis C virus infection, and increased recipient age. Most transplant patients present with pulmonary TB (51%), while 16% have extrapulmonary disease and 33% have disseminated TB. Only 64% of recipients with localized disease present with fever. Atypical radiographic presentations are common. In normal hosts, the risk of active TB is ~5% in the first 5–7 years after infection and ~0.1% per year thereafter.

Traditionally, macrophages have been thought to protect the host by producing fully formed granulomas with typical epithelioid macrophages "walling off" replicating mycobacteria using microbicidal activity limiting replication of intracellular and extracellular organisms. Host macrophages both block and facilitate persistent infection; pathogenic mycobacteria accelerate macrophage apoptosis while accelerating accumulation of uninfected macrophages, which provides a "safe harbor" for further replication and spread. In higher species, once bacilli are engulfed by phagocytes, the spread of bacilli occurs unless a specific Th1-type immune response develops, including IFNγ-producing CD4 and CD8 T cells. After renal transplantation most cases occur after 3–4 months and calcineurin phosphatase inhibition with either cyclosporin or tacrolimus advances its manifestation. Allograft loss can occur in about a third of patients from reduction of immunosuppression and rejection, drug interactions, and runaway disease, especially with delayed recognition and multiple comorbidities.

Transplant candidates should be screened for TB before transplantation. There are varying suggestions for testing for latent tuberculosis. Immunocompromised patients at risk for developing tuberculosis are poorly identified by both tuberculin skin test (TST) and Interferon gamma release assay (IGRA), also known as QuantiFERON-TB GOLD (QFT), especially in areas of high endemicity.[16,17] Serial IGRA studies show significant variability, but initial high magnitude response correlated with a consistent positivity.[17] IGRA-based Isoniazid Hydrochloride (INH) treatment with risk stratification by quantitative IGRA results appeared to have preventive benefits in a Korean study of TB in KTRs.[18] However the therapeutic toxicity and uncertainty of progression of latent TB limits this approach. In the United States, tuberculosis is one of the more common donor-derived bacterial infections.[19] Rifampicin-based therapy is effective and recommended post-transplantation but requires intense monitoring as it induces hepatic microsomal degradation of tacrolimus, cyclosporine, sirolimus, everolimus, prednisolone, and mycophenolate. The risk of rejection increases by 10%–20%. It is possible to use rifabutin or avoid the family of rifamycin, substituting with a quinolone. GeneXpert reliably identifies rifampicin and isoniazid resistance.

Aspergillus

Aspergillus is a ubiquitous, filamentous fungus. The spores inhaled into the lungs can cause invasive pulmonary aspergillosis (IPA) in the immunocompromised.

It has a 0.5%–3.5% prevalence in Spain and in India. These patients may present with fever, cough, and chest pain, especially if they are neutropenic. These infections generally occur 6 months after transplantation. Risk factors identified for IPA are chronic obstructive pulmonary disease, acute rejection, and delayed allograft function, and later infections are likely to occur in patients who have had CMV disease, tuberculosis, or de novo malignancy after transplantation.[20] The mortality rates are 30%–60% with a doubling the risk for graft loss. Early IPA and bilateral lung disease and metastatic lesions to critical areas are poor prognostic factors. Sputum yield for aspergillus is poor, while about half of those with bronchoalveolar lavage (BAL) will yield a positive culture which, and CT scan, which can increase the probability of IPA in KTs. A BAL galactomannan index value cutoff of at least 1.0, along with other fungal diagnostics, is recommended.[21] During colonization and recovery BAL aspergillus PCR may be positive but clinical features of infection with a positive test can help in clinical diagnosis. A negative PCR, BAL culture, and galactomannan improves the negative predictive value to 99%.[22]

A delayed diagnosis and treatment can result in higher morbidity and mortality. With emerging global resistance, speciation of clinically relevant isolates and antibiotic susceptibility testing, when possible, are important. Treatment with voriconazole (VCZ) with a loading dose of 6 mg/kg IV twice daily, or 400 mg twice daily orally during 24 h, then on 4 mg/kg IV twice daily intravenously or 200 mg twice daily orally is recommended. In CNS disease it is the preferred agent. However, in cases of relapse, major side effects with VCZ or on encountering aspergillus species with high minimum inhibitory concentrations (MIC) for azoles, liposomal amphotericin B 3–5 mg/kg daily is recommended. Generally, treatment is recommended for 12 weeks until resolution of clinical symptoms and radiological features have stabilized. A combination of these two classes of agents is not recommended unless it is salvage therapy.[23] Alternative agents are posaconazole and caspofungin.[24]

Nocardia

Nocardia is a gram-positive filamentous rod that, with inhalation causes pulmonary disease and dissemination in 0.2%–0.6% after 6 months in KTs. It manifests as central nervous system, joint, and subcutaneous infections mimicking the presentation of other opportunistic pathogens such as fungi. Risk associations include elderly recipients with deceased-donor transplantation, depleting antibody treatment, prior acute rejection, tacrolimus immunosuppression, and CMV viremia.[25] In the tropics, nocardia is a significant coinfection with CMV and tuberculosis and, chronic liver disease is an important risk factor for mortality.[26]

Microscopy of the infected specimen, commonly BAL, may show beaded branching filamentous gram and modified acid-fast stain-positive bacteria that are slow growing in culture. The treatment of choice is high-dose trimetho-prim/sulfamethoxazole (TMP/SMX), often used in various combinations with third-generation cephalosporins, carbapenems and amikacin. Lower dose TMP/SMX for PJP prophylaxis (see below) might in turn reduce the risk of nocardial infections.[27]

Cryptococcal Infection

In KTRs cryptococcosis is the second most common fungal infection with incidence of 0.3% to 5.8%.[28] Cryptococcal infections manifest a year after renal transplantation. Pulmonary infections are thought to derive from reactivation of a quiescent pulmonary focus through inhalation, though primary infection or reinfection have been documented with genotypic trails. Occasional cases of donor kidney transmission with very early presentation occur. Restricted pulmonary infection has a better prognosis, while CNS and disseminated infection has a higher mortality, as does infection with fluconazole-resistant strains of var.*gattii*.

In patients with disseminated disease or moderate to severe respiratory disease, an induction therapy for a minimum of 2 weeks with liposomal amphotericin 3–4 mg/kg/day and flucytosine 100 mg/kg/day, followed by a consolidation phase of fluconazole 6–12 mg/kg/day for 8 weeks and then a maintenance course of 3–6 mg/kg/day for 6–12 months is recommended.

Pneumocystis jirovecii Pneumonia (PJP)

Pneumocystis jirovecii (PJ) is a unicellular fungal organism found worldwide, with a high seroprevalence. The pneumonia is more often a *de novo* infection than with reactivation. The incidence is low (0.3%–2.6%) with prophylaxis but increases after its cessation, the late-onset PJP. The risk factors are age 65 years or older, lymphopenia (<500–1,000/mm^3) for at least 1 month, low gamma globulins, corticosteroid boluses, graft rejection, CMV viremia, and maintenance with sirolimus/everolimus.[29]

Patients present with shortness of breath with hypoxemia with nonproductive cough and high-grade fever. Though the latter two symptoms may be absent, some rapidly progress to respiratory failure. A third of patients may have a high serum lactate dehydrogenase and unexplained hypercalcemia. Confirmation of diagnosis needs visualization of the organism or a PCR of large-subunit ribosomal RNA of PJ in respiratory samples including BAL, lung biopsy, and induced sputum. With a high likelihood of infection, it is a discriminatory test. A negative test for serum beta D-glucan excludes the diagnosis in KTRs.[30] A combination of these tests gives a reliable diagnosis. Radiological features include bilateral pulmonary reticulation on chest X-ray, ground glass opacities, solid nodularity, and multifocal consolidation. Trimethoprim-sulfamethoxazole (TMP/SMX) is the drug of choice for PJ treatment and prophylaxis. Mild disease is treated for 3 weeks with oral TMP/SMX at a dose of two double-strength tablets (TMP 160 mg/SMX 800 mg) every 8 hours, and severe disease is treated intravenously at the same intervals with (TMP 20 mg per kg/SMX 100 mg per kg). Trimethoprim blocks proximal tubular secretion of creatinine, raising the possibility of rejection, but cystatin C, another measure of renal function, remains unchanged. Those intolerant of TMP/SMX can be treated with pentamidine, atovaquone, dapsone with trimethoprim, or primaquine. Pentamidine is used for 21 days. Moderate to severe disease requires oral prednisone 40–60 mg twice daily, started 72 hours prior to commencing treatment, continued for 5–7 days, then tapered over 2 weeks.

Prophylaxis with TMP/SMX is recommended for 6–12 months posttransplantation, and if the patient is intolerant, alternative agents such as atovaquone, dapsone (with normal G6PD enzyme), or monthly pentamidine inhalation are often used.

Late infections in KTRs remain an important point for intervention toward reducing morbidity and mortality, with improving awareness of such complications to patients and primary medical caregivers and early evaluation, diagnoses, and treatment.

Histoplasmosis

Histoplasmosis is an infection with a dimorphic fungus *Histoplasma capsulatum* endemic in Ohio and Mississippi river valleys in the United States.[31] Many kidney donors and recipients in this region have asymptomatic infection, often detected in chest CT scan as a small, healed granuloma. KTRs may develop primary infection, or direct transmission through the transplanted organ and often reactivation with immunosuppression. Respiratory symptoms such as cough, fever, and shortness of breath are the most common presentation. Diagnosis is often confirmed by presence of the organism through BAL, lung biopsy, and other organ biopsy. Histoplasma antigen can be detected in the urine as well. Antifungal treatment with itraconazole is very effective. Duration of the treatment varies, and it depends on severity of illness. Relapses are often seen, and hence long-term secondary prophylaxis is recommended while patient is on immunosuppression, without clear evidence. Itraconazole interacts with calcineurin inhibitors and hence, levels should be monitored carefully. Amphotericin is very effective as well and is not used as a primary agent due to its inherent nephrotoxicity.

Blastomycosis

Blastomycosis dermatitidis is a soil fungus and infection that can be serious in immunosuppressed KTRs.[32] It is largely asymptomatic and pulmonary involvement is common followed by other parts like skin, joint, and soft tissues. This infection is seen in upper midwestern states in the United States—Wisconsin, northern Illinois, and Minnesota. Diagnosis is confirmed by BAL or biopsy of lymph node, lung, soft tissue, or affected organ. Papanicolaou stain can document clusters of yeasts. The organism is 8 um and has a characteristic thick "double-contoured" cell wall differentiating inner and outer edges.[32] Mild disease can be treated with itraconazole, and severe disease should be treated with lipid formulation amphotericin followed by itraconazole. Alternative therapies include voriconazole, posaconazole, or fluconazole. Early detection and prompt treatment can decrease morbidity and mortality.

Coccidioidomycosis

Coccidioidomycosis is caused by *Coccidides immitis*, a fungal infection. It is often seen in desert region of the southwestern United States, Mexico, and central America. Pulmonary presentation is common with occasional isolated lymphadenopathy and rarely with dissemination to multiple organs.[33] Risk factors include diabetes, prior malignancy, HIV infection, collagen disease, and prior infection. Skin test, serological evaluation, and radiological examination are useful. Identification of spherules of *C. immitis* in any tissue is pathognomic of invasive coccidioidomycosis infection. Milder forms of disease can be treated with oral azoles (itraconazole, ketoconazole) and severe forms of disease should be treated with amphotericin. Early identification of the disease remains the key to preventing graft loss and mortality.

Immune Monitoring in Transplantation

Reconstitution of antipathogen immunity following organ transplantation provides long-term protection against recrudescence or primary acute infectious complications. Understanding of precise dynamics of this immune reconstitution can be helpful in clinical management of transplant patients especially in the context of antiviral therapeutic strategies, It is now well established that transplant recipients with robust antipathogen immunity can resist infectious complications, which can help to limit potential toxicities associated with long-term use of antiviral drug therapies. Emergence of novel immune monitoring technologies have allowed rapid assessment of immune reconstitution kinetics in transplant patients. However, clinical application of many of these immune monitoring technologies remains largely limited to advanced centers with dedicated immunodiagnostic capabilities. Traditionally, immunosuppressive drug therapy monitoring is used to assess immunocompetence of transplant patients.[34,35] While this strategy is quite effective in maintaining the graft integrity, there is now increasing realization that this approach does not take into consideration many other clinical variables that may modify the immune response of the patient and alter their susceptibility to specific pathogens. Monitoring of pathogen-specific immunity allows a more rigorous stratification of patients by their risk of developing infectious complications and this strategy is also helpful in regulating immunosuppressive and antiviral therapies.[36,37]

Antiviral prophylaxis has been successfully used as a preventive strategy for viral complications in transplant recipients. More recent clinical guidelines developed by various academic experts recommend routine surveillance of pathogen recrudescence in combination with preemptive antipathogen pharmaceutical intervention for use in preventing clinical disease.[38–40] There is now convincing evidence which clearly demonstrates that an effective immune reconstitution of antipathogen immunity in transplant recipients can spontaneously clear subclinical pathogen recrudescence without requiring pharmaceutical intervention. Studies have shown that impairment of T cell immunity can dramatically increases the risk of viral recrudescence, chronic pathogen persistence leading to end-stage organ disease.[41] This knowledge can be used to monitor transplant recipients and can alter clinical management and treatment options based on each patient's risk factors.

There are two broad approaches for clinical immune monitoring, referred to as global-immunity and pathogen-specific assays. Generally, nonpathogen immune monitoring is based on quantitative assessment of functional profile of immune system with no precise classification to specific antigens. These assays may include measurement of humoral immunity through analysis of serum immunoglobulin levels in peripheral blood or functional assessment of cellular immunity using a nonspecific mitogen stimulation of blood lymphocytes. In contrast, pathogen-specific immune assessment is specifically designed to measure the strength of antipathogen immunity using either whole pathogen, recombinant pathogen protein, or synthetic peptides as stimulants to activate pathogen-specific immune cells. In these assays pathogen-specific immunity is usually assessed by measuring IFN-γ or TNF following stimulation with known antigen(s). These immune monitoring strategies have been used to assess cellular immunity against EBV, BKPyV, and CMV. These studies have also shown that transplant recipients with strong antiviral immunity may be managed without preemptive therapy, or offered a shorter course of antiviral drugs if there is any evidence of viral recrudescence. On the other hand, preemptive antiviral therapy and rigorous virological monitoring may be essential for transplant recipients who fail to show robust antiviral immune reconstitution. As we progress with more reliable platform technologies for immune monitoring, this strategy will also improve the identification of patients who are at high risk of virus-associated complications and are likely to benefit from immune-based interventions such as adoptive T cell therapy rather than antiviral drugs. Summaries of assays used for assessing global and pathogen-specific immunity are outlined in Tables 9.2 and 9.3 respectively.

Adoptive Immunotherapy for Viral Complication in Transplant Recipients

Considering the importance of immune reconstitution in preventing or resolving viral complications in transplant recipients, adoptive immunotherapy based on in vitro expanded antigen-specific T cells has emerged as powerful tool for the treatment of pathogen-associated complications. Clinical management of infectious complications with pharmaceutical interventions used either prophylactically or therapeutically can offer short-term benefit; development of drug resistance, long-term toxicity, immunomodulatory impact, and allograft loss often lead to poor outcome for many patients. While newer drug formulations have recently entered clinical practice, lack of effective immune reconstitution can compromise their long-term benefit and lead to recrudescence of pathogen infection. These late-stage pathogen-associated complications are often difficult to manage with standard-of-care strategies.

Reconstitution of T cell immunity through the administration of antigen-specific T cells was initially pioneered in hematopoietic stem cell transplant

Table 9.2 Global Immunity Assessment for Infections in Transplant Recipients

Assays	Required sample	Assay time	Antigen composition	Functional readout	Cellular phenotype characterization	Target antigen identification	HLA identification	Advantages	Limitations
iATP in CD4+ T cells (ImmuKnow assay)	Whole Blood	18–24 h	N/A	Yes	No	No	No	FDA-approved commercial assay	Relatively high cost. Potentially biased by sample storage time
Peripheral blood lymphocyte subpopulations	PBMC	18–24 h	N/A	Yes	No	No	No	Commercially available. Can use Frozen PBMCs	Lack of technical standardization. No defined cutoff values.
Serum immunoglobulins	serum	6–8 h	N/A	No	No	No	No	Economical and easy to perform.	Lack of technical standardization
Serum complement factors (C3, C4, MBL)	serum	1–2 h	N/A	No	No	No	Yes	Economical and easy to perform.	Lack of technical standardization.
QuantiFERON Monitor	Whole blood	18–24 h	R848 and CD3 antibody	Yes	No	No	No	Economical and easy to perform.	Lack of technical standardization.

Table 9.3 Pathogen-Specific Immune Monitoring Assays for T-Cell-Mediated Immune Response in Transplant Recipients

Assays	Required sample	Assay time	Target antigen composition	Functional readout	Cellular phenotype characterization	Target antigen identification	HLA identification	Advantages	Limitations
QuantiFERON	Whole Blood	18–24 h	Defined T cell epitopes	Yes	No	No	No	Simple to perform and highly standardized. CE-approved commercial assay	Need whole blood and must be run with few hours of blood collection
ELISPOT	PBMC	18–24 h	Synthetic peptides or recombinant antigens	Yes	No	No	No	Commercially available. Can use Frozen PBMCs	Lack of technical standardization. No defined cutoff values.
Intracellular cytokine secretion	PBMC	6–8 h	Synthetic peptides	Yes	Yes	No	No	Commercially available. Can use Frozen PBMCs	Labor intensive. Lack of technical standardization.
MHC-peptide	PBMC	1–2 h	Individual peptides	No	Yes	Yes	Yes	Commercially available. Can use Frozen PBMCs	Labor intensive. Lack of technical standardization.

(HSCT) recipients and has been successfully used to treat multiple infectious complications including viral and fungal infections. In this case HSCT donor-derived peripheral blood mononuclear cells are used as source for in vitro expansion of antigen-specific T cells. Extension of this strategy to the organ transplant setting requires expansion of T cells of highly immunosuppressed transplant recipients, who generally show severe lymphopenia. Furthermore, manufacturing of autologous T cells from solid organ transplant recipients also raises the risk of expansion of alloreactive T cells, which may impact on the engrafted organ following adoptive immunotherapy. A modified T cell expansion protocol to overcome this limitation successfully used autologous EBV-specific T cells to treat EBV-associated PTLD in a lung transplant recipient. This strategy has since been successfully used in a large cohort of organ transplant recipients although these patients had received multiple lines of pharmaceutical interventions. Generally, adoptive immunotherapy was safe with no evidence of any adverse impact on engrafted organ and only grade 1 and 2 adverse events potentially associated with T cell infusion. More importantly, 11 of the 13 treated patients showed complete or partial resolution of clinical symptoms, including resolution or reduction in DNAemia and CMV-associated end-organ disease and/or the cessation or reduced use of antiviral drugs. Similar autologous T cell therapies have also been successfully used for the treatment of other viral infections including BK polyomavirus, adenovirus, and HHV6. A summary of clinical studies using autologous virus-specific T cells is summarized in Table 9.4.

While autologous T cell therapies have provided encouraging clinical responses in both HSCT and organ transplant recipients, delivery of these cell therapies to critically ill patients remains highly challenging. One of the major limitations includes prolonged manufacturing time, which limits their wider use for patients with end-stage organ disease. To overcome this limitation, ex vivo enrichment of virus-specific T cells has been used in the HSCT setting, however, this strategy requires a large volume of blood and high precursor frequency of antigen-specific T cells. Furthermore, the high cost of consumables and lack of access to unrelated HSCT donors also limits use of this approach in the clinical setting. Over the last decade, there has been an increasing interest in the use of allogenic virus-specific T cell therapies which can be premanufactured and stored as a bank to be offered to patients.

In clinical studies allogenic virus-specific T cell therapies were initially tested for EBV-associated PTLD and shown to be safe and efficacious. These observations have now been extended to other viral infections as well. Interestingly, these banked allogeneic virus-specific T cells can also be used for delivering chimeric antigen receptors targeting nonviral antigens. Some of the major challenges in delivering allogeneic virus-specific T cells in the

Table 9.4 Summary of Clinical Studies Based on Allogeneic Virus-Specific T Cell Therapies

Disease indication	Patient cohort (numbers)	Clinical response	Adverse events	Reference
EBV-PTLD	SOT (8)	3 CR 5 NR	None	Lancet, 360 (9331) (2002), pp. 436–442;
EBV-PTLD	SOT (2) HL (1) NHL (1)	SOT - 1CR, 1 SD HL - 1 PR NHL - 1 NR	None	Br J Haematol, 118 (3) (2002), pp. 799–808
EBV-PTLD	SOT (31) HSCT (2)	12 CR 9 PR 12 NR (5 not treated)	1 acute GvHD	Blood, 110 (4) (2007), pp. 1123–1131
EBV-PTLD	SOT (20) HSCT (28) Other (11)	SOT- 10 CR, 5 PR, 5 NR HSCT - 8 CR, 5 PR, 15 NR Other - 5 CR, 2 PR, 4 NR	2 acute GvHD (skin only)	Haematologica, 104 (8) (2019), pp. e356–e359
EBV-PTLD	SOT (13) HSCT (33)	SOT - 2 CR, 5 PR, 1 SD, 5 NR HSCT - 19 CR, 1 PR, 3 SD, 9 NR	1 acute GvHD	J Clin Invest, 130 (2) (2020), pp. 733–747
Multivirus infections (EBV, AdV, and CMV)	HSCT (50)	EBV - 2 CR, 4 PR, 3NR AdV - 7 CR, 7 PR, 3 NR CMV – 9 CR, 8 PR, 2 NR	8 acute GvHD	Blood, 121 (26) (2013), pp. 5113–5123
Multivirus infections (CMV, EBV, AdV, BKV, and HHV6)	HSCT (38)	CMV - 10 CR, 11 PR EBV - 2 CR AdV - 6 CR, 2 PR, 1 NR BKV - 12 CR, 4 PR HHV6 - 0 CR, 3 PR	3 acute GvHD 3 acute GvHD reactivation	J Clin Oncol, 35 (31) (2017), pp. 3547–3557
Multivirus infections (CMV, EBV, and AdV)	HSCT (30)	CMV - 22 CR, 6 NR EBV - 0 CR, 1 NR AdV - 1 CR	2 acute GvHD	Blood Adv, 1 (24) (2017), pp. 2193–2205

(continued)

Table 9.4 Continued

Disease indication	Patient cohort (numbers)	Clinical response	Adverse events	Reference
BKV viremia and hemorrhagic cystitis	HSCT (38) SOT (3)	HSCT – 27 CR, 4 PR, 7 NR SOT – 0 CR, 3 PR	1 acute GvHD	Blood Adv, 4 (22) (2020), pp. 5745–5754
CMV	HSCT (10)	7 CR 3 PR	None	Blood Adv, 3 (17) (2019), pp. 2571–2580
AdV	HSCT (23)	13 CR 6 PR 4 NR	1 acute GvHD	Blood Adv, 5 (17) (2021), pp. 3309–3321
BKV-associated hemorrhagic cystitis	HSCT (59)	CR 40 PR 5 NR 5	1 acute GvHD 1 acute GvHD reactivation	J Clin Oncol, 39 (24) (2021), pp. 2710–2719
EBV- and CMV-associated complications	HSCT (30)	CMV – 23 CR, 4 PR EBV – 3 CR	4 acute GVHD	Blood Adv, 6 (17) (2022), pp. 4949–4966
CMV-associated complications	HSCT (31)	CR 25 PR 6	3 acute GvHD	Cell Mol Immunol, 19 (4) (2022), pp. 482–491

clinical setting include HLA matching of banked T cells with patient's HLA and the potential risk of graft-vs.-host disease from adoptively transferred T cells. Interestingly, multiple clinical studies have shown that matching of two HLA class I alleles (including one with antiviral specificity) is sufficient for optimal clinical efficacy. Moreover, adoptive immunotherapy with partially matched virus-specific T cells is generally safe with rare grade 1 or 2 graft-vs.-host disease. A summary of clinical studies on allogeneic virus-specific T cells is provided in Table 9.5.

Conclusion

Late post-transplant infections are common, secondary to viral, fungal, and bacterial infection. Risk factors vary according to the type of infection. Long-term cumulative immunosuppression along with deficiency in cellular and humoral immunity play an important role in the pathogenesis of various infections. Advances in microbiological techniques to characterize microbes, awareness of

Table 9.5 Summary of Clinical Studies Based on Autologous Virus-Specific T Cell Therapies

Disease indication	Patient cohort (numbers)	Clinical response	Adverse events	Reference
EBV-PTLD	SOT (5; 1 patient treated with autologous EBV-specific T cells	Complete resolution of PTLD	None	Proc Natl Acad Sci U S A. 1999;96: 10391–10396
EBV-PTLD	SOT (1)	Complete resolution of PTLD	None	Transplantation 75(9):p 1556–1560, May 15, 2003.
EBV-PTLD	SOT (23; 7 patients treated with autologous EBV-specific T cells)	Stable decrease in viral load in 5 of 7 treated patients	None	Blood. 2002;99: 2592–2598.
EBV-PTLD	SOT (35; 12 treated with autologous EBV-specific T cells)	PTLD resolved in 2 patients NO PTLD emerged in 10 patients	None	Blood 2006 Nov 1;108(9):2942–2949.
CMV	SOT (1) treated with autologous CMV-specific T cells	Complete resolution of CMV replication	None	Am J Transplant (2009) 9:1679–1684.
Drug-resistant CMV infection	SOT (1) treated with autologous CMV-specific T cells	Complete resolution of CMV replication	None	Clin Transl Immunol (2015) 4:e35.
Drug resistant CMV infection	SOT (1) treated with autologous CMV-specific T cells	Partial resolution of CMV replication	None	J Hear Lung Transplant (2016) 35:685–687.
Drug resistant CMV-associated complications	SOT (22; 13 patients treated with autologous CMV-specific T cells)	11 patients showed either complete or partial response	None	Clin Infect Dis (2019) 68:632–640.

various infections, and newer antimicrobial agents, especially antiviral agents, have improved the outcome of post-transplant infections without jeopardizing kidney allograft function. However, the peril of irreversible graft failure and mortality persists. Innovative approaches such as adoptive T-cell therapy will open newer horizons to treating post-transplant viral infections.

References

1. Razonable RR, Humar A. Cytomegalovirus in solid organ transplant recipients— guidelines of the American Society of Transplantation Infectious Diseases Community of Practice. *Clin Transplant*. 2019;33(9):e13512.
2. Helantera I, Kyllonen L, Lautenschlager I, Salmela K, Koskinen P. Primary CMV infections are common in kidney transplant recipients after 6 months valganciclovir prophylaxis. *Am J Transplant*. 2010;10(9):2026–2032.
3. Puttarajappa C, Bhattarai M, Mour G, et al. Cytomegalovirus infection in high-risk kidney transplant recipients receiving thymoglobulin induction-a single-center experience. *Clin Transplant*. 2016;30(9):1159–1164.
4. Kumar D, Chin-Hong P, Kayler L, et al. A prospective multicenter observational study of cell-mediated immunity as a predictor for cytomegalovirus infection in kidney transplant recipients. *Am J Transplant*. 2019;19(9):2505–2516.
5. Jarque M, Crespo E, Melilli E, et al. Cellular immunity to predict the risk of cytomegalovirus infection in kidney transplantation: a prospective, interventional, multicenter clinical trial. *Clin Infect Dis*. 2020;71(9):2375–2385.
6. John GT, Manivannan J, Chandy S, Peter S, Jacob CK. Leflunomide therapy for cytomegalovirus disease in renal allograft recipients *Transplantation*. 2004;77(9):1460–1461.
7. Hariharan S. BK virus nephritis after renal transplantation. *Kidney Int*. 2006;69(4):655–662.
8. Weist BJ, Schmueck M, Fuehrer H, Sattler A, Reinke P, Babel N. The role of CD4(+) T cells in BKV-specific T cell immunity. *Med Microbiol Immunol*. 2014;203(6):395–408.
9. Comoli P, Cioni M, Basso S, et al. Immunity to polyomavirus BK infection: immune monitoring to regulate the balance between risk of BKV nephropathy and induction of alloimmunity. *Clin Dev Immunol*. 2013;2013:256923.
10. Kant S, Brennan DC. Donor derived cell free DNA in kidney transplantation: the circa 2020–2021 update. *Transpl Int*. 2022;35:10448.
11. Menter T, Mayr M, Schaub S, Mihatsch MJ, Hirsch HH, Hopfer H. Pathology of resolving polyomavirus-associated nephropathy. *Am J Transplant*. 2013;13(6):1474–1483.
12. Nickeleit V, Singh HK, Randhawa P, et al. The Banff Working Group classification of definitive polyomavirus nephropathy: morphologic definitions and clinical correlations. *J Am Soc Nephrol*. 2018;29(2):680–693.
13. Kable K, Davies CD, O'Connell PJ, Chapman JR, Nankivell BJ. Clearance of BK virus nephropathy by combination antiviral therapy with intravenous immunoglobulin. *Transplant Direct*. 2017;3(4):e142.
14. Le J, Durand CM, Agha I, Brennan DC. Epstein-Barr virus and renal transplantation. *Transplant Rev (Orlando)*. 2017;31(1):55–60.

15. John GT, Shankar V, Abraham AM, Mukundan U, Thomas PP, Jacob CK. Risk factors for post-transplant tuberculosis. *Kidney Int.* 2001;60(3):1148–1153.
16. Sester M, van Leth F, Bruchfeld J, et al. Risk assessment of tuberculosis in immunocompromised patients: a TBNET study. *Am J Respir Crit Care Med.* 2014;190(10):1168–1176.
17. Roth PJ, Grim SA, Gallitano S, Adams W, Clark NM, Layden JE. Serial testing for latent tuberculosis infection in transplant candidates: a retrospective review. *Transpl Infect Dis.* 2016;18(1):14–21.
18. Kim H, Kim SH, Jung JH, et al. The usefulness of quantitative interferon-gamma releasing assay response for predicting active tuberculosis in kidney transplant recipients: a quasi-experimental study. *J Infect.* 2020;81(3):403–410.
19. Ison MG, Nalesnik MA. An update on donor-derived disease transmission in organ transplantation. *Am J Transplant.* 2011;11(6):1123–1130.
20. Lopez-Medrano F, Fernandez-Ruiz M, Silva JT, et al. Multinational case-control study of risk factors for the development of late invasive pulmonary aspergillosis following kidney transplantation. *Clin Microbiol Infect.* 2018;24(2):192–198.
21. Husain S, Camargo JF. Invasive aspergillosis in solid-organ transplant recipients: guidelines from the American Society of Transplantation Infectious Diseases Community of Practice. *Clin Transplant.* 2019;33(9):e13544.
22. Florent M, Katsahian S, Vekhoff A, et al. Prospective evaluation of a polymerase chain reaction-ELISA targeted to aspergillus fumigatus and aspergillus flavus for the early diagnosis of invasive aspergillosis in patients with hematological malignancies. *J Infect Dis.* 2006;193(5):741–747.
23. Ullmann AJ, Aguado JM, Arikan-Akdagli S, et al. Diagnosis and management of aspergillus diseases: executive summary of the 2017 ESCMID-ECMM-ERS guideline. *Clin Microbiol Infect.* 2018;24(Suppl 1):e1–e38.
24. Walsh TJ, Anaissie EJ, Denning DW, et al. Treatment of aspergillosis: clinical practice guidelines of the Infectious Diseases Society of America. *Clin Infect Dis.* 2008;46(3):327–360.
25. Gibson M, Yang N, Waller JL, et al. Nocardiosis in renal transplant patients. *J Investig Med.* 2022;70(1):36–45.
26. John GT, Shankar V, Abraham AM, Mathews MS, Thomas PP, Jacob CK. Nocardiosis in tropical renal transplant recipients. *Clin Transplant.* 2002;16(4):285–289.
27. Singh N, Husain S. Infections of the central nervous system in transplant recipients. *Transpl Infect Dis.* 2000;2(3):101–111.
28. Ponzio V, Chen Y, Rodrigues AM, et al. Genotypic diversity and clinical outcome of cryptococcosis in renal transplant recipients in Brazil. *Emerg Microbes Infect.* 2019;8(1):119–129.
29. Kaminski H, Belliere J, Burguet L, et al. Identification of predictive markers and outcomes of late-onset *Pneumocystis jirovecii* pneumonia in kidney transplant recipients. *Clin Infect Dis.* 2021;73(7):e1456–e1463.
30. Karageorgopoulos DE, Qu JM, Korbila IP, Zhu YG, Vasileiou VA, Falagas ME. Accuracy of beta-D-glucan for the diagnosis of *Pneumocystis jirovecii* pneumonia: a meta-analysis. *Clin Microbiol Infect.* 2013;19(1):39–49.
31. Peddi VR, Hariharan S, First MR. Disseminated histoplasmosis in renal allograft recipients. *Clin Transplant.* 1996;10(2):160–165.
32. Gauthier GM, Safdar N, Klein BS, Andes DR. Blastomycosis in solid organ transplant recipients. *Transpl Infect Dis.* 2007;9(4):310–317.

33. Blair JE, Logan JL. Coccidioidomycosis in solid organ transplantation. *Clin Infect Dis.* 2001;33(9):1536–1544.
34. Fishman JA, Emery V, Freeman R, et al. Cytomegalovirus in transplantation—challenging the status quo. *Clin Transplant.* 2007;21(2):149–158.
35. Humar A. Reactivation of viruses in solid organ transplant patients receiving cytomegalovirus prophylaxis. *Transplantation.* 2006;82(Suppl 2):S9–S14.
36. Fernandez-Ruiz M, Kumar D, Humar A. Clinical immune-monitoring strategies for predicting infection risk in solid organ transplantation. *Clin Transl Immunology.* 2014;3(2):e12.
37. Lisboa LF, Kumar D, Wilson LE, Humar A. Clinical utility of cytomegalovirus cell-mediated immunity in transplant recipients with cytomegalovirus viremia. *Transplantation.* 2012;93(2):195–200.
38. Kotton CN, Huprikar S, Kumar D. Transplant infectious diseases: a review of the scientific registry of transplant recipients published data. *Am J Transplant.* 2017;17(6):1439–1446.
39. Kotton CN, Kumar D, Caliendo AM, et al. Updated international consensus guidelines on the management of cytomegalovirus in solid-organ transplantation. *Transplantation.* 2013;96(4):333–360.
40. Kotton CN. CMV: prevention, diagnosis and therapy. *Am J Transplant.* 2013;13(Suppl 3):24–40; quiz 40.
41. Crough T, Khanna R. Immunobiology of human cytomegalovirus: from bench to bedside. *Clin Microbiol Rev.* 2009;22(1):76–98.

10

Cancers after Kidney Transplantation

Nida Saleem, Germaine Wong, and Jeremy Chapman

Cancer—an expected, but unwanted complication after kidney transplantation!

Introduction

Cancer, infections, and cardiovascular diseases (CVDs) are known to be the mortality-defining outcomes after kidney transplants. However, there has been marked improvement in medical management and preventive strategies, resulting in a decline in infectious and CVD complications. CVD and post-transplant infections are discussed in Chapters 8 and 9. There has been a progressive rise in cancer incidence after transplant, owing to improved post-transplant survival and the longer-term adverse effects of immunosuppression.[1] In Australia and worldwide, cancer is one of the common causes of death in kidney transplant recipients. Kidney transplant patients consider cancer the most feared outcome because cancer impacts survival and the quality of life. In this chapter, we will discuss cancer epidemiology, risk factors, pathogenesis, surveillance, and management strategies in kidney transplant recipients.

Cancer Epidemiology in Kidney Transplantation

The cumulative incidence of solid-organ cancers reaches 10%–15% by 15 years post-transplantation. Skin cancers are frequent with up to 60% cumulative incidence in Europe, Australia, and New Zealand.[2] Overall, cancer risk in kidney transplant recipients is at least 2–3 times higher than in the age- and gender-matched general population,[3,4] but this varies significantly based on age, ethnicity, immunosuppression used, and a range of other factors such as virus exposure history and vaccination status. Compared to the general population, the relative risk of cancer-related death is more than 2.5 times higher.[2]

Origin of Cancers

Individuals are at risk of post-transplant cancer either from recurrence of pre-existing cancers, cancer that is transmitted from the organ donor, or de novo cancers developing post-transplantation.

Recurrence of Pre-Existing Cancers

Excluding patients from transplantation when they have an active cancer is standard clinical practice. There is a group of cancers that are associated with, or cause, kidney failure, including myeloma and a variety of urothelial cancers. While cancer may have been treated, there remains a potential of recurrence post-transplant and the mortality risk from the recurrent cancer is 1.5–3 times higher than in recipients without a prior cancer history.

The Kidney Disease Improving Global Outcomes (KDIGO) guidelines recommend postremission waiting times of 2–5 years before transplantation—largely depending on the primary organ involved, cancer stage, and its type—to reduce the recurrence risk.[5] While no waiting time is advised for several cancers, such as small isolated renal cell tumors, nonmelanoma skin cancers (NMSCs), and stage 1 medullary, papillary, low-grade prostate, and follicular thyroid cancers, the KDIGO guidelines recommend not transplanting people with metastatic carcinoma, invasive melanoma, and stage 4 thyroid and anaplastic cancers. Table 10.1 summarizes these recommendations.

Donor-Related Cancers

Cancer diagnosed post-transplant may be composed of donor cells not originating from the recipient. These cancers may either be "donor-transmitted" or "donor-derived." Donor-transmitted cancers are preexisting in the donated organ, while donor-derived cancers originate from donor tissue but develop de novo in the allograft post-transplantation. Careful donor workup of both deceased and living donors is designed to exclude such donor-transmitted cancers, despite which there remains an estimated incidence of around 0.01%–0.05% of transplants.[6]

A systemic review of case reports, case series, and registries showed that renal cell carcinoma (RCC) was the most common donor-transmitted cancer, followed by melanoma, lymphoma, and lung cancer.[7] The risk of actual cancer transmission depends on the type and extent of cancer, with higher rates and worse prognoses associated with donor lung cancer, melanoma, and

Table 10.1 Recommended Waiting Time between Cancer Remission and Kidney Transplantation

Cancer types	Stage	Recommended waiting time
Breast	Early	At least 2 years
	Advanced	At least 5 years
Colorectal	Dukes A/B	At least 2 years
	Duke C	2–5 years
	Duke D	At least 5 years
Bladder	Invasive	At least 2 years
Kidney	Incidentaloma (<3 cm)	No waiting time
	Early	At least 2 years
	Large and invasive	At least 5 years
Uterine	Localized	At least 2 years
	Invasive	At least 5 years
Cervical	Localized	At least 2 years
	Invasive	At least 5 years
Lung	Localized	2–5 years
Testicular	Localized	At least 2 years
	Invasive	2–5 years
Melanoma	Localized	At least 5 years
	Invasive	Contraindicated
Prostate	Gleason ≤6	No waiting time
	Gleason 7	At least 2 years
	Gleason 8–10	At least 5 years
Thyroid	Papillary/Medullary/ Follicular Stage 1	No waiting time
	Stage 2	At least 2 years
	Stage 3	At least 5 years
	Stage 4	Contraindicated
	Anaplastic	Contraindicated
Hodgkin lymphoma	Localized	At least 2 years
	Regional	3–5 years
	Distant	At least 5 years

(continued)

Table 10.1 Continued

Cancer types	Stage	Recommended waiting time
Non-Hodgkin lymphoma	Localized	At least 2 years
	Regional	3–5 years
	Distant	At least 5 years
PTLD	Nodal	At least 2 years
	Extranodal and cerebral	At least 5 years

Source: Content extracted from reference 5.

choriocarcinoma. In contrast, organ donation from donors with RCC without capsular invasion, NMSCs, and low-grade primary central nervous tumors, except medulloblastoma, is generally accepted because of the low chance of cancer in the donated tissue due to the low metastatic potential of these tumors.[1]

De Novo Cancers

De novo cancers account for most cancers that occur in kidney transplant recipients. These are the most common post-transplant cancers and are associated with the highest mortality risk, with a standardized mortality risk (SMR) of 2.6, comparing transplant recipients with the age- and sex-matched general population. The cumulative incidence of cancer increases from 4%–5% after 5 years, to 10% after 10 years, and more than 25% after 20 years of transplant.

The observational and registry data from Australia, North America, New Zealand, and Europe all show higher incidences of NMSCs and lip cancers in the White populations.[2] In contrast, among Asian and Black populations in North America, Japan, Korea, and China, the incidence of skin cancer is very low (0.06%). There are also national variations, for example in the incidence of urothelial transitional cell carcinoma among the Chinese population, perhaps due to higher dietary exposure to Chinese herbal medication containing aristocholic acid.[8] Japanese and Korean studies have reported a higher incidence of renal and gastrointestinal cancers, respectively.[8]

The first detailed analysis of specific cancers in a large cohort of renal transplant recipients was from the Australia and New Zealand Dialysis and Transplant (ANZDATA) registry.[9] The study compared renal transplant recipients to the general population and demonstrated the great range of site-specific standard incidence ratios (SIRs) for cancers in dialysis and transplant recipients. Higher SIRs observed for cancers such as melanoma, lip cancer, and lymphoma contrast with modestly elevated levels for colon cancer and no increase for prostate and breast cancers.[2,9] Careful analysis of the pattern of excess risk demonstrated the association with cancers known or suspected of having a viral etiology, such as human papillomavirus (HPV)–related cervical cancers (5–10 times increased risk). Epstein-Barr virus (EBV)–related post-transplant lymphoproliferative disease (PTLD; 15 times increased risk), and human herpesvirus-8 (HHV-8)–related Kaposi sarcomas (300 times increased risk) provide the extreme outlier examples.[2] Based on the results of the published data,[1] Table 10.2 summarizes

Table 10.2 Factors Influencing Post–Renal Transplant Cancer Risk

Factors	Change in risk
Patient-related factors	
1. Old age (>50 versus <35 years)	3–6 times increase
2. Gender (male versus female)	20%–30% increase
3. White versus non-White ethnicity	20%–35% increase
Medical history	
4. Smoking	2–3 times
5. Time on dialysis (>4.5 years versus <1.5 years)	40% increase
6. Prior history of cancer	40% increase
7. Diabetes mellitus	20%–40% decrease
8. Polycystic kidney disease	20% decrease
Transplant factors	
9. PRA score (80% versus 0%)	2 times increase
10. HLA-DR mismatches (2 versus 0)	25% increase
11. Deceased expanded criteria donor versus living donor	50% increase
12. Donor and recipient CMV status	No difference
Immunosuppression	
13. Azathioprine	2–9 times increase in SCC
14. T-cell-depleting agents	~30%–80% increase in NHL
15. IL-2r inhibitors	No increase
16. mTOR inhibitors	30%–50% decrease

Source: Content extracted from reference 1.
Abbreviations: PRA: panel reactive antibody, HLA: human leukocyte antigen, CMV: cytomegalovirus, SCC: squamous cell carcinoma, NHL: non-Hodgkin lymphoma, mTOR: mammalian target of rapamycin, IL-2: interleukin-2

factors influencing cancer risk in the post-transplant period and the magnitude of increased risk.

Pathogenesis of Cancer after Transplantation

The precise mechanisms for the increased occurrence of cancer post-transplant remain unclear. Several studies have attributed the loss of immune surveillance playing a significant role in cancer pathogenesis.[10] Several possible pathogenic mechanisms are presented in Table 10.3. Furthermore, several mechanistic hypotheses have been proposed to explain the process by which immunosuppression leads to an increase in specific cancers, as shown below.

Table 10.3 Mechanisms for the Pathogenesis of Increased Cancer Risk after Renal Transplantation

Mechanisms	Descriptions
Altered immune phenotype	
i. *Suppression of innate immunity:*	Natural killer (NK) cells play a significant role in the early recognition and control of viral infected and tumor cells and chronic immunosuppression is known to suppress the function and number of natural killer and dendritic cells
ii. *Increase in immunosenescent T-cells:*	Kidney transplant recipients overexpress immunosenescent T-cells. A study has shown a link between CD-57 overexpressing aged T-cells and squamous cell carcinoma with reduced immunorecognition of viral and tumor antigens, thus, promoting cancer development.[32]
iii. *Increase in regulatory T-cells (Treg):*	Upregulation of Treg in kidney transplant recipients has been linked to cancer development.[1] Treg cells may contribute to tumor progression by reducing the antitumor response through suppression of effector T cell proliferation, thus allowing tumor cells to escape from immune control.
Activation of pathogenic pathways	
i. *Loss of immune control over the oncogenic viruses*	For example, virus-associated cancers like PTLD—Epstein-Barr virus (EBV), Kaposi sarcoma—human herpes virus-8 (HHV-8), and urogenital cancers—human papillomavirus (HPV).[2]
ii. *Accumulation of mutations:*	Due to loss of immune-mediated DNA damage repair. For example, a deficient immune system can no longer repair phototoxic medication or UV radiation-induced DNA damage in skin cancers.[2]
iii. *Activation of the oncogenic RAS-RAF pathway:*	Induced by cyclosporine[1] leading to increased RCC risk.

Role of Specific Immunosuppressive Drugs

The exact type of drug as well as the cumulative dose of immunosuppression may determine the frequency of specific cancers in renal transplant recipients.[10] No conclusive clinical evidence is available regarding the oncogenic potential of a particular immunosuppressive medication. There are, however, some data that assist clinical decision-making and some animal studies that have exposed several pathogenic mechanisms.

Calcineurin inhibitors (CNIs) increase the expression of transforming growth factor-beta (TGF-beta) and vascular endothelial growth factor (VEGF), which have been shown to enhance tumor growth and angiogenesis, respectively.[11,12] Blockade of signaling pathways via calcineurin and nuclear factor of activated T cells (NFAT), CNIs indirectly lead to the loss of activation of p53, which is a tumor suppression gene. Cyclosporine also promotes IL-6 expression, which in turn supports B cell proliferation and increases the risk of PTLD.[1] It also leads to defective DNA repair, inducing T cell apoptosis and inhibiting apoptosis in other cells. Azathioprine promotes the occurrence of NMSC by sensitizing the skin to UV radiation and increasing the accumulation of 6-thioguanine in the DNA[10] but also lowers levels of NK cells and naive B cells.

T-cell-depleting agents like antithymocyte globulin (ATG) used for both induction and acute rejection treatment are known to be associated with increased cancer risk.[13] The exact mechanism by which short-term exposure leads to increased cancer occurrence years later is largely unknown. Viral replication with immunosuppression has been postulated for EBV-related PTLD.

Patient and Allograft Outcomes in Kidney Transplant Recipients with Cancer

The primary causes of death with a functioning graft within the 1st year post-transplant are CVD (31%), infections (31%), and cancer (7%). However, beyond the 1st year post-transplant, cancer becomes the leading cause of mortality (29%) for patients with a functioning graft, as cancer increases with time and the impact of dialysis-associated CVD and infections associated with high early levels of immunosuppression, wane.[11]

Not only is the incidence of cancer increased but also many studies have shown that tumors in the post-transplant period tend to display a more aggressive course than in the general population. Observational data show that cancer-associated mortality risk is 1.8–1.9 times that of the age- and sex-matched general population. Among cancer types, the risk of death is highest among melanoma, non-Hodgkin lymphoma, and urogenital cancers, with the risk of cancer mortality more than 10 times higher compared to the age- and sex-matched general population.[2]

Several potential explanations can be hypothesized for this high mortality risk, including enhanced oncogenesis reflecting enhanced tumor growth rates, poor levels of screening and preemptive therapies, limited cancer therapeutic options in transplant recipients, and concurrent comorbidities.

Specific Cancers

Skin Cancers

Skin cancers are the most common cancers in the renal transplant population. Squamous cell carcinoma (SCC), basal cell carcinoma (BCC), Kaposi sarcomas, and melanomas are the most reported skin cancers, with keratinocyte cancers accounting for 90%–95% of these cancers. In contrast to the general population, SCC incidence exceeds BCC by 4:1 in kidney transplant recipients.[14] The overall risk of post-transplant SCC is 250 times, Kaposi sarcoma is at least 100 times, and melanoma is five to eight times more frequent than in the general population.[15] Melanoma and spindle cell cancers have the highest mortality risk, but SCC is also much more dangerous than in the normal population especially when the tumors are multiple across chronically sun-damaged skin, as found in people who have prolonged sun exposure most of their lives. BCC, on the other hand, remains benign even in the transplant recipient.[16]

The complex interaction of factors plays a significant role in these skin cancer pathogenesis, including male gender, advanced recipient age, excessive ultraviolet (UV) radiation exposure, fair skin color, prolonged transplant duration, pretransplant skin cancer, and HPV infection. Specific immunosuppressives, including cyclosporine and azathioprine, are known to be pathogenic.[2] CNIs are also known to play a significant role in the HHV-8 virus-mediated Kaposi sarcoma pathogenesis.[2]

Management of skin cancers depends on their type, biology, and invasiveness.[2] For SCC in situ, published data recommend either surgical excision or electro dissection and curettage. Any lesion suspicious of being invasive needs a biopsy. The current standard of care for BCC is surgical excision alone. If the biopsy shows SCC, then surgery with margin clearance is the gold standard treatment, performed through Mohs micrographic surgery or surgical excision.[15] Studies also recommend radiotherapy as an alternative for inoperable SCC, while adjuvant radiotherapy is appropriate for positive margins or perineural involvement.[15] Chemoprophylaxis has also been recommended for multiple (more than five SCCs per year), early onset, and aggressive SCCs. These include therapies like retinoids, nicotinamide, and capecitabine.[2] For metastatic SCC, systemic chemotherapy is accepted, and immunotherapy may be beneficial in certain cases.[15]

Immunosuppression modulation is also recommended, based on the cancer risk and the graft type and circumstances. Reduction in overall immunosuppression and conversion to an mTOR inhibitor has been tested and demonstrated to be effective at least in reducing 1- to 3-year cancer recurrence rates.[15,17]

For Kaposi sarcoma, the reduction of CNIs and conversion to mTOR inhibitors have been proven as successful management strategies.[17] For Kaposi lesions nonresponsive to immunomodulation, treatment options include surgical excision, radiotherapy, cryotherapy, or laser ablation.[15]

Depending on the stage and histological grade of cancer, surgical intervention with wide excision and adequate margin clearance, combined with standard-of-care lymph node tracing and oncotherapy remain the standard therapeutic options for transplant recipients with melanoma. Checkpoint inhibitors offer a promising treatment for advanced-stage melanoma, However, this treatment is associated with a heightened risk of acute rejection (by approximately 50%–60%) and allograft loss (see "Newer Anticancer Agents and Kidney Transplant Immunosuppression" below). Novel approaches with adoptive cell therapies are under investigation.[18]

Lymphoma

PTLD and other forms of lymphoma are both frequent and associated with high mortality rates of up to 50%. The cumulative incidence of PTLD with 10 years of kidney transplant is around 1%–2% in adults and 3% in pediatric transplant recipients. Pediatric transplant recipients have 30 times greater PTLD risk compared to the age- and sex-matched general population.[19]

PTLD has a bimodal occurrence, with early onset occurring within 1–2 years post-transplant and then a later phase of tumors occurring over the longer term. Early onset PTLDs account for 90% of cases, which are strongly associated with de novo EBV infection and use of T-cell-depleting agents. These lymphomas often involve extranodal sites such as brain, lungs, and GI tract. Late-onset PTLDs occur approximately 7–10 years post-transplant, are associated with the use of CNIs, and are EBV-negative in 40%–50% of cases.[20] Clinical presentation varies from asymptomatic mononucleosis to advanced lymphoma. The WHO classifies lymphomas into four major categories: early lesions, monomorphic, polymorphic, and non-Hodgkin lesions. Polymorphic PTLDs are mostly

EBV-positive and early onset. Monomorphic PTLDs are usually of B cell origin, mostly diffuse large B cell lymphomas, and occasionally Burkitt lymphoma.[19]

The risk factors for PTLD vary with the time since the transplant. The recipient's (-) and donor's (+) EBV statuses, with resultant EBV infection, are the most significant determinants of early-onset PTLD. Use of T-cell-depleting agents (ATG) and their inherent ability to depress T cell surveillance against EBV, leads to early-onset PTLD. Late-onset incidence increases with prolonged CNI exposure and diabetes mellitus.[21] Other risk factors include male gender and use of the costimulatory blocker belatacept, in an EBV-naive recipient. In contrast, antiproliferative therapy does not seem to pose an increased risk. According to Australian data, there has been an 8% reduction in PTLD risk since 2000, possibly due to increasing anti-CD25 therapy and reduced use of ATG for induction, lower rejection rates, and lower CNI target levels.[21]

The treatment goal of PTLD is to obtain a disease cure through the reduction of immunosuppression to a level that does not significantly increase rejection risk. In the absence of good evidence, discontinuation of antimetabolites and reduction of CNIs are common. Published data show an improved 5-year survival rate of 60% with conventional chemotherapy (cyclophosphamide, vincristine, doxorubicin, prednisone) and rituximab. Rituximab (anti-CD20) therapy has proved more effective in tumors that are both EBV-positive and CD20-positive.[2]

More experimental treatments include EBV-directed cytotoxic T-cell therapy[19] and chimeric antigen receptors (CAR)-T therapy.[20] EBV-directed cytotoxic T-cell therapy is indicated for EBV-positive PTLD, refractory to other chemotherapeutic agents. However, CAR-T cell therapy remains challenging in transplant recipients owing to an increased risk for rejection.

Cervical Cancer

The incidence of cervical cancer in the renal transplant recipient is 5 to 10 times greater than in the general population likely related to loss of immune control against neoplastic cells and impaired immunity against HPV. Cervical cancer accounts for 3% of post-transplant malignancy and is the second most common malignancy in female recipients after skin cancers. Cytological screening and evaluation of preinvasive lesions through a Papanicolaou (PAP) smear has significantly reduced the cancer burden.

HPV-16 and -18 are implicated in up to 70% of cervical cancers in the transplant population. HPV bivalent (HPV-16 and -18 strains) and quadrivalent (against HPV-6, -11, -16, and -18 strains) vaccines have proven beneficial in HPV naive women, with less effectiveness in HPV-exposed females. Since other

HPV strains cause 30% of cervical cancers, continuous cervical cancer screening in vaccinated transplant women is still recommended.[22]

Native Kidney Cancer

Renal cell cancer (RCC) is substantially increased both in patients on dialysis and after transplantation compared to the normal population.[9] In the transplanted population there is a 5- to 10-fold increase in all urogenital cancers compared to the general population, with cancer in the native kidneys accounting for most of this risk. Clear cell and papillary RCCs are the most common native RCCs (32% and 28%, respectively).[23] Most kidney masses are diagnosed incidentally as small, localized, early lesions in the native kidneys on abdominal imaging, with a low chance of metastasis of < 2%. Acquired cystic kidney disease (ACKD) of the native kidney is a known risk factor for developing post-transplant RCC, leading some programs to screen these kidneys using ultrasound.[24] A prolonged duration of dialysis by >3 years increases the risk for ACKD. Other risk factors include male gender, smoking, long analgesic exposure, and African ethnicity.[2]

De novo native RCC should be managed based on stage and standard risk stratification. For localized RCC in dysfunctional native kidneys, total nephrectomy is curative.[24] Observational data suggest that reducing immunosuppression and initiating tyrosine kinase inhibitors and immunotherapy may benefit managing metastatic RCC.[25]

Other Common Solid Organ Cancers

The risk of colonic and lung malignancy is 2–3 times greater than in the age- and sex-matched general population, while breast and prostate cancer does not occur with an increased risk among renal transplant recipients.[9] Gastrointestinal and respiratory tract tumors may have a more aggressive course in transplant recipients, with 40% metastatic at the diagnosis,[25] but it is hard to exclude bias in these analyses.

Most transplant programs tend to reduce immunosuppression after the diagnosis of cancer. There is a better rationale for this approach in tumors with a high incidence compared to the general population, such as lymphoma and Kaposi sarcoma, than for those with no increases such as breast and prostate. Indeed, one observational study has shown no significant increase in the rejection risk or cancer-free survival with immunosuppression dose reduction in solid organ cancers.[26] The conversion of CNIs to mTOR inhibitors or low-dose CNIs with mTOR inhibitors is certainly of proven benefit for the management of Kaposi sarcoma and NMSCs,[17] and there is a rationale for using this approach in RCC. However, more long-term clinical studies of immunomodulation are warranted to establish the balance of risks for preventing graft rejection while retarding the progression of neoplastic diseases.

Hematological Cancers

Although quite rare in renal transplant recipients, post-transplant leukemias are five times more common than in the age- and sex-matched general population and have a 1.6-fold greater relative risk compared to the patients on the wait list. Multiple myeloma may cause or contribute to end-stage kidney disease (ESKD) and has both a high post-transplant recurrence rate and a high de novo diagnosis rate.[27] Advanced age and T-cell-depleting induction immunosuppressive therapy significantly increase the risk of occurrence for both malignancies. Ten-year post-transplant survival is dismal at only 26% and 39% for post-transplant myeloma and leukemia, respectively.[27]

In the past, multiple myeloma was traditionally considered a contraindication for renal transplant due to the higher risk of disease relapse and allograft loss. However, the FDA has approved many drugs that have, between them, improved median myeloma survival from 20 months to 8 years, including proteasome inhibitors, monoclonal antibodies, and immunomodulatory agents. Kidney transplantation can thus be contemplated for ESKD patients with myeloma but only with great care to assess the effectiveness of each individual's treatment regimens.[20] A US-based study recommends a waiting time of 1 year after achieving complete remission or very good partial remission post–stem cell transplantation, before a kidney transplant and the use of monoclonal antibodies (anti-CD38 therapy, daratumumab) and proteasome inhibitors (bortezomib, ixazomib) as a possible maintenance agent for post–renal transplant myeloma management.[20]

Cancer Screening

Routine cancer screening is an accepted practice for appropriate cancers in the general population. In renal transplant recipients, many guidelines recommend, in the absence of high-quality data, similar screening strategies for colorectal, breast, and cervical cancers as for the general population. Additionally, guidelines also recommend annual skin cancer screening by a dermatologist, especially in high-risk cases. Screening for lung, hepatocellular, bladder, and native kidney cancers, is usually recommended only in select high-risk populations. These are discussed in Chapter 3, "Wellness after Kidney Transplantation," as well. Table 10.4 summarizes several evidence-based guidelines.

Table 10.4 Recommendations for Post-Transplant Cancer Screening

Cancer type	Screening recommendations	Screening modality	Screening frequency
Breast	-Women aged 40 to 49 if preferred	Mammography	Yearly
	-Women aged 50 to 74	Mammography	Biennially
Colorectal	-Both males and females, aged 50–75years	Fecal immunochemical testing (FIT) OR	Biennially
		Sigmoidoscopy Complete colonic exam	Every 5 yearly
	-Positive FIT	by colonoscopy	
Liver	For those with known cirrhosis	Liver ultrasound and alpha-fetoprotein screening	6 monthly or annually
Cervical	Females from 25 to 74 years	Papanicolaou (PAP) test OR	Every three yearly
		HPV testing	Every 5 yearly
Lung	People at high risk for lung cancer -Aged 55 to 80 years -Smoking history of at least 30 pack-years -Current smokers or have quit within the past 15 years	Low-dose CT scan chest	Annually
Prostate	Male, aged 55 to 69, if they wish	Prostate-specific antigen (PSA)	Periodically
Kidney	-Family history of renal cancer - Personal history of acquired cystic disease (ACKD) -Analgesic nephropathy -Long-term smokers -Prolonged dialysis duration	Ultrasound native kidneys	Routinely
Bladder	-Previously exposed to chemotherapeutic agents such as cyclophosphamide -Regular users of analgesics -Heavy smokers (≥ 30 pack-year history)	Urine cytology and cystoscopy	Routinely
Skin	All transplant recipients	Self-examination Examination by a dermatologist	Routinely Annually
PTLD	-high risk (donor EBV seropositive/ recipient seronegative).	EBV by NAT	Once in the first week after transplant, monthly for the first 3–6 months, and every 3 monthly till 1-year post-transplant

Source: Content extracted from references 2, 5.

Newer Anticancer Agents and Kidney Transplant Immunosuppression

Several novel therapeutic approaches and new drugs have shown promising results for managing malignancies in the general population but need careful application to the transplant population. These include immune checkpoint inhibitors ICIs), CAR-T cell therapy, and monoclonal antibodies for myeloma.

Immune Checkpoint Inhibitors

Immunotherapy with ICIs targets cytotoxic T-lymphocyte antigen-4 (CTLA-4), program cell death receptor, and its ligand 1 (PD/PDL1). CTLA-4 blocks the costimulatory signal (CD28 on T cells and B7 on antigen-presenting cells) required for T cell activation. These inhibitors thus promote antitumor T cell function by activating this costimulatory pathway. Tumor cells express the PD receptor, which on binding to PDL1 on T-cells, inhibits T cell proliferation and cytokine production. Blocking this PD/PDL1 axis promotes an antitumor T cell response.[28]

ICIs have proven to be highly effective for immunocompetent patients, with the FDA approving them for treating several cancers including melanoma, cutaneous squamous cell carcinoma, Merkel cell carcinoma (MCC), non-small-cell lung cancer, head and neck squamous cell carcinoma, and renal cancer in the general population. However, most trials excluded the transplant population because of association with increased allograft rejection risk and graft loss, with the risk higher with PD/PDL1 inhibitors than with CTLA-4.[29]

Few studies have used these therapies in transplant recipients, and those that have are small cohort studies or case reports in advanced stage of malignancies. A recent analysis of such cases showed a 68% mortality rate, 49% of recipients had rejection, predominantly T-cell-mediated vascular rejection (Banff 2A and 2B), with PD/PDL1 inhibitors and 30% with CTLA-4 inhibitors.[29]

Concomitant management of immunosuppression and ICI has been studied with promising preliminary results with the use of mTOR inhibitors leading to reduction in rejection risk from 36% to 20%.[30] Belatacept therapy needs to be avoided in patients treated with ICI as it can render ICI ineffective, though prospective studies and trial-based evidence are still needed.[29]

Monoclonal Antibody Therapy in Multiple Myeloma

In 2015, the FDA approved two monoclonal antibodies, daratumumab (anti-CD38) and elotuzumab (anti-SLAMF7), for the management of multiple myeloma based on clinical trial results. Both CD38 and SLAMF7 are antigens highly expressed on the surface of myeloma cells, and antibodies to these antigens promote apoptosis of malignant plasma cells.[28] Botta et al.,[31] in an analysis of 18 trials, concluded that daratumumab, combined with lenalidomide and dexamethasone, ranked first among other regimens in terms of activity, efficacy, and tolerability. Several trials have proven them to be efficacious in refractory or relapsing myeloma, high-risk smoldering myeloma, and even newly diagnosed myeloma.[28] The data on renal transplant recipients is limited to case reports and small series. A study suggests that, in addition to proteasome inhibitors, anti-CD38 monoclonal antibodies may play a role in maintenance therapy for myeloma post renal transplant, but with a risk of T-cell-mediated rejection through inhibition of regulatory T-cells.[20]

CAR-T Therapy

CAR-T cells are a manufactured cell product derived from T lymphocytes engineered to express chimeric antigen receptors (CARs) against cancer cells. CAR-T cells targeting B cell maturation antigen (BCMA) have been approved by the FDA for managing multiple myeloma, acute lymphocytic leukemia, and diffuse large B cell lymphoma (DLBL) in the nontransplant population.[20] CAR-T therapy in solid organ transplant patients remains challenging because of a presumed greater risk of rejection and concerns that concomitant immunosuppression would increase the chance of manufacturing failure of autologous CAR-T therapy.[20] This therapy also has several potential adverse effects, including cytokine release syndrome, neurotoxicity, increased infections, acute kidney injury, capillary leak syndrome, low cardiac output, and bone marrow suppression.

Future Research

Most published data today focus on post-transplant cancer types, their incidence, mortality, pathogenesis, risk factors, and on screening modalities. Opportunities for clinical trials are limited, however, further studies are needed to identify mechanisms of cancer pathogenesis, effective cancer screening strategies, and the optimal treatment approaches with different immunosuppression regimens on cancer incidence and outcome. Trial-based evidence is needed to identify the role of effective immunosuppression in the context of immunomodulation and the utility of novel cancer therapies (CAR-T therapy, ICIs, monoclonal antibodies) in renal transplant recipients to promote cancer control and avoid allograft rejection. A multinational trials consortium is needed to address these questions.

Conclusion

Renal transplantation provides the best treatment modality for patients with ESKD. However, immunosuppression increases in long-term risks of cancer contributing to morbidity and mortality. A proactive approach to cancer risk stratification, post-transplant drug management, routine cancer screening, and effective cancer management is necessary to prolong the survival of renal transplant recipients. Multidisciplinary decision-making with oncologists, surgeons, radiotherapists, and transplant nephrologists remains an optimal approach for kidney transplant patients with cancer.

References

1. Au E, Wong G, Chapman JR. Cancer in kidney transplant recipients. *Nat Rev Nephrol*. 2018;14(8):508–520.
2. Al-Adra D, Al-Qaoud T, Fowler K, Wong GJ. De novo malignancies after kidney transplantation. *Clin J Am Soc Nephrol*. 2022;17(3):434–443.
3. Engels EA, Pfeiffer RM, Fraumeni JF, et al. Spectrum of cancer risk among US solid organ transplant recipients. *JAMA*. 2011;306(17):1891–901.
4. Huo Z, Li C, Xu X, et al. Cancer risks in solid organ transplant recipients: results from a comprehensive analysis of 72 cohort studies. *Oncoimmunology*. 2020;9(1):1848068.
5. Chadban SJ, Ahn C, Axelrod DA, et al. KDIGO clinical practice guideline on the evaluation and management of candidates for kidney transplantation. *Transplantation*. 2020;104(4S1):S11–S103.
6. Hedley JA, Vajdic CM, Wyld M, et al. Cancer transmissions and non-transmissions from solid organ transplantation in an Australian cohort of deceased and living organ donors. *Transpl Int*. 2021;34(9):1667–1679.
7. Xiao D, Craig J, Chapman J, Dominguez-Gil B, Tong A, Wong GJ. Donor cancer transmission in kidney transplantation: a systematic review. *Am J Transplant*. 2013;13(10):2645–2652.
8. Zhang J, Ma L, Xie Z, et al. Epidemiology of post-transplant malignancy in Chinese renal transplant recipients: a single-center experience and literature review. *Med Oncol*. 2014;31(7):32.
9. Vajdic CM, McDonald SP, McCredie MR, et al. Cancer incidence before and after kidney transplantation. *JAMA*. 2006;296(23):2823–2831.

10. Sprangers B, Nair V, Launay-Vacher V, Riella LV, Jhaveri KD. Risk factors associated with post–kidney transplant malignancies: an article from the Cancer-Kidney International Network. *Clin Kidney J.* 2018;11(3):315–329.
11. Hariharan S, Israni AK, Danovitch GD. Long-term survival after kidney transplantation. *NEJM.* 2021;385(8):729–743.
12. Geissler EK. Post-transplantation malignancies: here today, gone tomorrow? *Nat Rev. Clin. Oncol.* 2015;12(12):705–717.
13. Lim WH, Turner RM, Chapman JR, et al. Acute rejection, T-cell-depleting antibodies, and cancer after transplantation. *Transplantation.* 2014;97(8):817–825.
14. Chapman JR, Webster AC, Wong GJ. Cancer in the transplant recipient. *Cold Spring Harb Perspect Med.* 2013;3(7):a015677.
15. Mittal A, Colegio OJ. Skin cancers in organ transplant recipients. *Am J Transplant.* 2017;17(10):2509–2530.
16. Garrett GL, Blanc PD, Boscardin J, et al. Incidence of and risk factors for skin cancer in organ transplant recipients in the United States. *JAMA.* 2017;153(3):296–303.
17. Lim WH, Russ GR, Wong G, Pilmore H, Kanellis J, Chadban SJ. The risk of cancer in kidney transplant recipients may be reduced in those maintained on everolimus and reduced cyclosporine. *Kid International.* 2017;91(4):954–963.
18. Dafni U, Michielin O, Lluesma SM, et al. Efficacy of adoptive therapy with tumor-infiltrating lymphocytes and recombinant interleukin-2 in advanced cutaneous melanoma: a systematic review and meta-analysis. *Ann Oncol.* 2019;30(12):1902–1913.
19. Petrara MR, Giunco S, Serraino D, Dolcetti R, De Rossi A. Post-transplant lymphoproliferative disorders: from epidemiology to pathogenesis-driven treatment. *JCl.* 2015;369(1):37–44.
20. Murakami N, Webber AB, Nair VJ. Transplant onconephrology in patients with kidney transplants. *Adv Chronic Kidney Dis.* 2022;29(2):188–200. e1.
21. Francis A, Johnson DW, Teixeira-Pinto A, Craig JC, Wong GJ. Incidence and predictors of post-transplant lymphoproliferative disease after kidney transplantation during adulthood and childhood: a registry study. *NDT.* 2018;33(5):881–889.
22. Webster AC, Wong G, Craig JC, Chapman JR. Managing cancer risk and decision making after kidney transplantation. *Am J Transplant.* 2008;8(11):2185–2191.
23. Hernández-Gaytán CA, Rodríguez-Covarrubias F, Castillejos-Molina RA, et al. Urological cancers and kidney transplantation: a literature review. *Curr Urol Rep.* 2021;22(12):1–10.
24. Dahle DO, Skauby M, Langberg CW, Brabrand K, Wessel N, Midtvedt K. Renal cell carcinoma and kidney transplantation: a narrative review. *Transplantation.* 2022;106(1):e52–e63.
25. Krishnan A, Wong G, Teixeira-Pinto A, Lim WH. Incidence and outcomes of early cancers after kidney transplantation. *Transpl Int.* 2022;35:10024.
26. Hope CM, Krige AJ, Barratt A, Carroll RP. Reductions in immunosuppression after haematological or solid organ cancer diagnosis in kidney transplant recipients. *Transpl Int.* 2015;28(11):1332–1335.
27. Caillard S, Agodoa LY, Bohen EM, Abbott KC. Myeloma, Hodgkin disease, and lymphoid leukemia after renal transplantation: characteristics, risk factors and prognosis. *Transplantation.* 2006;81(6):888–895.
28. Abramson HN. Monoclonal antibodies for the treatment of multiple myeloma: an update. *Int J Mol Sci.* 2018;19(12):3924.

29. Delyon J, Zuber J, Dorent R, et al. Immune checkpoint inhibitors in transplantation—a case series and comprehensive review of current knowledge. *Transplantation*. 2021;105(1):67–78.

30. Esfahani K, Al-Aubodah T-A, Thebault P, et al. Targeting the mTOR pathway uncouples the efficacy and toxicity of PD-1 blockade in renal transplantation. *Nat Commun*. 2019;10(1):1–9.

31. Botta C, Ciliberto D, Rossi M, et al. Network meta-analysis of randomized trials in multiple myeloma: efficacy and safety in relapsed/refractory patients. *Blood Adv*. 2017;1(7):455–466.

32. Bottomley MJ, Harden PN, Wood KJ. CD8+ immunosenescence predicts post-transplant cutaneous squamous cell carcinoma in high-risk patients. *JASN*. 2016;27(5):1505–1515.

11

Recurrent and De Novo Diseases after Kidney Transplantation

Craig P. Coorey and Steven J. Chadban

Recurrent Disease—what goes around comes around!

Introduction

For most patients with end-stage kidney disease (ESKD), kidney transplant (KT) is the treatment of choice. KT provides a replacement kidney and immunosuppression, but in most cases does not ameliorate the underlying cause of kidney failure. As a result, both glomerular and systemic diseases can recur after KT, leading to graft dysfunction and failure with concurrent extra-renal morbidity and possibly death. Although less common, there are diseases that can occur de novo post transplantation that may also damage the kidney allograft.

Definition of Recurrent and De Novo Diseases

Recurrence of disease post-transplantation is best defined as the histological occurrence in the kidney allograft of the primary disease that caused the patient's kidney failure. For diagnostic certainty, the disease that caused ESKD should be biopsy proven, and diagnosis of disease recurrence would then require a biopsy of the kidney allograft to confirm the same disease is present. This assumes that the donor kidney was free of disease at the time of transplantation, which is not always true, as there have been reports of deceased donor (DD) kidneys being transplanted with undiagnosed glomerular diseases.

Less rigorous definitions of recurrence include clinical recurrence (symptoms and signs suggestive of disease recurrence, such as proteinuria, hematuria, and kidney dysfunction) or immunological recurrence (newly positive or up-trending pathological autoantibodies or markers suggestive of disease recurrence). Both clinical and immunological recurrence may not necessarily correlate with histopathological recurrence. For example, there may be a "silent" histopathological recurrence detected on protocol kidney biopsy without any clinical or immunological features of disease. The most rigorous definition of recurrence, combining histopathological diagnosis plus graft failure attributed to recurrence, has been employed in some registry studies and provides the ultimate measure of recurrence and its impact.[1]

"De novo diseases" refers to diseases that occur after KT that were not known to be present pretransplant. Several de novo diseases have a substantially different pathophysiology and clinical course post-transplantation compared to pretransplant. Additionally, a recurrent disease may be incorrectly diagnosed as a de novo disease if the patient was not formally diagnosed with the disease prior to transplantation, particularly if the patient was asymptomatic of disease or presented late and was labeled as ESKD of unknown cause.

If a patient experiences allograft loss and concurrently has either a recurrent or de novo disease, a decision needs to be made whether the recurrent or de novo disease is the primary cause of graft loss. Alternative causes of graft loss need to be considered, such as rejection and chronic allograft nephropathy. Making this distinction can be particularly challenging in a patient who has had a long duration of time since transplant, where there may be multiple disease processes leading to graft failure.

Prevalence, Incidence, and Impact of Recurrent and De Novo Diseases

In general, all glomerular and systemic diseases that cause ESKD can recur post-transplantation, however there is wide variability in the frequency of recurrence, timing of recurrence, and risk of allograft loss secondary to disease recurrence (Table 11.1).

Both recurrent and de novo disease may be triggered by factors such as changes in immunosuppression, adverse effects of medications, infections in the post-transplant period, or comorbid diseases or can be idiopathic. Patients may have a predisposition for disease recurrence based on genetic and comorbid factors.

The chance of recurrence generally increases with time post-transplant. Important exceptions include diseases where the presence of an abundant immunological or metabolic mediator, unappreciated at the time of transplant, can cause recurrent disease very soon after transplantation. Prime examples are focal segmental glomerulosclerosis (FSGS; immunological) and oxalosis (metabolic), both of which can cause severe graft dysfunction within days of transplantation. Some systemic diseases that may cause kidney damage, such as diabetes mellitus, are not resolved and may be exacerbated by transplantation thereby incurring risk of recurrence in the graft.

Table 11.1 Select Recurrent and De Novo Diseases Post-KT Including Frequency, Timing, and Risk of Allograft Loss

Disease type	Frequency of disease recurrence post-transplantation	Timing of disease recurrence post-transplantation	Risk of allograft loss if there is disease recurrence in the allograft
Recurrent primary FSGS	9%–55%	Early (days to months)	Up to 50%, often rapid
Recurrent IgA nephropathy	8%–60%	Late (years)	<10% on registry studies, slowly progressive
Recurrent primary membranous nephropathy	Up to 50%	Variable, early or late	Up to 50%, progressive
Recurrent MPGN	Variable depending on subtype, up to 67%	Middle to late	Up to 60%, progressive
Recurrent SLE	Variable depending on study, <5% to 54%	Variable, early or late	Rare
Recurrent AAV	<10% in current era	Both early (days to months) and late (years)	7%–36%
Recurrent scleroderma	Rare	Early (months)	Rare
Recurrent anti-GBM disease	<4%	Variable, early or late	Up to 33% on registry studies
Recurrent complement-mediated TMA	Variable depending on mutation, from <5% to >90%	Early (months)	Up to 100% depending on the mutation
Recurrent diabetes mellitus	Difficult to ascertain	Late (years)	Likely low
Recurrent hyperoxaluria	High	Early	32% in a registry study
De novo anti-GBM in Alport's syndrome	2%–3%	Early (within first year)	Difficult to determine
De novo primary membranous	<10%	Late (years)	Difficult to determine
De novo minimal change disease	Rare	Early (within first month)	Unlikely

Abbreviations: FSGS: focal segmental glomerulosclerosis, MPGN: membranoproliferative glomerulonephritis, SLE: systemic lupus erythematosus, AAV: ANCA-associated vasculitis, GBM: glomerular basement membrane, TMA: thrombotic microangiopathy.

An improved understanding of pathophysiology and advances in management have led to reductions in the incidence and impact of several recurrent diseases. For some of the rarer diseases, there is currently only limited data available regarding incidence, clinical course, and management, mostly confined to case reports and small case series. For these diseases, the literature may be biased toward reporting more severe cases of disease and so it can be difficult to gauge the true epidemiology and trends over time of these diseases.

Recurrent Primary Glomerulonephritis

Primary Focal Segmental Glomerulosclerosis

Primary FSGS is one of the most common causes of nephrotic syndrome in adults and frequently progresses to ESKD. After KT, FSGS has a relatively high recurrence rate of 9%–55%. Recurrence typically occurs within several months of transplant and has been reported to occur within hours. Loss of a previous transplant from recurrence is the strongest predictor of recurrence, while older age of native disease onset, native kidney nephrectomies, and low body mass index are other associations.[2] In contrast to primary FSGS, the other forms of FSGS (secondary and genetic) very rarely recur after KT.

Recurrence is associated with a high risk of allograft loss, with a recent large international cohort study including 57 patients with recurrent FSGS reporting graft loss occurring in 22 (39%) patients over a median of 3.3 years follow-up.[2] Circulating glomerular permeability factors have long been postulated to be causative, though this has never been proven. The success of plasmapheresis in reversing recurrent FSGS provides circumstantial support. Possible candidates include cardiotrophin-like cytokine factor 1 (CLCF-1), calcium/calmodulin-dependent serine protein kinase (CASK),[3] nephrin autoantibodies,[4] and anti-CD40 antibodies.[5] It is presumed that deposition of the "permeability factor" triggers immune-mediated podocyte injury and consequent heavy proteinuria and glomerulosclerosis.

Standard of care treatment for FSGS recurrence involves plasmapheresis or immunoadsorption, which is thought to remove pathogenic circulating glomerular permeability factors. Plasmapheresis is typically continued for 9 cycles over 2–3 weeks, in addition to ongoing calcineurin inhibitor-based transplant immunosuppression including mycophenolate and prednisolone. CD20-directed antibodies such as rituximab have been increasingly used in management. A retrospective study in France of 148 patients with recurrent FSGS found there to be no survival advantage for giving rituximab upfront together with standard of care treatment but it may be useful if standard of care treatment fails or plasmapheresis is withdrawn early.[6] A case series of 27 patients with recurrent FSGS highlighted that some patients may need chronic treatment for primary FSGS recurrence and remain on plasmapheresis long-term to maintain remission.[7] Patients who are maintained on immunosuppression and plasmapheresis for extended periods of time are at an elevated risk of infection, which requires prudent monitoring and ongoing risk assessment. In an attempt to decrease the frequency of recurrence of FSGS post-transplantation, prophylactic therapy (such as plasmapheresis and/or rituximab) post-transplantation has been trialed but has not yielded consistent results to date.

Immunoglobulin A Nephropathy

Immunoglobulin A nephropathy (IgAN) recurrence post-transplantation has a variable disease presentation, commonly manifesting as asymptomatic proteinuria and slow graft dysfunction developing years after transplantation, and uncommonly with macroscopic hematuria, rapid loss of kidney function, and glomerular crescents on biopsy.[8] Histological recurrence is more frequent and earlier than clinical recurrence or graft failure. As a result, there have been wide estimates in the literature of the recurrence rate of IgAN, ranging from 8% to 60%, depending on the cohort, duration of follow-up, and use of clinical or histological criteria for a diagnosis. Recurrence of IgAN is associated with an increased risk of allograft loss. Registry data has demonstrated a risk of graft loss of between 5% and 10% within 10 years of transplantation,[1] with rates higher than 25% being reported in cohort studies.[9,10] However, given the delay in recurrence of IgAN, graft failure may be a combination of IgAN, rejection, and chronic alloimmune injury.

Risk factors for recurrence of IgAN include young recipient age at transplantation, rapid progression of IgAN in the native kidney, heavy proteinuria, and recurrence in a previous transplant. Specific immunosuppressive agents may be protective, particularly maintenance steroids, and potentially use of tacrolimus and basiliximab.[10,11]

Some studies have suggested a possible link between IgAN recurrence and donor-specific antibodies (either formed pretransplant or post-transplant), however these results have not been consistently replicated.

Novel biomarkers for IgAN are being investigated[8] including a proliferation-inducing ligand (APRIL), a cytokine of the tumor necrosis factor superfamily that has been implicated in the pathogenesis of IgAN. A study of 35 patients with IgAN who underwent KT reported that those with biopsy-proven IgA recurrence ($n = 14$) had increased serum APRIL level at 6 months post-transplantation and APRIL levels remained higher in the first 3 years compared to those who did not develop recurrence ($n = 21$).[12] A novel steroid budesonide, designed to deliver treatment targeting mucosal B cells in the ileum, responsible for production of galactose-deficient IgA antibodies has been approved in the United States for the treatment of native kidney IgAN. Its role in preventing or delaying the progression of recurrent IgAN remains to be determined.

Supportive therapy is the mainstay of management of KT recipients with IgAN recurrence, including management of proteinuria and hypertension with angiotensin-converting enzyme inhibitors or angiotensin receptor blockers. As steroid-free maintenance therapy has been strongly associated with graft failure from recurrence, steroids should not be ceased.[11] While addition of steroids to steroid-free patients with recurrence is logical, this strategy has not been tested in clinical trials. Escalating immunosuppression may be considered on a case-by-case basis depending on the clinical circumstances, particularly if there is rapidly progressive disease, but there is little evidence supporting this practice. Agents shown to prevent progression of native kidney IgAN, such as SGLT2-inhibitors, have not been tested for KT recipients after transplant.

Primary Membranous Nephropathy

Developments in our understanding of primary membranous nephropathy (MN) have identified a number of culprit antibodies thought to mediate this disease, particularly anti-phospholipase A2 receptor (PLA2R). Antibodies to other antigens that have been identified as triggers in both primary and secondary MN include thrombospondin type-1 domain-containing 7A (THSD7A), neural epidermal growth factor-like 1 protein (NELL-1), semaphorin 3B (Sema3B), protocadherin 7 (PCDH7), exostosin 1/exostosin 2 (EXT1/EXT2), neural adhesion molecule 1 (NCAM1), contactin 1 (CNTN1), protocadherin FAT-1, proprotein convertase subtilisin/kexin Type 6 (PCSK6), and neuron-derived neurotrophic factor (NDNF). Numerous case reports of post-transplant recurrent MN have demonstrated the presence of the same pathogenic antibody both pre- and post-transplant.

Recurrence rates of up to 50% have been reported, and recurrence is usually associated with proteinuria and/or rise in serum creatinine. Time to recurrence is variable, ranging from early recurrences, commonly within 3 months of transplantation, to late recurrences years later. Diagnosis is confirmed by kidney biopsy, and the culprit autoantibody may be detected in serum. Recurrence is associated with an increased risk of allograft failure, with an Australia and New Zealand Data (ANZDATA) Registry study of 167 patients with MN who underwent KT finding that 19 (11%) patients had disease recurrence after a median time of 3.6 years post-transplantation and of these, 9 (47%) patients experienced graft loss after a median time of 3 years after recurrence.[13]

Risk factors for recurrence of primary MN include high levels of proteinuria pretransplantation, shorter time from ESKD to transplant, and high anti-PLA2R titers pretransplantation and at the time of transplantation.[14] As such, screening for culprit autoantibodies such as anti-PLA2R antibodies at the time of transplant may be useful to identify patients at higher risk of disease recurrence post-transplantation.

Studies have suggested that specific alleles may predispose to primary MN, particularly at the HLA-D and PLA2R1 loci. To investigate their role in disease recurrence post transplantation, an international retrospective cohort study (Europe and Canada) of 105 donor-recipient pairs found several single nucleotide polymorphisms (SNPs) in these loci of the donor allograft that were associated with disease recurrence.[15]

Recurrence of primary MN is usually managed with rituximab in addition to supportive therapy, with proteinuria, eGFR and serum anti-PLA2R antibodies (if present) used to monitor response. The use of rituximab in addition to standard post-transplantation immunosuppression increases the risk of infections, which needs to be considered and monitored. Other options for management have limited evidence and include the proteosome inhibitor bortezomib. The use of prophylactic rituximab to prevent post-transplant recurrence has not been investigated.

Membranoproliferative Glomerulonephritis

Membranoproliferative glomerulonephritis (MPGN) is a pattern of glomerular injury that can be classified as either immune-complex-mediated, complement-mediated, or dysproteinemia. The complement-mediated forms include C3 glomerulopathies such as dense deposit disease and C3 glomerulonephritis. Patients with MPGN are at high risk of post-transplant recurrence, with a recent retrospective study in Spain of 220 KT recipients with MPGN as primary disease reporting a recurrence rate of 18% in those with the immune-complex-mediated form, 62% in those with the complement-mediated forms, and 67% in those with the dysproteinemic form.[16] In this study, recurrence occurred after a median of 16 months and 61% of those with recurrence incurred transplant failure. While recurrence is very common, and progressive loss of graft function is the rule, this may occur after many years and consequently transplantation in general remains worthwhile.

Risk factors for recurrence of MPGN include younger age of MPGN diagnosis, low serum C3 levels, higher proteinuria, and living related-donor kidneys.

Several HLA loci have also been implicated such as the HLA-B8DR3 haplotype. Evidence to support various management options is limited by a paucity of studies given the rarity of these conditions.

For the immune-complex-mediated forms, there is a lack of consensus regarding treatment. Case reports have described success with a combination of rituximab and plasmapheresis.[17] Other treatment strategies include immunosuppression with high-dose steroids and cyclophosphamide.

For recurrent C3 glomerulopathy, our knowledge of its management is largely derived from developments for treating C3 glomerulopathy in native kidneys. Targeted therapies have emerged based on inadequate regulation of the alternative complement pathway in these diseases.[18] Eculizumab has shown to be useful depending on the degree of dysregulation of the alternative pathway and terminal complement cascade, as measured by genetic and functional testing. In select patients, soluble membrane attack complex (sMAC) is a potential biomarker for monitoring while on treatment with eculizumab. Other treatments for C3 glomerulopathy that have been trialed include rituximab, plasma exchange, or aliskiren, with inconsistent results. Treatment for MPGN secondary to dysproteinemia is usually directed at the underlying plasma cell dyscrasia.

Systemic Inflammatory Diseases

Systemic Lupus Erythematosus

Kidney transplant is associated with a survival benefit in those patients with ESKD secondary to lupus nephritis, mainly driven by reductions in mortality from cardiovascular disease and infection.[19] Estimates of recurrence of lupus nephritis in the graft have varied, ranging from <5% to up to 54%, likely due to differences in the type of study (registry or cohort), histopathological classification system used, and duration of follow-up.[20] The timing of recurrence is variable, with both early (days) and late (years) recurrences reported. Most studies are consistent in demonstrating that lupus nephritis is rarely a cause of graft failure.[1] Patients with lupus nephritis are at increased risk of graft thrombosis, particularly those with significant antiphospholipid antibodies, lupus anticoagulant, and previous thrombotic events.

Small Vessel Vasculitis

Patients with antineutrophil cytoplasmic antibody (ANCA)-associated vasculitis (AAV) have a relatively low risk of recurrence in the kidney allograft post-transplantation, with recent studies suggesting rates lower than 10%, likely due to standard post-transplantation immunosuppression suppressing disease. The timing of disease recurrences can be early (days to months) or late (years) post-transplantation, with a median time of approximately 30 months.[21] Recurrence of AAV can manifest as renal-limited disease, extrarenal disease, or both renal and extrarenal disease. ANCA is usually present in serum at time of disease recurrence, but there have been case reports of recurrence without detectable serum ANCA.

Recurrence of AAV is associated with an increased risk of allograft loss. A registry study in the Netherlands reported allograft loss in 4 of 11 (36%) patients who had a renal recurrence of disease within 5 years of transplantation.[22] However, other registry studies have reported rates of graft loss lower than 10% from disease recurrence.[1]

Management of relapses may include glucocorticoids and cyclophosphamide with consideration of rituximab and plasmapheresis on a case-by-case basis. An ANZDATA registry study found that KT recipients who had primary disease AAV had a higher risk of dying with a functioning allograft compared to other etiologies of kidney failure, with mortality mostly driven by malignancy and infection likely because of immunosuppression.[23]

Scleroderma

Given its low prevalence, there is limited data on the outcomes of patients with scleroderma post-KT. A review of the United Network for Organ Sharing (UNOS) database from 1987 to 2004 reported recurrences of scleroderma renal crisis in the kidney allograft in 5 (1.9%) out of 260 KT recipients who had scleroderma.[24] The risk of recurrence appeared to increase if there was rapid progression to ESKD in the patient's native kidneys. It remains unknown whether the glucocorticoids used in transplantation play a significant role in disease recurrence.

Case reports indicate that disease mostly recurred within the first few months after transplantation but can occur 1–2 years later. In several reported cases, disease recurrence was preceded by diffuse skin thickening, new-onset anemia, and cardiac complications.

A European registry study of 57 patients with scleroderma who received a KT reported patient and graft 5-year survivals post-transplantation of 88.2% and 72.4% respectively, which was not different compared to matched controls without scleroderma receiving KT.[25] Graft loss is more likely to be secondary to acute and chronic rejection, as opposed to disease recurrence, which is a rare event.[24,26] Nevertheless, patients who are post-KT are still at risk of extrarenal manifestations of scleroderma.

There is limited evidence regarding management of recurrences of sclero-derma renal crisis post-transplantation, and its management appears to be largely guided by protocols for scleroderma renal crisis used in the nontransplant setting.

Anti–Glomerular Basement Membrane Disease

Recurrence of anti-GBM disease post-transplantation is now a rare event, with recent studies reporting recurrence rates of 1.9%–3.8%.[27,28] Time to recurrence is usually within 5 years of transplantation. When it does recur, there is a high risk of allograft loss, with an ANZDATA registry findings of graft loss in two patients out of six patients with disease recurrence.[29] Postulated risk factors for recur-rence include presence of anti-GBM antibodies at the time of transplantation and reductions in immunosuppression post-transplantation. Recurrence can be detected by reappearance of anti-GBM antibodies in serum and confirmed on kidney biopsy. There is limited data on management strategies for disease recur-rence, but an attempt to treat using high-dose steroids and cyclophosphamide appears prudent.

The presence of linear IgG staining in the allograft kidney biopsy without other features of glomerulonephritis or anti-GBM disease has been reported, and its significance is unclear.[27]

Complement-Mediated Thrombotic Microangiopathy

Complement-mediated thrombotic microangiopathy (TMA), previously known as atypical hemolytic uremic syndrome, occurs due to defects in alternative com-plement pathway regulation and can rapidly progress to kidney failure. Specific mutations and genetic variants of complement genes such as complement factor H (CFH) and membrane-cofactor protein (MCP) have been identified in at least half of affected patients.

The risk of recurrence post-transplantation has been shown to be largely dependent on the specific complement genetic abnormality, ranging from less than 20% in low-risk genetic abnormalities, such as MCP, which will be present on the transplanted kidney, to more than 80% in others.[30] In particular, the highest risk of recurrence has been seen in those patients with CFH mutations or gain of function mutations in C3 or factor B.[31] Living donor transplant carries significant risks of recurrence, unless extensive predonation genetic evaluations are conducted to exclude the presence of pathogenic mutations in the donor.

Recurrence of disease usually occurs within the 1st month but can occur up to several years later.[32] Recurrence can be detected by monitoring for declines in hemoglobin and platelets, reduced haptoglobin, raised lactate dehydrogenase and presence of red cell fragments on blood film review. Diagnosis is confirmed on kidney allograft biopsy showing changes consistent with TMA. In rare circumstances, kidney recurrence may occur in the absence of hematological and biochemical markers of TMA.

Historically, there was a very high risk of graft loss in disease recurrence, with estimates up to 100% depending on the genetic abnormality. The mainstay of treatment currently is the anti-C5 antibody eculizumab, which had substantially improved outcomes. However, it is unclear how long therapy with eculizumab needs to be maintained after KT, how it should be withdrawn, and what monitoring should be done, and further studies are needed. Prophylactic eculizumab is being increasingly used in several transplant centers, particularly in those patients who are at higher risk of recurrence.

Systemic Metabolic Disease

Diabetes Mellitus

Diabetic nephropathy (DN) is one of the leading causes of ESKD. Post-transplantation there is a risk of recurrence of DN in the allograft, however there is limited data available, and interpretation is complicated by the occurrence of post-transplantation diabetes mellitus. Recurrence is usually late. A cohort study of 164 patients with pretransplant diabetes mellitus reported mesangial matrix expansion on kidney allograft biopsy in 47.7% patients by 5 years.[33] The study also found that recurrence occurred despite intensive glycemic control, independent of post-transplant glycated hemoglobin levels.

Many studies reporting long-term transplant outcomes for people with diabetic kidney disease have reported increased mortality and cardiovascular morbidity post-transplantation compared to patients without pre-existing diabetes mellitus.[34] In this context, the risk of graft loss from recurrent DN is substantially less than the risk of premature mortality.

In patients with preexisting type 1 diabetes mellitus and ESKD, simultaneous pancreas-kidney transplantation has proven to have additional benefits in terms of glycemic control and very low risks of recurrence.[35]

Amyloidosis

Kidney transplant has emerged as a suitable treatment for selected patients with ESKD secondary to primary (AL) amyloidosis, particularly those who achieve hematological remission following specific therapy and who have little or no cardiac involvement.

A study of 49 patients in the United States with AL amyloidosis who underwent KT, with a median follow-up of 7.2 years, found clinical and histological
evidence of disease recurrence in 14 (29%) patients with a median time to recurrence of 3.7 years, of whom 4 had allograft loss secondary to amyloidosis.[36]
Median overall survival, graft survival, and amyloid recurrence times were longer
in those patients who had hematologic complete response or very good partial
response prior to KT compared to those with partial response or no response.

Another study of 60 patients in the United States with AL amyloidosis who
underwent KT reported disease recurrence in 13 (22%) patients over a median
follow-up of 61 months, with no allograft loss secondary to disease recurrence.[37]
This study also found improved outcomes in those patients who had complete
or very good partial hematologic response compared to partial response or no
response, but found the improved outcomes were independent of whether the
hematologic response was achieved before or after transplant.

Lastly, a retrospective study in the United Kingdom included 51 patients with
AL amyloidosis and 48 patients with systemic amyloid A (AA) amyloidosis who
underwent KT.[38] The etiology of AA amyloidosis in this cohort included inflammatory arthritis (42%), hereditary periodic fever syndrome (15%), chronic
infection (15%) and inflammatory bowel disease (10%). Of these patients with
AA amyloidosis, 79% had received specific treatment prior to transplantation
(such as chlorambucil, anakinra, tocilizumab, infliximab, colchicine) while 21%
only had supportive therapy. There was disease recurrence in 9 (19%) patients of
those with AA amyloidosis and in 7 (14%) patients of those with AL amyloidosis,
over a median follow-up of 6.1 years post-transplantation. Among the 9 patients
with recurrent AA amyloidosis, allograft loss occurred in 4 (44%) patients at a
median of 4 years post-transplantation and recurrence was associated with elevated serum amyloid A concentration.

Hyperoxaluria

Hyperoxaluria can be primary in which there is an inborn error of hepatic metabolism of oxalate, or secondary if there is another disease process leading to
oxalosis, most commonly leading to excessive enteric absorption. Hyperoxaluria
leads to calcium oxalate kidney stone formation and nephrocalcinosis,
predisposing to ESKD. Prior to transplantation, such patients may have developed a large total body oxalate burden and kidney-alone transplantation may
result in rapid mobilization of systemic oxalate, rapid deposition within the
transplanted kidney, and allograft failure within weeks of transplantation.

Type I primary hyperoxaluria is the most common primary hyperoxaluria,
resulting from deficient alanine–glyoxylate aminotransferase enzyme activity in the liver. Historically, ESKD caused by this disease has been managed

with combined liver-kidney transplantation, however there are now newer therapeutics under investigation such as small interfering RNA treatments that may ameliorate the need for liver transplantation.[39]

Enteric oxalosis is caused by excessive absorption of oxalate from the gastrointestinal tract, typically occurring post–gastric bypass surgery or after extensive bowel resection.

Kidney transplant performed without the knowledge of the etiology of ESKD can result in recurrence of oxalosis in the allograft. Not surprisingly, enteric oxalosis is not corrected by liver or kidney transplantation and a very high risk of recurrence is incurred after KT. Strategies to clear oxalate with intensive dialysis before and after transplantation, coupled with a very low oxalate diet, may enable successful KT in some cases.

An ANZDATA registry study of 19 patients with ESKD secondary to hyperoxaluria (primary or secondary) who underwent KT found allograft failure occurred in 9 (47%) patients over a median follow-up of 9 years post-transplantation, with the causes of allograft failure being disease recurrence (6 patients, 67%), acute rejection (1, 11%), and chronic allograft nephropathy (2, 22%).[40] Risk factors for allograft failure were receiving a KT alone (compared to both kidney and liver) and transplantation after more than 1 year of renal replacement therapy.

Fabry Disease

Fabry disease is an X-linked lysosomal disorder involving a defect in α-galactosidase leading to accumulation of globotriaosylceramide and multisystem dysfunction, resulting in ESKD by the fifth decade. Enzyme replacement therapy can be used to slow progression of disease, but KT remains the gold standard treatment when the disease progresses to ESKD. Fabry disease is not thought to clinically recur in the allograft but there have been reports of histopathological recurrence. Graft survival has been shown to be like matched controls without Fabry disease.[41] It is suggested that patients continue taking enzyme replacement therapy after KT for the extrarenal manifestations of Fabry disease. Cardiovascular diseases have been shown to be a major cause of mortality post-transplantation, and vigilance is required.

Cystinosis

Cystinosis results from loss of function of cystinosin, resulting in accumulation of free cystine in lysosomes and multisystem toxicity. KT is considered curative for the renal manifestations of cystinosis given the presence of functioning cystinosin in the allograft. A retrospective study of 30 patients with cystinosis who underwent KT reported excellent outcomes, with a 10-year graft survival of 86.5%.[42] However, transplant recipients remain at risk of other progressive extrarenal manifestations of cystinosis.

Select De Novo Diseases

Anti-GBM Disease after Transplant in Patients with Alport's Syndrome

Patients with Alport syndrome generally have excellent overall and graft survival post-KT. However, there is a 2%–3% risk of de novo anti-GBM disease occurring within the 1st year after transplant.[43] This is thought to arise because of exposure to collagen IV α5 chain in the transplanted kidney, which may serve as a neoantigen that stimulates development of autoantibodies. Risk factors for occurrence include X-linked collagen IV mutations (and therefore males), progression to ESKD before age 40, and sensorineural deafness. A rise in serum creatinine should prompt testing for serum anti-GBM antibodies and allograft biopsy to confirm the diagnosis. Treatment should include plasma exchange until anti-GBM antibody negative, and consideration of augmentation of immunosuppression to include cyclophosphamide for 6 months. Despite treatment, there is a substantial risk of graft loss and risk of recurrence in subsequent transplants.

De Novo Membranous Nephropathy

De novo primary MN has been described with an incidence of 1%–2% post-KT in adult recipients.[14] It is considered to have a different pathological mechanism and clinical course compared to recurrent primary MN, typically occurring later post-transplantation in younger patients.[44] Serum anti-PLA2R antibodies are not typically present, however circulating immune complexes are. Risk factors include hepatitis B and C infection, malignancy, renal infarction, ureteral obstruction, and antibody-mediated rejection. In addition to anti-PLA2R antibodies, cases have also been described with antibodies to THSD7A and NELL-1 antigens.[45]

Diagnosis is confirmed by kidney biopsy showing basement membrane IgG deposits and changes typical of primary membranous nephropathy, however there is less likely to be severe foot-process effacement. In some cases, mesangial hypercellularity and focal and segmental distribution of deposits are apparent.

There is an associated increased risk of graft loss, but given that it can co-occur with antibody-mediated rejection, it is difficult to quantify the allograft loss attributed to de novo primary MN. A multicenter case series that included 27 KT recipients with de novo MN reported inferior graft survival compared to those patients with recurrent MN (hazard ratio 3.2).[44] Management may include a combination of steroids, rituximab, plasma exchange, and intravenous immunoglobulin.

De Novo Minimal Change Disease

De novo minimal change disease is a rare occurrence post-transplantation with data limited to case reports and small series.[46,47] Disease onset is usually within one month of transplantation, presenting with nephrotic-range proteinuria with or without a raised creatinine. Diagnosis is confirmed by kidney biopsy. Other causes of proteinuria in the post-transplant period need to be first ruled out, such as FSGS. Treatment is not evidence-based but may involve management of proteinuria and consideration of high-dose steroids. Most patients have a remission from disease without any long-term sequalae.

Future Directions

An emerging area is the development of risk prediction tools that can identify patients who are at a higher risk of disease recurrence post-KT. This may involve novel serum or urine markers as well as genetic markers such as single nucleotide polymorphisms from both the donor and recipient. Use of machine learning and artificial intelligence may assist in developing models based on big data, particularly genetic and epigenetic sequencing data. If such risk prediction models are used prior to transplant, they may potentially assist with selection of living donors and may guide post-transplant care.

One caveat in identifying patients at a higher risk of recurrence is that we would ideally need evidence-based therapeutic strategies that could be given in the peritransplant period to either reduce the risk of recurrence or minimize the impact of disease recurrence. Very little evidence currently exists to support such strategies, and this is an emerging area of need.

A challenge for research in this area is the relatively low numbers of patients who are at risk of or develop recurrent or de novo glomerular diseases post-transplant, and the sparse geographical distribution of such patients. National registries have yielded excellent information on incidence, risk factors, and consequences of recurrence, but cannot be used in their current observational form to define effective therapies. To prove prevention or treatment strategies, randomized clinical trials will be required. Achieving adequate recruitment and follow-up in clinical trials will require multicenter, multinational collaborations. Development of such collaborations and, ideally, well characterized cohorts of patients is the next step required to build a platform for meaningful research into prevention and management of recurrent disease.

Conclusion

Disease recurrence after KT is a significant contributor to morbidity and mortality for ESKD patients after KT. Despite this, KT remains the preferred modality of kidney replacement therapy for the majority. With advances in the field of glomerulonephritis through characterization of the pathophysiological mechanisms and mediators of recurrence, there is improved capacity to prevent, predict, diagnose, and manage disease recurrence post KT. This will lead to further improvements in long-term survival.

References

1. Briganti EM, Russ GR, McNeil JJ, Atkins RC, Chadban SJ. Risk of renal allograft loss from recurrent glomerulonephritis. *N Engl J Med.* 2002;347(2):103–109.
2. Uffing A, Pérez-Sáez MJ, Mazzali M, et al. Recurrence of FSGS after kidney transplantation in adults. *Clin J Am Soc Nephrol.* 2020;15(2):247–256.
3. Beaudreuil S, Zhang X, Herr F, et al. Circulating CASK is associated with recurrent focal segmental glomerulosclerosis after transplantation. *PLoS ONE.* 2019;14(7):e0219353.
4. Hattori M, Shirai Y, Kanda S, et al. Circulating nephrin autoantibodies and posttransplant recurrence of primary focal segmental glomerulosclerosis. *Am J Transplant.* 2022;22(10):2478–2480.
5. Delville M, Sigdel TK, Wei C, et al. A circulating antibody panel for pretransplant prediction of FSGS recurrence after kidney transplantation. *Sci Transl Med.* 2014;6(256):256ra136.
6. Lanaret C, Anglicheau D, Audard V, et al. Rituximab for recurrence of primary focal segmental glomerulosclerosis after kidney transplantation: results of a nationwide study. *Am J Transplant.* 2021;21(9):3021–3033.
7. Uffing A, Hullekes F, Hesselink DA, et al. Long-term apheresis in the management of patients with recurrent focal segmental glomerulosclerosis after kidney transplantation. *Kidney Int Rep.* 2022;7(6):1424–1427.
8. Wyld ML, Chadban SJ. Recurrent IgA nephropathy after kidney transplantation. *Transplantation.* 2016;100(9):1827–1832.
9. Moroni G, Longhi S, Quaglini S, et al. The long-term outcome of renal transplantation of IgA nephropathy and the impact of recurrence on graft survival. *Nephrol Dial Transplant.* 2013;28:1305–1314.

‛10. Uffing A, Pérez-Saéz MJ, Jouve T, et al. Recurrence of IgA nephropathy after kidney transplantation in adults. *Clin J Am Soc Nephrol.* 2021;16(8):1247–1255.

11. Clayton P, McDonald S, Chadban S. Steroids and recurrent IgA nephropathy after kidney transplantation. *Am J Transplant.* 2011;11(8):1645–1649.

12. Martín-Penagos L, Benito-Hernández A, San Segundo D, et al. A proliferation-inducing ligand increase precedes IgA nephropathy recurrence in kidney transplant recipients. *Clin Transplant.* 2019;33(4):e13502.

13. Yang WL, Bose B, Zhang L, et al. Long-term outcomes of patients with end-stage kidney disease due to membranous nephropathy: a cohort study using the Australia and New Zealand Dialysis and Transplant Registry. *PloS ONE.* 2019;14(8):e0221531.

14. Leon J, Pérez-Sáez MJ, Batal I, et al. Membranous nephropathy posttransplantation: an update of the pathophysiology and management. *Transplantation.* 2019;103(10):1990–2002.

15. Berchtold L, Letouzé E, Alexander MP, et al. HLA-D and PLA2R1 risk alleles associate with recurrent primary membranous nephropathy in kidney transplant recipients. *Kid Int.* 2021;99(3):671–685.

16. Caravaca-Fontán F, Polanco N, Villacorta B, et al. Recurrence of immune complex and complement-mediated membranoproliferative glomerulonephritis in kidney transplantation. *Nephrol Dial Transplant.* 2022;38(1):222–235.

17. Yango AF, Fischbach BV, Ruiz R, Mudrovich S, Klintmalm G. Treatment of recurrent, post-kidney transplant membranoproliferative glomerulonephritis with plasmapheresis and rituximab: a case report and literature review. *Clin Nephrol.* 2019;91(1):52.

18. Bomback AS, Smith RJ, Barile GR, et al. Eculizumab for dense deposit disease and C3 glomerulonephritis. *Clin J Am Soc Nephrol.* 2012;7(5):748–756.

19. Jorge A, Wallace ZS, Lu N, Zhang Y, Choi HK. Renal transplantation and survival among patients with lupus nephritis: a cohort study. *Ann Intern Med.* 2019;170(4):240–247.

20. Contreras G, Mattiazzi A, Guerra G, et al. Recurrence of lupus nephritis after kidney transplantation. *J Am Soc Nephrol.* 2010;21(7):1200–1207.

21. Nachman PH, Segelmark M, Westman K, et al. Recurrent ANCA-associated small vessel vasculitis after transplantation: a pooled analysis. *Kid Int.* 1999;56(4):1544–1550.

22. Göçeroglu A, Rahmattulla C, Berden AE, et al. The Dutch Transplantation in Vasculitis (DUTRAVAS) Study: outcome of renal transplantation in antineutrophil cytoplasmic antibody–associated glomerulonephritis. *Transplantation.* 2016;100(4):916–924.

23. Kuhnel L, Hawley CM, Johnson DW, Gobe GC, Ellis RJ, Francis RS. Allograft failure in kidney transplant recipients who developed kidney failure secondary to ANCA-associated vasculitis. *Clin Transplant.* 2021;35(4):e14235.

24. Pham PT, Pham PC, Danovitch GM, et al. Predictors and risk factors for recurrent scleroderma renal crisis in the kidney allograft: case report and review of the literature. *Am J Transplant.* 2005;5(10):2565–2569.

25. Hruskova Z, Pippias M, Stel VS, et al. Characteristics and outcomes of patients with systemic sclerosis (scleroderma) requiring renal replacement therapy in Europe: results from the ERA-EDTA registry. *Am J Kidney Dis.* 2019;73(2):184–193.

26. Gibney EM, Parikh CR, Jani A, Fischer MJ, Collier D, Wiseman AC. Kidney transplantation for systemic sclerosis improves survival and may modulate disease activity. *Am J Transplant.* 2004;4(12):2027–2031.

27. Coche S, Sprangers B, Van Laecke S, et al. Recurrence and outcome of anti-glomerular basement membrane glomerulonephritis after kidney transplantation. *Kidney Int Rep.* 2021;6(7):1888–1894.
28. Singh T, Kharadjian TB, Astor BC, Panzer SE. Long-term outcomes in kidney transplant recipients with end-stage kidney disease due to anti-glomerular basement membrane disease. *Clin Transplant.* 2021;35(2):e14179.
29. Tang W, McDonald SP, Hawley CM, et al. Anti-glomerular basement membrane antibody disease is an uncommon cause of end-stage renal disease. *Kidney Int.* 2013;83(3):503–510.
30. Loirat C, Fremeaux-Bacchi V. Hemolytic uremic syndrome recurrence after renal transplantation. *Pediatr Transplant.* 2008;12(6):619–629.
31. Le Quintrec M, Zuber J, Moulin B, et al. Complement genes strongly predict recurrence and graft outcome in adult renal transplant recipients with atypical hemolytic and uremic syndrome. *Am J Transplant.* 2013;13(3):663–675.
32. Noris M, Remuzzi G. Thrombotic microangiopathy after kidney transplantation. *Am J Transplant.* 2010;10(7):1517–1523.
33. Coemans M, Van Loon E, Lerut E, et al. Occurrence of diabetic nephropathy after renal transplantation despite intensive glycemic control: an observational cohort study. *Diabetes Care.* 2019;42(4):625–634.
34. Lim WH, Wong G, Pilmore HL, McDonald SP, Chadban SJ. Long-term outcomes of kidney transplantation in people with type 2 diabetes: a population cohort study. *Lancet Diabetes Endocrinol.* 2017;5(1):26–33.
35. Redfield RR, Scalea JR, Odorico JS. Simultaneous pancreas and kidney transplantation: current trends and future directions. *Curr Opin Organ Transplant.* 2015;20(1):94.
36. Angel-Korman A, Stern L, Sarosiek S, et al. Long-term outcome of kidney transplantation in AL amyloidosis. *Kid Int.* 2019;95(2):405–411.
37. Heybeli C, Bentall A, Wen J, et al. A study from The Mayo Clinic evaluated long-term outcomes of kidney transplantation in patients with immunoglobulin light chain amyloidosis. *Kid Int.* 2021;99(3):707–715.
38. Law S, Cohen O, Lachmann HJ, et al. Renal transplant outcomes in amyloidosis. *Nephrol Dial Transplant.* 2021;36(2):355–365.
39. Devresse A, Cochat P, Godefroid N, Kanaan N. Transplantation for primary hyperoxaluria type 1: designing new strategies in the era of promising therapeutic perspectives. *Kidney Int Rep.* 2020;5(12):2136–2145.
40. Heron VC, Kerr PG, Kanellis J, Polkinghorne KR, Isbel NM, See EJ. Long-term graft and patient outcomes following kidney transplantation in end-stage kidney disease secondary to hyperoxaluria. *Transplant Proc.* 2021;53(3):839–847.
41. Ersözlü S, Desnick RJ, Huynh-Do U, et al. Long-term outcomes of kidney transplantation in Fabry disease. *Transplantation.* 2018;102(11):1924–1933.
42. Cohen C, Charbit M, Chadefaux-Vekemans B, et al. Excellent long-term outcome of renal transplantation in cystinosis patients. *Orphanet J Rare Dis.* 2015;10:90.
43. Kashtan CE. Renal transplantation in patients with Alport syndrome: patient selection, outcomes, and donor evaluation. *Int J Nephrol Renovasc Dis.* 2018;11:267–270.
44. Batal I, Vasilescu ER, Dadhania DM, et al. Association of HLA typing and alloimmunity with posttransplantation membranous nephropathy: a multicenter case series. *Am J Kidney Dis.* 2020;76(3):374–383.

45. Münch J, Krüger BM, Weimann A, et al. Posttransplant nephrotic syndrome resulting from NELL1-positive membranous nephropathy. *Am J Transplant.* 2021;21(9):3175–3179.
46. Zafarmand AA, Baranowska-Daca E, Ly PD, et al. De novo minimal change disease associated with reversible post-transplant nephrotic syndrome: a report of five cases and review of literature. *Clin Transplant.* 2002;16(5):350–361.
47. Mochizuki Y, Iwata T, Nishikido M, Uramatsu T, Sakai H, Taguchi T. De novo minimal change disease after ABO-incompatible kidney transplantation. *Clin Transplant.* 2012;26:81–85.

12

Behavior and Psychosocial Functioning after Kidney Transplantation

Jennifer L. Steel and Daniel Cukor

Disorders of human behavior, impacting kidney transplant survival!

Contribution of Psychosocial and Behavioral Conditions to Survival Post–Renal Transplant

Psychosocial and behavioral factors are considered among the determinants of health and are critical in the development and progression of chronic disease. Psychosocial factors, including anxiety, post-traumatic stress disorder (PTSD), and depression, and behavioral factors, such as diet, physical activity, and substance use, may contribute to the development of end-stage renal disease. These psychosocial and behavioral factors remain important for quality and quantity of life post–renal transplant. While psychosocial factors such as depression, sleep, anxiety, and substance use have been shown to contribute to increased risk of mortality in other chronic diseases, there is a paucity of research linking these factors to post–kidney transplant survival.

Of the research that has been performed, several of these psychosocial and behavioral factors have been associated with poorer survival in renal transplant recipients (Figure 12.1). In a meta-analysis, depression was shown to increase the risk of graft loss and mortality across all solid organ transplant recipients.[1] Anxiety, albeit less studied, has been shown to increase the risk of mortality among kidney transplant recipients.[2] Behavioral factors including sleep disorders and fatigue were found to be associated with increased risk of all-cause mortality post–kidney transplantation.[3,4] Tobacco use has long been known to increase the risk of cancer, cardiovascular disease, and mortality across all solid organ transplant recipients.[5] While the rates of drug use in kidney transplant recipients is low, marijuana use post-transplant has been associated with increased death-censored graft failure, but not mortality.[6] Prescription opioid use has also been shown to be linked to a higher risk of complications, graft loss, and mortality. The relationship between opioids and

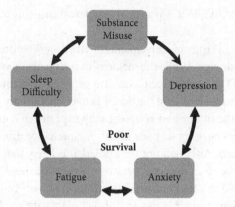

Figure 12.1 Psychosocial and behavioral factors associated with poorer survival after renal transplant.

poor outcomes are associated with the dose of the opioids and is like what has been observed in other transplant recipients. No studies were found in the literature regarding other types of drug use (e.g., cocaine, IV drug use) and survival. Behavioral factors such as nonadherence to immunosuppressive medications, pain, and maintenance of a healthy weight (e.g., exercise and diet) are also critical in long-term quality of life and survival. They are discussed in detail in Chapters 3 and 13, respectively. In this chapter we discuss psychological adjustment post-transplant and psychological disorders most common in patients post–renal transplant (e.g., depression and anxiety, post-traumatic stress disorder, substance abuse, fatigue and sleep disorder).

Long-Term Psychosocial Adjustment Post–Kidney Transplant

Living and Deceased Donor Kidney Recipients

The receipt of a life-saving or life-enhancing organ is unique to transplant. The gift is experienced in different ways depending on if it is a living donor (LD) versus deceased donor (DD) organ. DD organ transplants have continued to grow while the number of LD organ transplant has remained stable over the last decade. Most LD and DD transplant recipients report gratitude for the gift. However, those who have received a DD have reported feelings of guilt for having to have someone die for them to be able live. Some donors also report the development of new preferences or personality traits that they believe may have been from the DD. While it is possible, very few transplant recipients meet the DD family.

In contrast, the LD transplant recipients often know their donor, both directed and nondirected donors. While the majority of recipients meet their donor after the transplant, LD transplant recipients also experience gratitude for the organ they receive and while knowing the donor is overwhelmingly positive there are instances where the donor and recipient may experience conflict, particularly if the recipient is engaging in poor health maintenance after transplant (e.g., smoking, poor diet). Although not yet studied, it is likely that having a LD may improve adherence to immunosuppressive medications and reduce poor life-style behaviors, and as a result may enhance long-term survival. The rates of psychosocial and behavioral problems and/or disorders have not been well studied in renal transplant recipients.

Psychological Disorders Common in Renal Transplant Recipients

Renal transplant patients have higher rates of psychological disorders when compared to the general population. Table 12.1 depicts the estimated rates based on current evidence.

Depression and Anxiety

Depression and anxiety are the most common mental health challenges among kidney transplant recipients. The prevalence rates vary by the type of assessment,

Table 12.1 Rates of Psychosocial and Behavioral Conditions in Renal Transplant Recipients

Psychosocial or behavioral condition	Rates
Depression	20%–40% w/ symptoms; 10% w/diagnosis
Anxiety	10%–30%
Post-Traumatic Stress Disorder	Unknown
Fatigue	20%–60%
Sleep Problems	40%–60%
Substance Misuse	<1%

with self-report measures indicating higher levels of symptoms of depression and anxiety, as opposed to interview-based or clinician assessments, which are more focused on the diagnosis of anxiety or depression. The rates of psychological distress are estimated to be between 20% and 40%, and the rates of a diagnosable major depressive disorder closer to the 10% range. These estimates are significantly below the rates observed in patients being treated with hemodialysis, but higher than the general population. Anxiety is less widely studied and is often comorbid with depression, further complicating its assessment. The rates of elevated anxiety symptoms are estimated to be 10%–30% in kidney transplant recipients, which is also lower than people treated with hemodialysis but higher than the general population.

There is scant evidence for the treatment of depression or anxiety that is specific to the kidney transplant recipient. There are no controlled pharmacological trials in this population, but trials in earlier stage chronic kidney disease (CKD) and with patients who are dialysis-dependent have shown mixed results, with the CAST trial showing no benefit for sertraline over placebo in non-dialysis-dependent patients with CKD, and the ASCEND trial demonstrating an effect for sertraline in dialysis-dependent patients with end-stage kidney disease (ESKD), but with an increase in serious side effects.[7]

While antidepressant use may be effect in ESKD, in a retrospective analysis of a national US transplant registry, antidepressant use in the 1st year after transplant has been associated with higher risk of death and graft failure.[8] The cost-benefit analysis for antidepressant use in patients with kidney transplants is far from clear, and clinical trials are desperately needed. The psychosocial treatments of depression and anxiety do not result in serious side effects as with pharmacological treatments. Cognitive-behavioral therapy, mindfulness-based stress reduction, and problem-solving therapy have all been shown to reduce depression and anxiety, at least in the short term, in kidney transplant recipients. Larger clinical trials with longer follow-up periods are needed to better understand the magnitude and duration of these effects.

Post-Traumatic Stress Disorder

The most common event resulting in PTSD in kidney transplant patients is medical trauma, which is defined as set of psychological and physiological responses to pain, injury, serious illness, medical procedures, and/or frightening treatment. While patients may have been exposed to other traumatic events (e.g., combat, assault) and develop PTSD, we will focus on medical trauma due to the prevalence in those who have been treated with dialysis and/or are transplant recipients.

Approximately 20%–30% of patients who have been in the intensive care unit and 15%–25% of children and 30%–33% of adults experience psychosocial and behavioral consequences associated with a traumatic medical experience. The factors that make a medical experience traumatic include: (1) the nature of the illness, (2) the feeling of shock and/or loss of sense of control, (3) life-altering complications or an unexpected medical intervention, (4) the noise and disruptions in routine associated with a long hospitalization, (5) hallucinations caused by delirium, and (6) perceived or actual mistreatment by medical providers.

Symptoms of PTSD are the most common consequence of medical trauma, but people also suffer from depression, anxiety, substance use, and legal and re-lationship problems as a result of medical trauma. Treatment of medical trauma may include the standard of care for the presenting symptom or disorder (e.g., PTSD, depression) but if possible, having a provider who is knowledgeable about medical trauma and in the case of PTSD understanding of the theory of the enduring somatic threat (e.g., internal threat versus external threat) is im-portant for the efficacy of the treatment. There are no estimates for the rates of medical trauma in kidney transplant recipients, but having chronic incurable disease, the many exposures to the medical system (e.g., surgeries, dialysis) and the existential threat to life, all place people with kidney transplants at greater risk for significant traumatic reactions. Only one study has been conducted fo-cused on PTSD and survival, and it did not find that those who had a history of PTSD were at greater risk for complications, graft rejection, or increased risk of mortality.

Substance Use

The rates at which people with kidney transplants use or misuse alcohol or substances are not known. Analyses conducted on the United State Renal Data System (USRDS) suggest very low rates of alcohol dependence (<1%) at the time of ESKD diagnosis, but transplant recipient substance abuse at time of transplan-tation was associated with a small but significant increased risk of death after transplantation. Two small European prospective studies in kidney transplant recipients both identified alcohol use to be common, but there were low rates of problematic alcohol consumption and no observable relationships between alcohol use and negative health outcomes. The rate of recreational marijuana use is not well documented in kidney transplant recipients, but some estimates suggest current use is rare (3%–5%). Retrospective analyses have not identified increased rejection risk with recreational marijuana use in small samples.[6] The impact of the growing legalization of recreational marijuana in the United States on the kidney transplant recipient is unclear but should certainly be carefully monitored.

Fatigue and Sleep Difficulties

Fatigue is difficult to define but is often thought of as extreme tiredness not resulting from mental or physical exertion and comprises physical, psychological, and emotional components. Similarly, sleep quality can be defined in a variety of ways but comprises both a subjective sense of having had restorative sleep and objective parameters of sleep success (sleep efficiency, sleep latency, number of awakenings, etc.).

The relationship between fatigue, sleep difficulty, and psychological distress is complex, with both fatigue and tiredness leading to psychosocial sequela and increased psychological distress causing patients to be more tired and sleep less well. The prevalence of fatigue in people with kidney transplants has only been reported in a few studies and varies between 20% and 60%, making it one of the most identified challenges to quality of life. The rates of sleep difficulty are also varied in the literature, with most studies reporting 40%–60% of kidney transplant recipients with self-reported poor sleep quality.

Study of the treatments for fatigue and sleep difficulty are underdeveloped. Regular exercise, behavioral activation, and pacing have all been shown to be effective in addressing distress caused by fatigue in other medical populations, but there is limited information available that is specific to the kidney transplant population. Similarly, pharmacological treatments of sleep difficulty in mixed populations have low rates of success, high rates of unwanted side-effects, and may be associated with risks for falls or other medical complications, but again, there is limited data specific to the kidney transplant population. Cognitive-behavioral therapy for insomnia, relaxation training, and stress reduction all hold promise to increase energy and promote sleep health as well as minimize the impact of fatigue and sleep difficulty on quality of life (Table 12.2).

New Directions in Long-Term Renal Transplant Recipient Care

Side Effects of Medications

Patients with end-stage renal disease who undergo kidney transplantation report an improved quality of life post-transplant, but patients still report symptoms and side effects from medications affecting their overall quality of life. The science of

Table 12.2 Hypothesized Mechanisms of Psychological and Behavioral Factors on Kidney Transplant Outcome

Depression	**Hypothesized Link to Survival:** Depression is marked by lack of motivation, and for the kidney transplant recipient this may be of particular concern, as their ability to committedly take their immunosuppressant medication and engage in other health behaviors may be reduced. Studies have shown a relationship between increased depression and reduced medication adherence. Inflammation has also been hypothesized as a potential mediator of depression and survival, however this has not been studied in renal transplant recipients.
	Example: Ms. D was adjusting well to her life post-dialysis until her husband passed away. She made it through the initial grief stages with support of her family, but then depression set in and continued for the next two years. She was no longer able to reliably care for herself, letting her diet and personal care suffer. She began missing doses of her medication and despite showing signs of rejection, she did not contact the transplant team due to her depression.
Anxiety	**Hypothesized Link to Survival:** People with high levels of anxiety can be high or low utilizers of healthcare and as a result may avoid necessary medical appointments or procedures or may inundate their healthcare providers with somatic concerns, making it difficult to identify critical healthcare concerns that may be treatable.
	Example: Mr. A accepted his third kidney offer, after 7 years on peritoneal dialysis. He is extremely involved in his treatment and wants the physician to allow him to titrate his immunosuppression based on how he feels. He would often "be creative" with his dialysis treatment and insists he knows his body best, the loss of control over his treatment was challenging for him, and he calls the office nearly daily, but as he began to reject the kidney the nurse did not take his symptoms seriously due to his frequent complaints.
Fatigue	**Hypothesized Link to Survival:** Decreased physical activity can lead to muscle atrophy and increased body mass index, which leads to multiple chronic medical conditions (e.g., cancer, cardiovascular disease).
	Example: One of Ms. F's greatest motivations to get off dialysis was her constant fatigue. She has been extremely disappointed with her lack of energy level, now going on 2 years post-transplant. She acknowledges she feels better now than she did on dialysis but was hoping to feel like "herself" of when she began dialysis, nearly 12 years ago. She has gained 50 pounds and has now requires three blood pressure medications and has developed diabetes.
Poor sleep	**Hypothesized Link to Survival:** Chronic sleep difficulties and sleep apnea are independent predictors of mortality, which may be due to underlying cardiovascular abnormalities or the fatigue, mood changes, and psychosocial isolation all associated with poor sleep. Inflammation has also been hypothesized as a potential mediator between sleep and mortality in other chronic diseases and the general population.

Table 12.2 Continued

	Example: Mr. C experienced chronic fatigue and had difficulties maintaining alertness during the day. His wife complained of his snoring and mentioned his sleepiness and snoring to his doctor. He was referred to a sleep disorders center and was diagnosed with sleep apnea. While he was prescribed a continuous positive airway pressure (CPAP) device, he did not use it. As a result, Mr. C died of cardiovascular disease that may have been preventable.
Substance misuse	**Hypothesized Link to Survival:** Depending on the substance and its amount, there could a direct biological pathway between overuse and death (e.g., IV drug use) and increased risk of cancer or other medical problems such as in the case of tobacco use (e.g., COPD).
	Example: Mr. C had worked in the steel mills and smoked since he was a teenager. While he was successful in quitting prior to transplant as he would not be listed unless he stopped smoking, once he was transplanted, he started to smoke again. He went on to develop lung cancer and died approximately 2 years after transplantation.

symptom clusters has emerged in the last two decades in the hopes of identifying common underlying biological mechanisms associated with the symptoms to develop targeted treatments. While symptom clusters have been identified and biological and genetic underpinnings have been examined, symptom clusters have been less studied in the context of kidney transplantation. Of the studies that do exist, 62 symptoms were included and the clusters that were identified included (1) emotional-sleep, (2) pain-gastrointestinal, (3) immune-related symptoms, (4) fatigue, and (5) visual dysfunction. Future research is warranted to better understand the symptoms clusters patients experience and lead to poorer quality of life post-transplant. Treatment of these symptoms is needed to improve the quality of life of the recipient and possibly survival.

Care for Transplant Patients' Caregivers

Although patients are required to identify a caregiver prior to listing for transplant, due to the importance of support, there is a paucity of research regarding family caregivers and kidney transplantation.[9] Caregiving has been associated with increased risk of cardiovascular disease and while the transplant recipient may have improved quality of life after transplant, research suggests that caregivers of kidney transplant recipients are significantly affected, with lower levels of life satisfaction before and after transplant. Similarly, caregivers of pediatric kidney transplant patients also report stress and burden persisting after transplant. While family caregiving has been extensively studied in those caring for people diagnosed with dementia and more recently cancer, there remains a paucity of research regarding the needs of family caregivers of renal transplant candidates.

Palliative Care

While kidney transplantation has been performed for over seven decades, new areas continue to emerge. While at some point, every kidney transplant recipient will die, referral by the transplant team for palliative care or hospice for transplant recipients is not common, despite the close follow-up of recipients and the frequency of hospitalization for kidney transplant recipients (e.g., six times higher than the general population). This may be in part because the patient, family, and transplant team remain hopeful that they will receive another organ in the case of failing allograft. Even if a patient returns to dialysis, nephrology referrals to palliative care or hospice are more common and interventions are being developed specifically for patients with end-stage renal disease on hemodialysis.

Conclusion

The evaluation and treatment of psychosocial and behavioral factors are important both pre- and post-transplant to improve long-term outcomes. While much research has been performed in this area, there remains much to do in the context of psychosocial and behavioral functioning in renal transplant recipients to improve quality and quantity of life.

References

1. Dew MA, Rosenberger EM, Myaskovsky L, et al. Depression and anxiety as risk factors for morbidity and mortality after organ transplantation: a systematic review and meta-analysis. *Transplantation*. 2015;100(5):988–1003.
2. Schouten RW, Haverkamp GL, Loosman WL, et al. Anxiety symptoms, mortality, and hospitalization in patients receiving maintenance dialysis: a cohort study. *Am J Kidney Dis*. 2019;74(2):158–166.
3. Yang XH, Zhang BL, Gu YH, Zhan XL, Guo LL, Jin HM. Association of sleep disorders, chronic pain, and fatigue with survival in patients with chronic kidney disease: a meta-analysis of clinical trials. *Sleep Med*. 2018;51:59–65.
4. Lubas MM, Ware JC, Szklo-Coxe M. Sleep apnea and kidney transplant outcomes: findings from a 20-year (1997–2017) historical cohort study. *Sleep Med*. 2019;63:151–158.

5. Bossola M, Arena M, Urciuolo F, et al. Fatigue in kidney transplantation: a systematic review and meta-analysis. *Diagnostics.* 2021;11(5):833.

6. Vaitla PK, Thongprayoon C, Hansrivijit P, et al. Epidemiology of cannabis use and associated outcomes among kidney transplant recipients: a meta-analysis. *J Evid Based Med.* 2021;14(2):90–96.

7. Mehrotra R, Cukor D, Unruh M, et al. Comparative efficacy of therapies for treatment of depression for patients undergoing maintenance hemodialysis: a randomized clinical trial. *Ann Intern Med.* 2019;170(6):369–379.

8. Lentine KL, Naik AS, Ouseph R, et al. Antidepressant medication use before and after kidney transplant: implications for outcomes–a retrospective study. *Transplant International.* 2018;31(1):20–31.

9. Rodrigue JR, Dimitri N, Reed A, et al. Spouse caregivers of kidney transplant patients: quality of life and psychosocial outcomes. *Prog Transplant.* 2010;20(4):335–342.

13

Social Determinants Impacting Transplant Outcomes

Akhil Sharma and Allyson Hart

Education, Environment and Economics impacting kidney transplant outcomes!

Introduction

While the transplant community celebrates improvements in long-term kidney allograft outcomes, research and policy are increasingly focused on further improving long-term patient and graft outcomes. In addition, frustrations remain regarding the persistence of gaps in outcomes based on socioeconomic factors and other social determinants of health (SDoH). While research and advancements in medical factors, such as improved immunosuppression, cancer treatments, and cardiovascular disease management, are all critical to achieving this goal, SDoH, which are one of the largest contributors to poor outcomes, are less well studied by the transplant research community. In this chapter, we will review SDoH, describe how they impact kidney transplant (KT) recipient outcomes, and discuss strategies and additional research priorities to realize the full promise of better KT outcomes for patients with kidney disease.

Definitions and Classification of Social Determinants of Health

The US Department of Health and Human Services Healthy People 2030 defines SDoH as "the conditions in the environments where people are born, live, learn, work, play, worship, and age that affect a wide range of health functioning, and quality-of-life outcomes and risks." These determinants are classified into five categories:

- Education Access and Quality: Language and literacy; early childhood education; primary, secondary, and higher education; vocational training,

- Healthcare Access and Quality: Health insurance, health system and provider accessibility, health literacy and numeracy, quality of healthcare,
- Neighborhood and Built Environment: Housing safety, access to nutritious food and recreation, transportation and isolation, social order and walkability, and environmental exposures,
- Social and Community Context: Social norms, network and culture, mistrust, community engagement, segregation and discrimination, media, and technology access, and•Economic Stability: Income, employment, housing stability, and food security (Figure 13.1).[1]

While race and ethnicity are not social determinants per se, marginalized communities bear a disproportionate burden of social determinants,[2] therefore equity in KT outcomes is inextricably linked to SDoH.

While healthcare providers are typically focused on the biologic basis of disease and treatments that can be prescribed or provided within healthcare

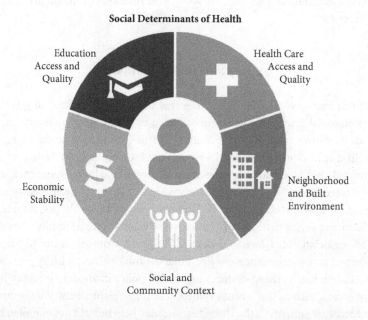

Figure 13.1 Framework for Social Determinants of Health: Healthy People 2030. U.S. Department of Health and Human Services, Office of Disease Prevention and Health Promotion.

settings, only a minority of premature deaths can be attributed to genetic pre-disposition or the provision of healthcare.[3] At least 50% of premature deaths are attributable to SDoH. Cardiovascular disease (CVD) remains one of the highest risk factors for morbidity and mortality in KT recipients, and SDoH play a key role in the risk of CVD. In one meta-analysis of more than 1.7 million participants in 48 clinical trials spanning 7 high-income World Health Organization (WHO) member countries, employment classification alone conferred a cardiovascular risk equivalent to traditional risk factors. Lower occupational position (classified as high, intermediate, or low) was associated with a 2.1-year decrease in life-years, compared to 1.6 years for hypertension and 3.9 years for diabetes.[4] For KT recipients, realizing optimal long-term outcomes requires expansion of our healthcare lens to include these important factors. While many SDoH are beyond the traditional purview of transplant providers, others are more amenable to intervention and advocacy on the part of healthcare providers and organizations. The adverse medical outcomes of greatest importance to long-term patient and allograft survival and their con-nection to potentially modifiable social determinants of health are illustrated in Table 13.1.

Key Social Determinants

The full impact of SDoH on KT recipient outcomes is difficult to quantify, as data on social determinants are not collected by large transplant registries. Using crude measures, such as socioeconomic status (SES) index scores by zip code, Axelrod et al. demonstrated a dose-response increase in both death and death-censored graft failure among both deceased donor and living donor recipients in the United States, with a 15%–30% increase in death and death-censored graft loss in the lowest versus highest SES index score quartiles.[5] The precise role of the influence of access to health insurance is also unclear. Mixed results from studies of the association between measures of SES and KT outcomes in countries with universal access to healthcare suggest that insurance access is likely part, but not all, of the issue.[6-8] These studies suggest that policy changes to improve health-care access, such as the recent expansion of immunosuppressive drug coverage for Medicare patients in the United States, may help but will not completely mit-igate the impact of SDoH on allograft outcomes. Health literacy is another po-tentially modifiable target for interventions to improve outcomes. Lower health literacy has been associated with decreased access to transplant; however, studies in outcomes among KT recipients are lacking. Determinants, such as social sup-port, may impact the perception of treatment burden in patients with KT. While quality of life is improved for most KT recipients compared to dialysis, treatment burdens remain high and therefore are likely impacted by SDoH.[9] However,

Table 13.1 Adverse Long-Term Biological Outcomes in Kidney Transplant Recipients and Their Association with Potentially Modifiable Social Determinants of Health

Adverse biological outcomes in kidney transplant recipients	Social determinants of health amenable to interventions and policy changes
Allograft Rejection secondary to inadequate immunosuppression	Economic Stability: Ability to afford copays, insurance premiums for medications
	Healthcare Access and Quality: Access to providers, clinical pharmacists, health literacy
	Education Access and Quality: Language and literacy
	Neighborhood and Built environment: transportation, availability of pharmacies
	Social and Community Context: Social support with adherence to medications
Cardiovascular Disease	Economic Stability: Ability to afford copays, insurance premiums, healthy foods
	Healthcare Access and Quality: Access to providers, health literacy
	Education Access and Quality: Language and literacy
	Neighborhood and Built environment: Access to healthy food, access to safe exercise spaces
	Social and Community Context: Engagement in civic participation, addressing stressors associated with incarceration and discrimination
Cancer	Economic Stability: Ability to afford copays, insurance premiums for preventive screenings and early detection
	Healthcare Access and Quality: Access to providers, health literacy to understand recommended screenings
	Education Access and Quality: Language and literacy to understand recommended screenings
	Neighborhood and Built environment: Access to healthy food, screening for environmental risk factors for cancers, access to safe exercise spaces
	Social and Community Context: Social support with adherence to medications, exposure to tobacco

more research is needed, especially in underserved populations, on the precise role factors such as social support, education, and health literacy and economic factors—such as difficulty affording medication copays—play in disparities in post-transplant morbidity and mortality.

Current Assistance Available to Address Social
Determinants of Health

While there has been a growing focus on identifying and addressing SDoH in management of chronic kidney disease and KT, unfortunately, there are limited evidence-based interventions that available currently to address these issues that lead to disparities in healthcare. When targeting different key SDoH, healthcare systems and providers are limited in scope to what they can truly intervene on. Thus, while all SDoH are important and can interplay with one another, the current assistance available often addresses the healthcare access and quality aspects.

The largest mechanism for assistance available to patients post-KT comes in the form of access to healthcare. Many countries have universal access to healthcare, though as previously noted, this alone does not address SDoH sufficiently to reduce health disparities. However, ensuring access is a key first step. The United States made important policy progress toward expanding healthcare access for KT patients when the House of Representatives (H.R.) 133 bill, which included H.R. 5534, was signed into law on December 27, 2020. H.R. 5534 will extend Medicare coverage for immunosuppressive medications for post-KT patients in select situations beyond the current provided 36-month coverage as of January 2023. The extension of coverage has been proposed to be cost-effective.[10] This a key first step toward improving access to necessary care for post-KT patients to help improve long-term KT survival, but importantly will not address the challenges associated with copays and insurance premiums that are not addressed by this legislation.[8] Still, healthcare access and healthcare expenditure are by no means the end-all-be-all solutions to addressing SDoH. It is well known that United States experiences lower life expectancy and higher infant mortality rate compared to like countries despite higher expenditure, which likely affects transplant care and outcomes as well. Taken altogether, SDoH has vast impact on our healthcare outcomes in all countries despite differences in healthcare expenditure and healthcare delivery. Thus, additional interventions will be required given the vast impact that SDoH has on our healthcare outcomes.

In addition to healthcare policy assistance, there are nonprofit organizations that offer assistance for patients after KT. While these interventions are not evidence-based with regard to long-term outcomes, these organizations are important partners to healthcare systems in helping address disparities created by SDoH. In the United States, there are a variety of organizations (as listed on kidney.org) that provide the opportunity for some financial assistance to help cover medications, premiums, and transportation costs. Many of these organizations also offer the ability for patients and their families to connect with one another, which can potentially create an additional layer of necessary support, and patient-designed education regarding KT. Given high costs associated with transplantation, both short and long term, the role of organizations providing aid, both as direct financial support for patients and in health policy advocacy, is even more important in countries where costs of healthcare are still largely out-of-pocket. For example, in India, the Multi-Organ Harvesting Aid Network (MOHAN) Foundation has worked to improve access to transplantation and offers financial support for patients in the form of grants.

Given the impact SDoH can have on health outcomes and the resulting disparities, the lack of current evidence-based assistance is disappointing to say the least. As noted previously, further research on the precise impact of key aspects of SDoH beyond healthcare access in KT patients is needed.

Addressing Social Determinants of Health Post–Kidney Transplant

As a field, there is tremendous opportunity to learn more about how SDoH impact the long-term outcomes of KT patients specifically; a focused research in this area will serve as springboard to designing evidence-based interventions, both at the individual and population level. Here we break down potential areas of interest and barriers that may be faced when progressing the KT field to address SDoH (Figure 13.2)

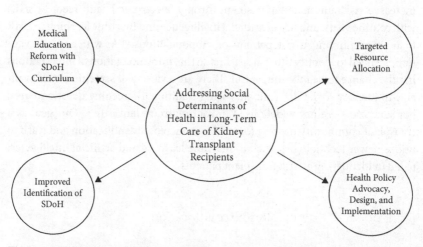

Figure 13.2 Strategies to address social determinants of health in the long-term care of kidney transplant recipients.

Education

Recognition of the impact of SDoH on health outcomes has certainly grown recently. Likewise, the importance of incorporating SDoH into curricula at all levels of learning for current and future healthcare providers has become a point of emphasis. The specifics of the optimal educational approach to improve equity remains up for debate, but the call for transformational change in our medical education has been proposed.[11] There is at least preliminary evidence to suggest including SDoH longitudinal curricula in our medical education is improving provider confidence in working with the underserved.[12] Similarly, as a transplant community, we need to incorporate formalized curricula into our training programs for transplant nephrologists and surgeons.

Identification

The importance of simply identifying and acknowledging SDoH in our routine clinical care of post-KT patients is an essential first step to tackling this issue. While we do an excellent job of reviewing medications, vital signs, and labs with our patients at routine visits, we often do not explore important SDoH such as health literacy, housing, and financial strain. Barriers for screening include lack of time and personnel as well as financial considerations from healthcare business models. Potential suggestions for improving SDoH identification include enhanced recognition prior to transplant (coordination with dialysis unit and transplant social workers during evaluation and while on wait list) for those at increased risk, automated assessment through electronic health record (EHR) with routine visits, and use of artificial intelligence and machine learning in EHR to aid in identifying at-risk patients or subpopulations.[13] As with any intervention, we need to identify those at risk first so that implementation of interventions has the chance to be most impactful. There are a variety of screening tools available to identify social determinants using traditional screening questionnaires, but such tools are not widely used in routine transplant care.[14] Our goal as a transplant community moving forward is to increase identification and learn to utilize newer technologies, such as machine learning and artificial intelligence, to aid in identifying at-risk transplant patients.

Resource Allocation

With improved identification of SDoH, we can better allocate resources to those at increased risk. While there are limited evidence-based approaches to address SDoH post-KT, we can adopt practices used in other aspects of healthcare that have been successful. Specifically, patient care navigators have been shown to improve process measure outcomes in a variety of chronic diseases and also in reducing healthcare utilization while increasing access to necessary resources.[15] Given the complexity of post-transplant care, patients can get lost in fragmented care with multiple specialties and healthcare systems; implementing patient care navigators may help improve efficiency and quality of the post-transplant healthcare that we deliver. Additionally, engagement of healthcare systems to form partnerships with community-based organizations led by community care health workers may better help address aspects of SDoH outside the scope of healthcare access and delivery, which also has been shown in other chronic disease states.

Addressing Policy

The impact SDoH has on long-term care of KT recipients is wide-reaching, and many key determinants will need to be addressed from a population standpoint. Using the recent passage of H.R. 5534 as a representative model, advocating for policy changes locally and nationally is an important step that we can take to address SDoH from a population standpoint. To best advocate for meaningful changes in policy, research to identify the key aspects of SDoH to target is imperative, as previously noted. With this knowledge, we need to translate our research findings in a multidisciplinary approach (healthcare systems, community health programs, lawmakers, payors) into implementation of policy changes with measurable outcomes that will improve long-term care of KT recipients.

Barriers

As with any intervention in healthcare, both at the individual and population level, limited resources, including time, personnel, and financial support, are the usual constraints in translating key findings into actual clinical practice and healthcare policy. To best overcome these barriers, the multiple stakeholders (healthcare systems, providers, community health organizations, patients, payors) need to align incentives to truly address the health of individuals and the population. To address SDoH directly, the way we deliver healthcare must be reimagined.

Conclusion

Advances in the care of KT patients have resulted in improved outcomes. Understandably, there has been an increased focus on improving long-term outcomes for KT recipients. As with other aspects of healthcare, health outcomes after KT are also largely influenced by aspects beyond traditional medical factors, such as SDoH, and these aspects extend beyond access to transplantation and quality care. In the KT field, research focused on SDoH remains limited and constitutes an unmet need that warrants further exploration. To truly realize the promise of better long-term outcomes for KT patients, we must focus on SDoH and identify key elements that are most influential and impactful. These should be individualized for each patient, and a concurrent approach toward designing interventions that target some of the vital SDoH in a collaborative fashion will be beneficial. A multipronged approach and collaborative work toward developing and implementing policies could improve better overall health of KT patients and will improve long-term survival.

References

1. Healthy People 2030. *Social determinants of health*. health.gov. https://health.gov/healthypeople/priority-areas/social-determinants-health. Accessed April 10, 2023.
2. Ndugga N, Artiga S. *Disparities in health and health care: 5 key questions and answers*. KFF. https://www.kff.org/racial-equity-and-health-policy/issue-brief/disparities-in-health-and-health-care-5-key-question-and-answers/. Accessed April 10, 2023.
3. Hall YN. Social determinants of health: addressing unmet needs in nephrology. *Am J Kidney Dis*. 2018;72(4):582–591.
4. Stringhini S, Carmeli C, Jokela M, et al. Socioeconomic status and the 25 × 25 risk factors as determinants of premature mortality: a multicohort study and meta-analysis of 1·7 million men and women. *Lancet*. 2017;389(10075):1229–1237.
5. Axelrod DA, Dzebisashvili N, Schnitzler MA, et al. The interplay of socioeconomic status, distance to center, and interdonor service area travel on kidney transplant access and outcomes. *Clin J Am Soc Nephrol*. 2010;5(12):2276–2288.
6. Laging M, Kal-van Gestel JA, van de Wetering J, IJzermans JNM, Weimar W, Roodnat JI. Understanding the influence of ethnicity and socioeconomic factors on graft and patient survival after kidney transplantation. *Transplantation*. 2014;98(9):974–978.
7. Mistretta A, Veroux M, Grosso G, et al. Role of socioeconomic conditions on outcome in kidney transplant recipients. *Transplant Proc*. 2009;41(4):1162–1167.
8. Hart A, Gustafson SK, Wey A, et al. The association between loss of Medicare, immunosuppressive medication use, and kidney transplant outcomes. *Am J Transplant*. 2019;19(7):1964–1971.
9. Lorenz EC, Egginton JS, Stegall MD, et al. Patient experience after kidney transplant: a conceptual framework of treatment burden. *J Patient Rep Outcomes*. 2019;3(1):8.
10. Kadatz M, Gill JS, Gill J, Formica RN, Klarenbach S. Economic evaluation of extending medicare immunosuppressive drug coverage for kidney transplant recipients in the current era. *J Am Soc Nephrol*. 2020;31(1):218–228.
11. Sharma M, Pinto AD, Kumagai AK. Teaching the social determinants of health: a path to equity or a road to nowhere? *Acad Med*. 2018;93(1):25–30.
12. Denizard-Thompson N, Palakshappa D, Vallevand A, et al. Association of a health equity curriculum with medical students' knowledge of social determinants of

health and confidence in working with underserved populations. *JAMA Netw Open*. 2021;4(3):e210297.

13. Han S, Zhang RF, Shi L, et al. Classifying social determinants of health from unstructured electronic health records using deep learning-based natural language processing. *J Biomed Inform*. 2022;127:103984.

14. Andermann A. Screening for social determinants of health in clinical care: moving from the margins to the mainstream. *Public Health Rev*. 2018;39:19.

15. McBrien KA, Ivers N, Barnieh L, et al. Patient navigators for people with chronic disease: a systematic review. *PLoS ONE*. 2018;13(2):e0191980.

14

Simultaneous Liver and Kidney Transplantation

Michele Molinari and Ty B. Dunn

Understanding the complexities involved in dual liver
and kidney transplantation !

Introduction

Simultaneous liver and kidney transplant (SLKT) is performed with increasing frequency as the number of patients with liver and renal failure has grown significantly after the incorporation of the Model for End-Stage Liver Disease (MELD). The aim of the current chapter is to provide the readers a succinct overview of the epidemiology, the most common indications, and the criteria used to select patients who require SLK transplantation. Their unique medical and surgical challenges and outcomes will also be presented.

Simultaneous Liver and Kidney Transplantation

The first SLKT was performed by Margreiter and colleagues[1] at the University of Innsbruck, Austria, in 1983. Since then, the outcomes of patients undergoing SLKT have improved significantly, and it is a relatively common procedure performed in select patients with simultaneous liver and renal disease. In the United States, after the implementation of the MELD for the allocation of liver grafts, the frequency of SLKT has doubled, from 4.6% (years 2002–2004) to 9.0% (years 2020–2022) (Table 14.1). The degree of renal dysfunction plays an important role in the calculation of the MELD score, and more patients with renal failure are listed for liver transplantation.[2] Increasing frequency of SLKT has also been reported in other continents as well.[3-6]

The most common clinical scenarios of patients who might benefit from SLKT are:

Table 14.1 Number of SLKT, Kidney Transplants Alone, Liver Transplants Alone, and the Percentage of Simultaneous Liver-Kidney Transplants Performed in the United States, 2002–2022

	2002–2004	2005–2007	2008–2010	2011–2013	2014–2016	2017–2019	2020–2022
SLKT	737	1,186	1,129	1,369	1,915	2,143	2,336
KTA (Deceased Donor)	26,567	31,164	31,617	33,074	37,251	42,297	55,918
LTA (Deceased Donor)	16,168	18,712	18,180	18,308	20,714	23,936	26,007
Percentage of SLKT (%)	4.6	6.3	6.2	7.5	9.2	9.0	9.0

Abbreviations: SLKT = simultaneous liver and kidney transplant; KTA = kidney transplant alone; LTA = liver transplant alone; Percentage of SLKT = ((number of SLKT)/(number of LTA))*100.

Source: Data from OPTN (Organ Procurement and Transplantation Network) website: https://optn.transplant.hrsa.gov/data/view-data-reports (Access date: 02-06-2023).

1. Presence of chronic liver disease with concurrent chronic kidney disease and eGFR below 30 mL/min/1.73 m^2,
2. Development of acute liver failure with rapid deterioration of renal function, and

3. Presence of persistent hepatorenal syndrome.
The Combination of Renal and Liver Disease

Renal impairment is common in patients with advanced liver disease and approximately 15%–20% of patients listed for liver transplantation in the United States have significantly impaired renal function[7,17] and that up to 50%–60% of patients on the wait list experience at least one episode of acute kidney injury (AKI) while awaiting transplant[8,9] (Table 14.2). Most patients with AKI waiting for a liver transplant,[9,10] however, do not require SLKT. In fact, in most patients the glomerular filtration rate (GFR) improves when appropriately resuscitated before or after liver transplantation. Shusterman et al.[11] reported 66%–78% of liver transplant recipients with preoperative AKI recovered their renal function within the first 3 months after liver transplantation. However, it is important to notice that the proportion of patients who experience complete resolution of their renal dysfunction/failure after liver transplant varies based on the chronicity of renal disease and the presence of other risk factors such as diabetes,

Table 14.2 Summary of the Criteria and Definitions Proposed by the International Club of Ascites to Determine Acute Kidney Injury (AKI) in Patients with Liver Disease (Updated in 2015).

Baseline serum creatinine	Value if serum creatinine obtained in the previous 3 months. In patients with more than one value, the serum creatinine closest to the hospital admission should be used. For patients without previous serum creatinine values, the value on admission should be used.
Definition of AKI	Increase of serum creatinine ≥0.3 mg/dL (≥26.5 μmol/L) within 48 hours Increase of serum creatinine ≥50% from baseline
Staging	1: increase of serum creatinine ≥0.3 mg/dL (≥26.5 μmol/L) or ≥1.5- to 2-fold from baseline 2: increase of serum creatinine >2- to 3-fold from baseline 3: increase of serum creatinine >3-fold from baseline or serum creatinine ≥4.0 mg/dL (353.6 μmol/L) with an acute increase ≥0.3 mg/dL (≥26.5 μmol/L), or initiation of renal replacement therapy
Response to treatment	No response: no regression of AKI Partial regression: decrease of serum creatinine >0.3 mg/dL above the baseline Full response: return of serum creatinine to a value within 0.3 mg/dL of the baseline value

hypertension, hypotension, or exposure to nephrotoxic medications or the use of intravenous radiological contrasts that can have profound lasting effects on their renal function.[12]

Risk Factors for Irreversible Renal Failure in Cirrhotic Patients

Liver transplant candidates who require dialysis for more than 90 days, and patients with prolonged AKI from acute tubular necrosis (ATN) are at significant risk of persistent renal impairment after liver transplantation. Yet, in most circumstances, the determination whether patients should be listed for liver transplant alone or combined with kidney transplantation, remains unclear.[7] Noninvasive tests are inadequate to determine whether the renal function will recover. Renal biopsies are rarely feasible in patients with liver decompensation due to the presence of coagulopathy and thrombocytopenia. Therefore, the determination whether a patient should be listed for SLKT depends on two main factors:

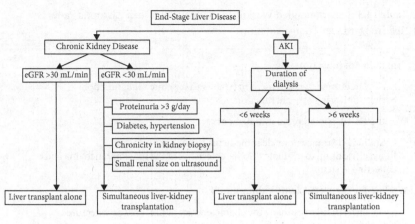

Figure 14.1 Algorithm for the selection of patients who should be considered for combined liver and kidney transplantation. The duration and etiology of renal dysfunction/failure are the main factors determining the need for renal transplantation.

1. the degree and duration of renal impairment, and
2. whether renal impairment is due to hepatorenal syndrome (HRS/ATN).[7,13]

Figure 14.1 represents the clinical algorithm largely accepted for the selection of patients who should be considered for SLKT based on the nature and duration of their renal dysfunction/failure.[14–16]

Workup and Criteria for Simultaneous Liver and Kidney Transplant

The recommended tests necessary to determine whether a patient should be listed for liver transplant only or SLKT are summarized in Table 14.3. Patients should undergo a renal ultrasound to rule out structural causes of kidney disease, a urinalysis to rule out the presence of proteinuria, pyuria, or hematuria, which are usually absent in patients with HRS, and the measurement of urine electrolytes, especially for patients producing less than 500 mL of urine per day. A formal policy that regulates the criteria for the listing of patients for SLKT was introduced in the United States in 2017. This policy was developed to reduce the significant variability in clinical practices among transplant centers.[3] The current policy requires that patients listed for SLKT satisfy the criteria reported in Table 14.4.

Table 14.3 Recommended Workup for Kidney Disease in Cirrhotic Patients Referred for Liver Transplantation

---

Evaluation of renal function

Serum creatinine measurement to establish a baseline renal function
Serial monitoring of renal function

Workup for suspected renal impairment

Cystatin C clearance or nuclear medicine renal function scan
Renal ultrasound to evaluate the characteristics of the renal parenchyma and collecting system

Workup for suspected acute kidney injury

Renal ultrasound to evaluate the characteristics of the renal architecture
Urinalysis
Urine electrolytes if the patient is oliguric (urinary output < 500 mL per day)
Native renal biopsy if safe
Clinical review of medications or other nephrotoxic agents and exclusion of shock

---

Table 14.4 UNOS Criteria for the Selection of Patients Who Can Be Listed for Simultaneous Liver-Kidney Transplantation in the United States

---

Medical eligibility for simultaneous liver-kidney transplantation in the United States: UNOS policy 2017 Transplant nephrology service needs to confirm the diagnosis of:

Documentation of at least one of the following:
1. Chronic kidney disease with estimated glomerular filtration rate (eGFR) ≤60 mL/min for > 90 consecutive days
    a) The candidate has started dialysis (Stage 5 of chronic kidney disease)
    b) eGFR ≤ 30 mL/min (Stage 4 of chronic kidney disease)
2. Acute kidney injury (AKI)
    a) Dialysis for ≥6 consecutive weeks (*)
    b) eGFR<25 mL/min for ≥6 consecutive weeks (eGFR documented every 7 days) (*)
    c) Any combination of a) or b) for ≥6 consecutive weeks (*)
3. Metabolic disease
    a) Hyperoxaluria
    b) Atypical hemolytic uremic syndrome (HUS) from mutations in factory H and possibly factor I
    c) Familial nonneuropathic systemic amyloid
    d) Methylmalonic aciduria

Legend: (*): before the implementation of the 6-week policy, most transplant centers used a 4-week duration of dialysis for SLKT.

Safety Net

Many patients with renal failure improve their renal function after liver transplantation. Hence, the Organ Procurement and Transplantation Network (OPTN) has introduced a rescue strategy to reduce the risk of performing unnecessary SLKTs. This strategy is commonly known as "Safety Net." Instead of listing patients for SLKT, transplant programs can now choose to perform liver transplantation alone and selectively proceed with renal transplantation only in patients with persistent renal failure after liver transplantation. This group of patients receive priority for deceased-donor renal grafts. To be eligible for the "Safety Net," patients must develop renal impairment after liver transplantation, or patients must be eligible for combined liver-kidney transplant before undergoing liver transplantation only. The criteria currently used for the "Safety Net" are the same used for the listing of patients in need of a kidney transplant but based on an eGFR of less than 20 mL/min or being on dialysis.[3]

Patients who received a SLKT also qualify for the "Safety Net" if they experienced a primary renal graft nonfunction.[3] The "Safety Net" eligibility is available between 60 to 365 days after liver transplantation.[3] Candidates who are eligible for the "Safety Net" but not listed for renal transplantation within the 1st year after liver transplantation can be approved only after their application is approved by the UNOS board.[3]

Induction Immunosuppression for Simultaneous Liver-Kidney Transplantation

Contrary to patients undergoing isolated renal transplantation,[17] induction immunosuppression is given only to a small group of patients undergoing isolated liver transplantation.[18] In 2015, 91% of renal transplant recipients received induction therapy in the form of T-cell-depleting agents or interleukin 2 receptor antagonist (IL2-RA)[19] in comparison to only 35% of liver transplant recipients.[18] For recipients of SLKT, the use of induction therapy has been more controversial as there is evidence that the liver reduces the risk of kidney rejection regardless of the level of calculated panel reactive antibody (cPRA), or presence of donor-specific antibodies (DSA) and positive crossmatch.[20] In a recent study of 5,172 SLKT recipients, Kamal et al.[17] found that at 5 years, patient survival was 74%, 71%, and 68% for SKLT recipients who received IL2-RA induction, no induction, and T-cell-depleting agents, respectively ($p < 0.001$). Liver and kidney allograft survivals at 5 years were 73% and 70%, respectively, for recipients who received IL2-RA induction; 70% and 68% for recipients who received no induction therapy; and 67% and 64% for recipients who received T-cell-depleting agents ($p < 0.001$). Multivariate analysis showed the type of induction therapy did not impact patient and graft survival. Based on Kamal's study and other groups,[7,21] current consensus is that the use of T-cell-depleting agent or IL2-RA induction immunosuppression is not recommended for SLKT due to the immunomodulatory effect of the liver graft.

Long-Term Immunosuppression after Liver-Kidney Transplantation

Although there are significant center-specific variations in the long-term immuno-suppression therapy used for recipients of SLKT[22] the most common regimen includes the use of calcineurin inhibitors (CNIs) in addition to an antimetabo-lite (mycophenolate mofetil or mycophenolic acid) and steroids.[23] A recent study by Kamal et al.[17] suggested that immunosuppression maintenance with CNIs in combination with low-dose steroids is associated with better patient and graft survival compared to other regimens. Further studies are necessary to determine the optimal long-term immunosuppression therapy for SLKT. Currently, some transplant centers use immunosuppression based on immunological risk profiles (pretransplant DSA against class II human leukocyte antigen [HLA], positive cross-match, high calculated panel reactive antibody [cPRA]).

Outcomes of Simultaneous Liver-Kidney Transplantation

There is growing evidence supporting the theory that transplanted liver may play a protective role in preventing renal allograft rejection in SLKT cases where the same donor is used. However, there is no definitive evidence demonstrating improved recipient or graft survival.[24] A study by Martin et al.[24] found that the survival rate of patients who underwent SLKT was similar to those who underwent liver transplant alone, with both groups having a 5-year survival rate of around 65%. In contrast, patients who underwent kidney after liver transplant or liver after kidney transplant had much lower 5-year patient survival rates of 27.6% and 53.3%, respectively.

Anesthesia Challenges for Patients with Renal and Liver Failure

The anesthetic management of patients undergoing SLKT can be challenging due to the complexity of the surgical procedure and the presence of multiorgan system failure in patients with ESLD and ESKD[25] ESLD can be associated with various complications, including hepatopulmonary syndrome, portopulmonary hypertension, hepatic hydrothorax, HRS, ascites, varices, coagulopathy, cardiomyopathy, encephalopathy, hyponatremia, and hypocalcemia. ESKD can cause hyperkalemia, platelet dysfunction, pulmonary edema, pericardial effusion, and coronary artery disease. The combination of these two diseases can lead to significant acidosis, anemia, and altered drug metabolism. Fluid overload is a major concern during SLKT, and restricted fluid replacement with a central venous pressure (CVP) of 5–7 mmHg is recommended in the preanhepatic phase. Continuous renal replacement therapy (CRRT) is indicated in certain recipients, in prolonged anhepatic phase, and in patients with severe acidosis, hyperkalemia, and fluid overload. However, Continuous Venous-Venous Hemodialysis (CVVHD) can be associated with various problems, including circuit or filter clotting, hypotension, air embolism, disconnection, hemorrhage, and postoperative vascular thrombosis. If the anhepatic phase is short and there are no signs of fluid overload, acidosis can be managed with boluses of sodium bicarbonate. Tranexamic acid is used to prevent postreperfusion fibrinolysis[23] and should be infused in the anhepatic phase and discontinued within 2 hours of liver reperfusion to avoid the possibility of hypercoagulation and hepatic artery thrombosis.

Donor Selection

With increasing number of patients waiting for transplantation, centers have explored the utility of donors after circulatory death (DCD) for candidates for SLKT. Two recent retrospective analyses of the UNOS data compared the outcomes of SLKT using DCD versus donors after brain death (DBD).[26] Although studies have demonstrated that patients receiving DCD organs had inferior graft survival for both organs and inferior patient survival,[26,27] in more recent years, the gap in survival between the two groups has become less clinically significant.[28]

Novel Approach in SLKT

Traditionally, combined liver and kidney transplantation were performed as a single continuous procedure during which the kidney transplant is performed immediately after the reperfusion of the liver graft. More recently, Ekser et al.[29] have proposed a new approach in which the renal graft procured from the same donor as the liver graft is maintained on hypothermic pulsatile perfusion pump until the hemodynamic instability and the coagulopathy following liver transplant recipients are resolved. Subsequent implantation of the kidney graft can be delayed until optimal circumstances are reached, on average 2 to 3 days after liver transplantation. Despite the significant increase in the mean cold ischemia of the kidney grafts (mean 50 ± 15 hrs. vs. 10 ± 3 hrs; $p < 0.0001$), Ekser and colleagues have observed a significant reduction in delayed graft function (DGF; 7% vs. 0%; $p < 0.06$) and perioperative mortality within the first 90 days (9% vs. 5%; $p = 0.50$), and lower serum creatinine levels at 1 year (1.33 mg/dL $\pm$ 0.44 vs. 1.15 ± 0.32; $p = 0.02$). Patient survival was also significantly improved with 1-year survival rate up to 91% in comparison to 83%, 3-year survival rate up to 87% in comparison to 78%, and 5-year survival rate up to 87% in comparison to 63% ($p = 0.01$).

Outcomes after SLKT

Recent analysis of national data indicated that the overall incidence of DGF after SLKT in the United States is 22%.[30] The main risk factors for DGF were history of pretransplant dialysis, elevated donor body mass index, donation after cardiocirculatory death, and duration of cold ischemia time.[30] The overall 1-year mortality after SLKT has continued to improve over the years. In an analysis of data from a consortium of six high-volume transplant centers, Cullaro et al.[4,16] have reported that 1-year postoperative mortality declined from 11% in 2002 to 4% in 2017 ($p < 0.001$). On the other hand, during the same period, the proportion of patients with DGF increased from 6% to 43% ($p < 0.001$).[4,16] Most recent studies on the long-term outcomes after SLKT report a 5-year patient survival ranging between 64%[7,8] to 88%[31] and graft survival rates range between 62% to 87% for the liver[11] and 59% to 88% for the kidney[26] (Table 14.5).

SLKT versus Liver Transplant Followed
by Kidney Transplant

There have been increasing concerns that due to the expanding number of patients listed for SLKT, the number of kidneys available for patients with renal disease will continue to decrease as kidneys are preferentially used for liver recipients. In some centers, mortality after SLKT at 1 year exceeds 20%.[11,32] Because of the increased risks of perioperative complications leading to graft loss or death after SLKT, some groups have proposed that patients should undergo liver transplantation first followed by a kidney transplant from a different donor at a later time. A Markov model developed by Kiberd et al.[33] onstrated that SLKT

Table 14.5 Patient Survival after Simultaneous Liver and Kidney Transplantation

Author (Ref.)	Journal	Year	n. pts	1 year	3 year	5 year
Becker et al.[1]	Liver Transplantation	2003	38	73.7%	73.7%	64.1%
Becker et al.[1]	Liver Transplantation	2003	47	-	-	-
Simultaneous	-	-	38	73.7%	73.7%	56.1%
Sequential	-	-	9	66.7%	53.3%	53.3%
Demirci et al.[2]	Liver Transplantation	2003	38	73.7%	-	64.1%
Creput et al.[3]	Am J Transplantation	2003	45	85.0%		-
Fong et al.[4]	Transplantation	2003	800	74.0%	-	64.0%
Simpson et al.[5]	Transplantation	2006	1136	80.0%	-	65.0%
Locke et al.[6]	Transplantation	2008	1032	82.0%		-
Schmitt et al.[7]	Transplant Intern	2009	959	79.4%	69.0%	-
Van Wagner et al.[8]	J Hepatology	2009	38	73.7%	-	68.1%
Martin et al.[9]	Liver Transplantation	2012	2327	81.8%	71.7%	64.1%
Liver transplant alone	-	-	-	84.4%	75.4%	68.4%
Simultaneous	-	-	-	81.8%	71.7%	64.1%
Liver after kidney transplant	-	-	-	71.0%	61.2%	54.2%
Kidney after liver transplant	-	-	-	33.4%	25.4%	22.0%
<3 months	-	-	-	36.5%	31.1%	28.1%
3–6 months	-	-	-	68.0%	52.0%	52.0%
>6–12 months	-	-	-	89.3%	82.8%	78.1%
>12 months	-	-	-	75.5%	53.9%	46.1%
Wadei et al.[10]	Liver Transplantation	2014	66	92.4%	90.5%	87.4%
Pineiro et al.[11]	Liver Transplantation	2020	88		-	-
Low immunological risk			68	94.0%	-	88.0%

(continued)

Table 14.5 Continued

Author (Ref.)	Journal	Year	n. pts	1 year	3 year	5 year
High immunological risk (*)			20	70.0%	-	57.0%
Cullaro et al.[12]	Liver Transplantation	2021	572	92.0%	87.0%	82.8%

[1] Becker T, Nyibata M, Lueck R, et al. Results of combined and sequential liver-kidney transplantation. *Liver Transpl.* 2003;9(10):1067–1078.

[2] Demirci G, Becker T, Nyibata M, et al. Results of combined and sequential liver-kidney transplantation. *Liver Transpl.* 2003;9(10):1067–1078.

[3] Creput C, Durrbach A, Samuel D, et al. Incidence of renal and liver rejection and patient survival rate following combined liver and kidney transplantation. *Am J Transplant.* 2003;3(3):348–356.

[4] Fong TL, Bunnapradist S, Jordan SC, Selby RR, Cho YW. Analysis of the United Network for Organ Sharing database comparing renal allografts and patient survival in combined liver-kidney transplantation with the contralateral allografts in kidney or kidney-pancreas transplantation. *Transplantation.* 2003;76(2):348–353.

[5] Simpson N, Cho YW, Cicciarelli JC, Selby RR, Fong TL. Comparison of renal allograft outcomes in combined liver-kidney transplantation versus subsequent kidney transplantation in liver transplant recipients: analysis of UNOS database. *Transplantation.* 2006;82(10):1298–303.

[6] Locke JE, Warren DS, Singer AL, et al. Declining outcomes in simultaneous liver-kidney transplantation in the MELD era: ineffective usage of renal allografts. *Transplantation.* 2008;85(7):935–942.

[7] *Schmitt TM, Kumer SC, Al-Osaimi A, et al. Combined liver–kidney and liver transplantation in patients with renal failure outcomes in the MELD era. Transpl Int. 2009;22:876–883. https://doi.org/ 10.1111/j.1432-2277.2009.00887.x*

[8] VanWagner LB, Holl JL, Montag S, et al. Blood pressure control according to clinical practice guidelines is associated with decreased mortality and cardiovascular events among liver transplant recipients. *Am J Transplant.* 2020;20(3):797–807.

[9] Martin EF, Huang J, Xiang Q, Klein JP, Bajaj J, Saeian K. Recipient survival and graft survival are not diminished by simultaneous liver-kidney transplantation: an analysis of the United Network for Organ Sharing database. *Liver Transpl.* 2012;18(8):914–929.

[10] Wadei HM, Bulatao IG, Gonwa TA, et al. Inferior long-term outcomes of liver-kidney transplantation using donation after cardiac death donors: single-center and Organ Procurement and Transplantation Network analyses. *Liver Transpl.* 2014;20(6):728–735.

[11] Pineiro GJ, Rovira J, Montagud-Marrahi E, et al. Kidney graft outcomes in high immunological risk simultaneous liver-kidney transplants. *Liver Transpl.* 2020;26(4):517–527.

[12] Cullaro G, Sharma ·P, Jo J, et al. Temporal trends and evolving outcomes after simultaneous liver kidney transplantation: Results from the US SLKT Consortium. Liver Transpl. 2021;27(11):1613–1622.

is associated with higher quality-adjusted life-years provided that 1-year postoperative mortality is less than 39%.

Conclusion

Renal dysfunction is common in patients with irreversible liver disease requiring liver transplantation. Over the last few decades, the number of SLKT performed in most countries has increased as organ allocation policies prioritize patients with the highest acuity of organ failure. Although the short- and long-term outcomes of SLKT have significantly improved over time, SLKT remains a high-risk procedure that requires careful patient selection and perioperative care. Compared to single-organ transplant, perioperative morbidity and mortality after SLKT is significantly higher. However, postoperative survival after SLKT is superior to the survival of patients who undergo liver transplantation only with maintenance dialysis for ESKD. Over time, there has been a trend toward avoidance of T cell depletion as induction therapy in recipients of SLKT, and a recent study has suggested that renal transplant surgery should be delayed until the hemodynamic instability and coagulopathy after liver transplantation are resolved. Areas where future studies are needed include the optimal long-term immunosuppression regimen and the long-term outcomes of recipients of organs from donation after cardiovascular death or high Kidney Donor Profile Index (KDPI) grafts.

References

1. Demirci G, Becker T, Nyibata M, et al. Results of combined and sequential liver-kidney transplantation. *Liver Transpl.* 2003;9(10):1067–1078.
2. Kamath PS, Wiesner RH, Malinchoc M, et al. A model to predict survival in patients with end-stage liver disease. *Hepatology.* 2001;33(2):464–470.
3. Drak D, Tangirala N, Fink M, et al. Trends and outcomes in simultaneous liver and kidney transplantation in Australia and New Zealand. *Transpl P.* 2021;53(1):136–140.
4. Mekahli D, van Stralen KJ, Bonthuis M, et al. Kidney versus combined kidney and liver transplantation in young people with autosomal recessive polycystic kidney disease: Data From the European Society for Pediatric Nephrology/European Renal Association-European Dialysis and Transplant (ESPN/ERA-EDTA) Registry. *Am J Kidney Dis.* 2016;68(5):782–788.
5. Kim M, Hwang S, Ahn CS, et al. Simultaneous liver-kidney transplantation: A single-center experience in Korea. *Ann Hepatobiliary Pancreat Surg.* 2020;24(4):454–459.
6. Ekser B, Contreras AG, Andraus W, Taner T. Current status of combined liver-kidney transplantation. *Int J Surg.* 2020;82:149–154.
7. Gleisner AL, Jung H, Lentine KL, Tuttle-Newhall J. Renal dysfunction in liver transplant candidates: Evaluation, classification and management in contemporary practice. *J Nephrol Ther.* 2012;Suppl 4(SI Kidney Transplantation):006. doi: 10.4172/2161-0959.S4-006. Epub 2012 Mar 30. PMID: 32874772; PMCID: PMC7457375.
8. Lum EL, Cardenas A, Martin P, Bunnapradist S. Current status of simultaneous liver-kidney transplantation in the United States. *Liver Transpl.* 2019;25(5):797–806.
9. Molinari M, Fernandez-Carrillo C, Dai D, et al. Portal vein thrombosis and renal dysfunction: A national comparative study of liver transplant recipients for NAFLD versus alcoholic cirrhosis. *Transpl Int.* 2021;34(6):1105–1122.
10. Angeli P, Gines P, Wong F, et al. Diagnosis and management of acute kidney injury in patients with cirrhosis: Revised consensus recommendations of the International Club of Ascites. *Gut.* 2015;64(4):531–537.
11. Shusterman B, McHedishvili G, Rosner MH. Outcomes for hepatorenal syndrome and acute kidney injury in patients undergoing liver transplantation: A single-center experience. *Transplant Proc.* 2007;39(5):1496–1500.

12. O'Riordan A, Wong V, McCormick PA, Hegarty JE, Watson AJ. Chronic kidney disease post-liver transplantation. *Nephrol Dial Transplant*. 2006;21(9):2630–2636.

13. Marik PE, Wood K, Starzl TE. The course of type 1 hepato-renal syndrome post liver transplantation. *Nephrol Dial Transplant*. 2006;21(2):478–482.

14. Eason JD, Gonwa TA, Davis CL, Sung RS, Gerber D, Bloom RD. Proceedings of Consensus Conference on Simultaneous Liver Kidney Transplantation (SLK). *Am J Transplant*. 2008;8(11):2243–2251.

15. Nadim MK, Davis CL, Sung R, Kellum JA, Genyk YS. Simultaneous liver-kidney transplantation: A survey of US transplant centers. *Am J Transplant*. 2012;12(11):3119–3127.

16. Nadim MK, Sung RS, Davis CL, et al. Simultaneous liver-kidney transplantation summit: Current state and future directions. *Am J Transplant*. 2012;12(11):2901–2908.

17. Kamal L, Yu JNW, Reichman TW, et al. Impact of induction immunosuppression strategies in simultaneous liver/kidney transplantation. *Transplantation*. 2020;104(2):395–403.

18. Kim WR, Lake JR, Smith JM, et al. OPTN/SRTR 2017 Annual Data Report: Liver. *Am J Transplant*. 2019;19 Suppl 2:184–283. doi: 10.1111/ajt.15276. PMID: 30811890.

19. Hart A, Smith JM, Skeans MA, et al. OPTN/SRTR 2015 Annual Data Report: Kidney. *Am J Transplant*. 2017;17 Suppl 1(Suppl 1):21–116.

20. Dar W, Agarwal A, Watkins C, et al. Donor-directed MHC class I antibody is preferentially cleared from sensitized recipients of combined liver/kidney transplants. *Am J Transplant*. 2011;11(4):841–847.

21. Askar M, Schold JD, Eghtesad B, et al. Combined liver-kidney transplants: Allosensitization and recipient outcomes. *Transplantation*. 2011;91(11):1286–1292.

22. Das A, Taner T, Kim J, Emamaullee J. Crossmatch, donor-specific antibody testing, and immunosuppression in simultaneous liver and kidney transplantation: A review. *Transplantation*. 2021;105(12):E285–E291.

23. Weeks SR, Luo X, Haugen CE, et al. Delayed graft function in simultaneous liver kidney transplantation. *Transplantation*. 2020;104(3):542–550.

24. Martin EF, Huang J, Xiang Q, Klein JP, Bajaj J, Saeian K. Recipient survival and graft survival are not diminished by simultaneous liver-kidney transplantation: An analysis of the united network for organ sharing database. *Liver Transpl*. 2012;18(8):914–929.

25. Randolph HS CL. *Anaesthesia for abdominal organ transplantation*. 8th ed. Elsevier Saunders Publishers; 2010.

26. Simpson N, Cho YW, Cicciarelli JC, Selby RR, Fong TL. Comparison of renal allograft outcomes in combined liver-kidney transplantation versus subsequent kidney transplantation in liver transplant recipients: Analysis of UNOS database. *Transplantation*. 2006;82(10):1298–1303.

27. Weeks SR, Luo X, Toman L, et al. Steroid-sparing maintenance immunosuppression is safe and effective after simultaneous liver-kidney transplantation. *Clin Transplant*. 2020;34(10):e14036. doi: 10.1111/ctr.14036. Epub 2020 Aug 2. PMID: 32652700.

28. Alhamad T, Spatz C, Uemura T, Lehman E, Farooq U. The outcomes of simultaneous liver and kidney transplantation using donation after cardiac death organs. *Transplantation*. 2014;98(11):1190–1198.

29. Croome KP, Mao S, Yang L, Pungpapong S, Wadei HM, Taner CB. Improved national results with simultaneous liver-kidney transplantation using donation after circulatory death donors. *Liver Transpl*. 2020;26(3):397–407.

30. Ekser B, Mangus RS, Fridell JA, et al. A novel approach in combined liver and kidney transplantation with long-term outcomes. *Ann Surg.* 2017;265(5):1000–1008.
31. VanWagner LB, Holl JL, Montag S, et al. Blood pressure control according to clinical practice guidelines is associated with decreased mortality and cardiovascular events among liver transplant recipients. *Am J Transplant.* 2020;20(3):797–807.
32. Davis CL, Feng S, Sung R, et al. Simultaneous liver-kidney transplantation: Evaluation to decision making. *Am J Transplant.* 2007;7(7):1702–1709.
33. Kiberd B, Skedgel C, Alwayn I, Peltekian K. Simultaneous liver kidney transplantation: A medical decision analysis. *Transplantation.* 2011;91(1):121–127.

15

Simultaneous Pancreas and Kidney Transplantation

Ty B. Dunn and Michele Molinari

*Kidney and Pancreas transplantation—to correct the primary
cause and modify the outcome!*

Introduction

End-stage kidney disease (ESKD) is a major health problem in the United States, with 130,522 new cases in 2020.[1] Diabetes is a major cause of kidney failure and contributing to 38% of candidates listed for kidney transplant.[2] Among the 42,231 candidates added to the kidney wait list in 2022, only 1,535 were people with Type-1 diabetes; a decreasing number likely due to improved long-term diabetes management in this select population. During the same time, just 888 patients with Type-1 and 421 with non-Type-1 diabetes were added to the kidney/pancreas wait list. As of early 2023, a total of 1,924 candidates were waiting for a simultaneous pancreas-kidney transplant (SPKT).

A total of 810 SPKT transplants were done in 2022, representing 4.1% of the 19,636 kidney transplants from deceased donors. One issue limiting the number of SPKTs is the availability of suitable donor pancreases. Only a small proportion of deceased donors (DDs) are fit to donate their pancreas because the donor must be relatively young, lean, and free from major hemodynamic instability or multiorgan failure. Important additional constraints are deficiencies in patient and provider awareness, deficiencies in the national organ transportation system, with waning expertise in the procurement and transplant of the pancreas.[3] In fact, of all DDs in 2022 (N = 14,905), only 8.7% of pancreases (n = 1,310) were recovered for the purpose of transplant, and of those, 28% were not utilized, further underscoring the gravity of the issues that impact SPKT transplantation in the United States (based on Organ Procurement and Transplantation Network [OPTN] data as of March 16, 2023).

The current chapter aims to review the most recent data on the incidence, selection, and outcomes of SPKT, with an emphasis on how this transplant option can improve the quantity and quality of life for patients with kidney disease due to insulin-dependent diabetes.

Simultaneous Pancreas and Kidney Transplantation

Kidney transplantation is a well-recognized treatment option for patients with ESKD. However, for patients with insulin-dependent diabetes as their primary cause of native kidney disease, often the focus is on obtaining a kidney transplant to reap the immediate benefits of avoiding or minimizing time on dialysis, since it is well known that people with diabetes have increased morbidity and mortality associated with longer dialysis duration.[4–7] These ESKD patients, when medically appropriate (and when no living kidney donor is available), can receive an SPKT, an option that offers the most immediate and durable control of their primary disease, which protects their new kidney from microvascular injury and recurrent diabetic nephropathy.[8,9]

Pancreas transplantation peaked in the United States in 2004, when 1,484 pancreas transplants were performed, with the majority of these (59.4%, $n = 881$) being SPKT transplants. Less frequently, isolated pancreas alone (PA) were used for pancreas after kidney (PAK) or pancreas transplant alone (PTA) transplant types. Over the past couple decades, the number of isolated pancreas transplants has steadily decreased, likely due to multiple factors including but not limited to advancements in diabetes care via improved insulin pump and monitoring technologies. In 2015 and 2019, major changes in the kidney and pancreas allocation policy in the United States disentangled pancreas from kidney allocation and then allowed ESKD patients with an estimated glomerular filtration rate (eGFR) of 20 mL/min or less and any type of insulin-dependent diabetes to qualify for SPKT, with the goal to increase utilization of all suitable pancreases, improve equity for non-Caucasian candidates, and to decrease the excess morbidity and mortality that differentially impacts people with insulin-dependent diabetes *and* ESKD, compared to those with ESKD alone (Figure 15.1).

Despite implementation of the Final Rule in 2009, which mandated that dialysis facilities refer ESKD patients for kidney transplantation, many patients with kidney failure and insulin-dependent diabetes are not routinely referred to a transplant center that performs pancreas transplant.[10] Many patients are not aware of the option of pancreas transplantation. Pancreas transplantation is a specialized field and is performed at only 48% (121/250) of active adult kidney transplant centers (based on OPTN data as of March 16, 2023). Moreover, 50% of active pancreas centers did fewer than six pancreas transplants in 2022 (United Network for Organ Sharing [UNOS] Benchmark Report: Pancreas, April 2023). Further underscoring the infrequency of the procedure, some areas of the United

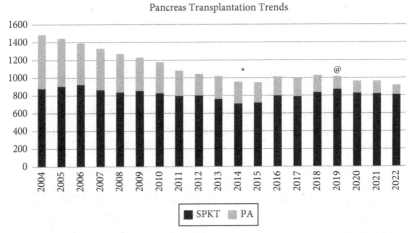

Figure 15.1 Trends in types of pancreas transplantation.
SPKT = simultaneous pancreas kidney transplant, PA = pancreas alone (after or
without a kidney transplant), * = allocation policy change where the kidney follows
the pancreas for candidates with type I and some with type II insulin dependent
diabetes (those with low C-peptide and limitations on body mass index [BMI]),
@ = allocation policy change removing BMI and C-peptide requirements altogether.

States have no pancreas transplant centers and have been described as "pancreas
deserts." Centers that do not offer pancreas in addition to kidney transplantation
are not mandated to educate or refer patients for pancreas transplant, therefore
patients are unlikely to be able to effectively advocate for themselves.[3]

Indications for SPKT

The indication for SPKT is driven by insulin-dependent diabetes with diabetic
nephropathy as the primary disease necessitating transplant. As such, it makes
great sense that individuals with insulin-dependent diabetes and ESKD be
carefully considered for pancreas transplantation and prioritized for access to
SPKT (or PAK if a living kidney donor is available).[11] Regardless of being highly
selected as fit for transplant, 22% of SPKT candidates on the waiting list will die
or be removed from the list within 3 years, underscoring the morbid combination of ESKD and diabetes.[12,13]

United Network for Organ Sharing (UNOS) SPKT listing criteria and wait time
qualification have moved away from an emphasis on the "type" of diabetes to recognize the imprecision and difficulties encountered in diabetes classification and
reporting, as well as the differential prevalence of non-Type-1 insulin-dependent

diabetes in non-Caucasian populations. At present, registrants with insulin-dependent diabetes may begin accruing waiting time for SPKT when GFR is 20 mL/min or less or upon dialysis initiation. SPKT candidates are increasingly classified as having Type-2 diabetes, up from 10% in 2010 to 22.9% in 2021.[12]

Selection of SPKT Candidates

Medical and surgical criteria for suitability for SPKT are more conservative than for kidney-only transplant, as the operation and recovery are of greater magnitude, necessitating sufficient cardiovascular performance status, lack of excess visceral obesity or frailty, solid social support, vetted compliance with their medical regimen, and other more nuanced surgical considerations (absence of significant aortoiliac vascular disease or a complex surgical abdomen).[14,15] Smoking cessation is a requirement in most programs, as smoking has a well-recognized negative impact on cardiovascular health—the predominant cause of death after transplant in patients with ESKD.[16]

The availability of a living kidney donor and the patient's anticipated timeline for progression toward starting dialysis is a major determinant in estimating the optimal path to transplant. Due to excessively long wait times for kidney-alone DD transplantation, patients with insulin-dependent diabetes are more likely to die waiting for a KAT for their ESKD caused by diabetes.[17] When no living kidney donor is available, it is a survival benefit for such candidates to receive a timely transplant of both the pancreas and the kidney from a DD. An important aspect of patient selection is an honest appraisal of a candidate's expected morbidity and mortality with SPKT in contrast to that expected from waiting for a DD kidney alone, especially in cases where age, BMI, or cardiac status may be outside a program's usual selection criteria. Iterative improvements in outcomes by era have prompted transplant programs to expand access to less traditional candidate phenotypes such as the older patient, the Type-2 patient, those with elevated BMI, and those with other comorbid conditions.[18,19]

Outcomes of SPKT

Pancreas transplantation has been associated with a significant rate of complications and morbidity as well as early graft loss, however these issues have faded with improvements in patient and graft survival after optimization of graft and candidate selection, operative techniques, and immunosuppression. Contemporary patient survival rates at 1- and 5-years post-transplant are 96%–98% and 90%, respectively.[3,20,21] Death-censored kidney graft survival after

SPKT is at 81.7% at 10 years, reflecting the excellent quality kidneys associated with SPKT and the prevention of recurrent diabetic nephropathy.[12] The first year of pancreas graft failure reported using the new definition (>0.5 units/kg/day insulin usage) was in 2021; the rate of graft loss of the pancreas in the first 90 days post-transplant for SPK (6%) was unchanged from prior, but for PAK (9%) and PTA (18%) was higher than reported under the old definition. These early failures are usually due to thrombosis, pancreatitis, or infection.[12] For those with functioning grafts at 1 year, the half-life of function for the kidney is more than 14 years (similar to outcomes of living donor kidney transplants) and for the pancreas as well, which is better than the average pancreas graft survival in PAK (9 years).[22] Medium- and longer-term data on excellent patient, kidney, and pancreas allograft outcomes, regardless of the "type" of diabetes has resulted in improved equity and access to kidney transplantation for patients with ESKD secondary to diabetic nephropathy.[23-26] Table 15.1 provides a summary of contemporary outcomes associated with each transplant type.[2,12,20,27-30] The first

Table 15.1 Rates of Technical Failure, Kidney and Pancreas Graft Survival, Risk of Rejection and Patient Survival Associated with the Various Transplant Options for Patients with Kidney Failure Due to Insulin-Dependent Diabetes

	Technical failure	Kidney graft survival	Pancreas graft survival	Risk of rejection	Patient survival
SPK	4%–6% pancreas 1%–2% kidney	1 yr 97% 10 yrs 81%	1 yr 92% 10 yr 58%	Low to medium	1 yr 97% 10 yrs 75%
PAK	6-9%	LD kidney >15 yrs, DD kidney 10–12 yrs	9 yrs	Medium	1 yr 96% 10 yrs 74%
LD-KTA	<1%	1&10 yrs: 97%/70% Average >15 yrs.	n/a	Low	1 yr 99% 10 yrs 85%
DD-KTA	1%	1&10 yrs: 91%/52% Average 9–11 yrs.	n/a	Low	1 yr 96% 10 yrs 75%

References:
OPTN/SRTR 2018 Annual Data Report: Kidney.[27]
OPTN/SRTR 2018 Annual Data Report: Pancreas.[28]
OPTN/SRTR 2020 Annual Data Report: Pancreas.[20]
OPTN/SRTR 2021 Annual Data Report: Kidney.[2]
OPTN/SRTR 2021 Annual Data Report: Pancreas.[12]
Gruessner et al.[29]

world consensus conference on pancreas transplantation was convened in Pisa in 2019 and provided a number of recommendations in support of the practice of pancreas transplantation as it pertains to improvements in long-term patient survival, quality of life, and the course of chronic complications of diabetes.[31,32]

Technical Challenges of SPKT

Most of the recent progress in decreasing surgical complications is related to the practice of more conservative graft selection and reducing cold ischemic time, which minimizes the risk of reperfusion pancreatitis and the ensuing potential downstream complications of thrombosis, reoperation, infection, and graft loss. Many centers have moved away from routine postoperative intravenous heparin anticoagulation to minimize the risk of bleeding. Some patient-specific situations can increase the technical challenges of surgery or even preclude an opportunity for SPKT. Most relevant to this is advanced aortoiliac calcific disease, which limits potential sites for transplant. In the most severe cases, the treatment focus is shifted away from SPKT and toward an opportunity for KTA, as it is far superior to remaining on dialysis. Patients with a complex surgical abdomen (prior operations including bowel resection or Roux-Y gastric bypass) can present challenges in both the operative time needed to prepare for organ implantation as well as an increased risk for enterotomy, prolonged ileus, or future bowel obstruction.

Organ Sources

Like other extrarenal combination transplants, the organ source is nearly always from a DD. Living donor segmental pancreas with (or without) kidney transplant was initially offered as a way to decrease the historically high rate of pancreas rejection and improve earlier access to pancreas transplant.[33–35] Modern immunosuppression, concerns for living donor safety after pancreas doantion, and the current allocation system have nearly eliminated the need for this procedure, which is rare worldwide and has not been done in the United.States since 2013 (based on OPTN data as of March 16, 2023).[32]

Pros and Cons of SPKT over Kidney Transplant Alone

With kidney transplantation comes the burden of immunosuppression, however patients with diabetes still have active primary disease. The slope of GFR decline is steeper in people with diabetes and chronic kidney disease compared to many other causes of renal failure, and can result in a shorter timeline until renal replacement therapy is required. There is demonstrated survival benefit for undergoing SPKT in candidates that have Type-1 diabetes compared to KTA or continuing on the waitlist.[13,36-42] Preemptive SPKT has been associated with a 17%–21% reduction in kidney allograft loss compared with those receiving SPKT after dialysis initiation.[4,29,43-46] Current policy allows the pancreas candidate to also be allocated the kidney if needed, which increases earlier access to kidney transplant for candidates who do not have a living donor; similarly, early referral increases the chance of obtaining a preemptive SPKT. Treating the primary disease with a pancreas transplant protects the new kidney from recurrent diabetic nephropathy and the ensuing earlier-than-average kidney graft failure.[47] In addition, the progression of peripheral vascular disease is decreased by SPKT compared to KTA.[48] While these benefits decrease the morbidity associated with diabetes and improves post-transplant patient survival and quality of life, the SPKT operation requires a longer recovery with more risk of readmission (mostly due to GI-associated issues and autonomic hypotension precipitated by euglycemia) than that experienced after KTA.[49] Unlike the retroperitoneal placement of the KTA, the pancreas is typically transplanted into the intra-abdominal space, which increases the risk of bowel obstruction and potential need for reoperation. Thrombosis and pancreatitis of the pancreas transplant are currently the main causes of early pancreas graft loss. These risks apply to PAK as well as SPKT, with thrombosis being a several-fold higher risk for pancreas than for KTA. Of all pancreas transplant types, SPKT has the lowest rate of early pancreas allograft loss.[12] Many patients like the idea of one operation that can simultaneously mitigate the risks of morbidity and mortality of two diseases, given that infection risks increase with taking on the burden of immunosuppression. While surgical complications have decreased significantly over time and now occur in a smaller subset of patients, they can be significant when they occur. Patients must weigh the small but real risk of complications or death when considering the potential longer-term gains that can be achieved through long-term euglycemia.[48] A summary of the pros and cons of each transplant type is provided in Table 15.2.

Diagnosis of Acute Rejection

Rates of clinical acute rejection have decreased significantly over time with the introduction of more effective immunosuppressive agents.[50] Most centers utilize T-cell-depletion induction therapy and tacrolimus, mycophenolic mofetil, and prednisone, with rejection rates currently at 10.6% for recipients of SPKT.[20] Rejection of the kidney and pancreas are concordant at least 60% of the time, but awareness of the possibility of discordant rejection is an important part of

Table 15.2 Pros and Cons of Transplant Types for People with Kidney Failure Due to Diabetes

	SPK	PAK	LD-KTA	DD-KTA
Pros	Freedom from insulin, Delays or avoids progression of diabetes, Increased access to Kidney transplant, One surgery, and Longest pancreas graft survival.	Freedom from insulin, Delays or avoids progression of diabetes, and May afford preemptive LD kidney transplant.	Smaller Operation, Lower immunosuppression, Less risk of surgical complications, and Shorter wait time	Smaller Operation, Lower immunosuppression, and Less risk of surgical complications
Cons	Longer surgery, Higher surgical complications, Longer recovery, Risk of reoperation, Medium immunosuppression burden, and Potential surgical complications	Two surgeries, Higher pancreas rejection and shorter pancreas graft survival, Risk of reoperation, Higher immunosuppression burden, and Potential surgical complications	Managing diabetes, and Progression of diabetic complications.	Managing diabetes Progression of diabetic complications, Recurrent diabetic nephropathy, Higher risk of needing kidney retransplant, and Longer wait time

optimal patient management.[51-53] The gold standard for the diagnosis of pancreas rejection requires tissue for examination, and this can be accomplished via percutaneous, laparoscopic, cystoscopic, and open techniques.[54] Some centers do not biopsy the pancreas because of a lack of institutional expertise for performing either ultrasound- or computed tomography–guided biopsy and/or interpretation of the biopsy, so instead rely on the serum creatinine in the SPKT recipient to alert for the concern for pancreas rejection, although creatinine is not a very sensitive marker and fluctuations in lipase can be multifactorial and less specific.[52,55] Surveillance biopsies are rarely practiced due to a perceived high risk/benefit ratio. Noninvasive detection of rejection in pancreas transplant is currently a significant unmet need, prompting an international survey of clinical monitoring practices.[56,57]

Long-Term Outcomes of SPKT

Compared to DD KTA and other combined transplants (simultaneous liver-kidney and simultaneous heart-kidney) the short- and long-term outcomes of SPKT are remarkably favorable. The sharpest decrease in pancreas graft survival occurs very early after transplant and is usually of a technical nature and has minimal impact on patient survival, with 3-month and 1-year pancreas graft survival around 92% with a gradual slope of graft loss thereafter. Kidney allograft survival is even better, around 98% at 1 year, rivaling outcomes associated with kidney transplants from living donors, This results in excellent long-term graft survival, with pancreas and kidney allografts lasting more than 14 years on average, which is quite comparable to the kidney graft survival rate seen after KTA from a living donor.[13,58] Data on the impact of pancreas transplant on quality of life is also favorable and is an area of active investigation.[59-61]

Special Considerations for SPKT

Since the 2019 policy change that allowed SPKT candidates to qualify for wait-time accrual with an eGFR of at least 20 and (simply) insulin-dependent diabetes, there has been an increase in recipients of SPKT who are characterized as having insulin-dependent diabetes not attributed to Type-1. This policy allows each patient with renal failure and insulin-dependent diabetes to be individually considered for SPKT, regardless of diabetes "type." A very small number of ESKD patients present with insulin-dependent diabetes due to pancreatectomy, chronic pancreatitis, or cystic fibrosis (3c or "pancreatogenic" diabetes) and may be suitable candidates for SPKT.[62]

Conclusion

Optimizing access to kidney transplant for ESKD patients with insulin-dependent diabetes is associated with improved equity, patient survival, quality of life, and importantly, improved life-years from DD kidney transplant. To that end, SPKT may decrease the need for kidney retransplantation compared to KTA, which is an important goal in the current climate of organ shortage. Unlike other kidney-inclusive multiorgan transplants available to patients without primary renal disease, current pancreas allocation policy achieves kidney transplant for ESKD patients via SPKT, and by utilizing a pancreas from the same donor confers better patient and kidney survival compared to DD KTA.

References

1. United States Renal Data System. 2022 USRDS annual data report: epidemiology of kidney disease in the *United States*. 2022. https://adr.usrds.org/2022.
2. Lentine KL, Smith JM, Miller JM, et al. OPTN/SRTR 2021 annual data report: kidney. *Am J Transplant*. 2023;23(2):S21–S120. https://doi.org/10.1016/j.ajt.2023.02.004.
3. Fridell JA, Stratta RJ, Gruessner AC. Pancreas transplantation: current challenges, considerations, and controversies. *J Clin Endocrinol Metab*. 2023;108(3):614–623. https://doi.org/10.1210/clinem/dgac644.
4. Becker BN, Rush SH, Dykstra DM, Becker YT, Port FK. Preemptive transplantation for patients with diabetes-related kidney disease. *Arch Intern Med*. 2006;166(1):44–48. https://doi.org/10.1001/archinte.166.1.44.
5. Helantera I, Salmela K, Kyllonen L, Koskinen P, Gronhagen-Riska C, Finne P. Pretransplant dialysis duration and risk of death after kidney transplantation in the current era. *Transplantation*. 2014;98(4):458–464. https://doi.org/10.1097/TP.0000000000000085.
6. Gill JS, Tonelli M, Johnson N, Kiberd B, Landsberg D, Pereira BJ. The impact of waiting time and comorbid conditions on the survival benefit of kidney transplantation. *Kidney Int*. 2005;68(5):2345–2351. https://doi.org/10.1111/j.1523-1755.2005.00696.x.
7. Prezelin-Reydit M, Combe C, Harambat J, et al. Prolonged dialysis duration is associated with graft failure and mortality after kidney transplantation: results from the French transplant database. *Nephrol Dial Transplant*. 2019;34(3):538–545. https://doi.org/10.1093/ndt/gfy039.
8. McCune K, Owen-Simon N, Dube GK, Ratner LE. The best insulin delivery is a human pancreas. *Clin Transplant*. 2023;37(4):e14920. https://doi.org/10.1111/ctr.14920.
9. Morath C, Zeier M, Dohler B, Schmidt J, Nawroth PP, Opelz G. Metabolic control improves long-term renal allograft and patient survival in type 1 diabetes. *J Am Soc Nephrol*. 2008;19(8):1557–1563. https://doi.org/10.1681/ASN.2007070804.
10. Centers for Medicare & Medicaid Services, Department of Health and Human Services. Medicare and Medicaid programs; conditions for coverage for end-stage renal disease facilities: final rule. *Fed Regist*. 2008;73(73):20369–20484.

11. Fridell JA, Stratta RJ. Modern indications for referral for kidney and pancreas transplantation. *Curr Opin Nephrol Hypertens.* 2023;32(1):4–12. https://doi.org/10.1097/MNH.0000000000000846.

12. Kandaswamy R, Stock PG, Miller JM, et al. OPTN/SRTR 2021 annual data report: pancreas. *Am J Transplant.* 2023;23(2):S121–S177. https://doi.org/10.1016/j.ajt.2023.02.005.

13. Sollinger HW, Odorico JS, Becker YT, D'Alessandro AM, Pirsch JD. One thousand simultaneous pancreas-kidney transplants at a single center with 22-year follow-up. *Ann Surg.* 2009;250(4):618–630. https://doi.org/10.1097/SLA.0b013e3181b76d2b.

14. Owen RV, Thompson ER, Tingle SJ, et al. Too fat for transplant? The impact of recipient BMI on pancreas transplant outcomes. *Transplantation.* 2021;105(4):905–915. https://doi.org/10.1097/TP.0000000000003334.

15. Parsons RF, Tantisattamo E, Cheungpasitporn W, et al. Comprehensive review: frailty in pancreas transplant candidates and recipients. *Clin Transplant.* 2023;37(2):e14899. https://doi.org/10.1111/ctr.14899.

16. Fridell JA, Gage E, Goggins WC, Powelson JA. Complex arterial reconstruction for pancreas transplantation in recipients with advanced arteriosclerosis. *Transplantation.* 2007;83(10):1385–1388. https://doi.org/10.1097/01.tp.0000261629.02700.ef.

17. Fridell JA, Niederhaus S, Curry M, Urban R, Fox A, Odorico J. The survival advantage of pancreas after kidney transplant. *Am J Transplant.* 2019;19(3):823–830. https://doi.org/10.1111/ajt.15106.

18. Budhiraja P, Heilman RL, Reddy KS, et al. Favorable outcomes in older recipients receiving simultaneous pancreas kidney transplantation. *Transplant Direct.* 2022;8(12):e1413. https://doi.org/10.1097/TXD.0000000000001413.

19. Messner F, Leemkuil M, Yu Y, et al. Recipient age and outcome after pancreas transplantation: a retrospective dual-center analysis. *Transpl Int.* 2021;34(4):657–668. https://doi.org/10.1111/tri.13845.

20. Kandaswamy R, Stock PG, Miller J, et al. OPTN/SRTR 2020 annual data report: pancreas. *Am J Transplant.* 2022;22(Suppl 2):137–203. https://doi.org/10.1111/ajt.16979.

21. Stratta RJ, Gruessner AC, Odorico JS, Fridell JA, Gruessner RW. Pancreas transplantation: an alarming crisis in confidence. *Am J Transplant.* 2016;16(9):2556–2562. https://doi.org/10.1111/ajt.13890.

22. Gruessner AC, Gruessner RW. Long-term outcome after pancreas transplantation: a registry analysis. *Curr Opin Organ Transplant.* 2016;21(4):377–385. https://doi.org/10.1097/MOT.0000000000000331.

23. Amara D, Hansen KS, Kupiec-Weglinski SA, et al. Pancreas transplantation for type 2 diabetes: a systematic review, critical gaps in the literature, and a path forward. *Transplantation.* 2022;106(10):1916–1934. https://doi.org/10.1097/TP.0000000000004113.

24. Pham PH, Stalter LN, Martinez EJ, et al. Single center results of simultaneous pancreas-kidney transplantation in patients with type 2 diabetes. *Am J Transplant.* 2021;21(8):2810–2823. https://doi.org/10.1111/ajt.16462.

25. Parajuli S, Mandelbrot D, Aufhauser D, Kaufman D, Odorico J. Higher fasting pretransplant C-peptide levels in type 2 diabetics undergoing simultaneous pancreas-kidney transplantation are associated with posttransplant pancreatic graft dysfunction. *Transplantation.* 2023;107(4):e109–e121. https://doi.org/10.1097/TP.0000000000004489

26. Alhamad T, Kunjal R, Wellen J, et al. Three-month pancreas graft function signif-icantly influences survival following simultaneous pancreas-kidney transplantation in type 2 diabetes patients. *Am J Transplant*. 2020;20(3):788–796. https://doi.org/10.1111/ajt.15615.

27. Hart A, Smith JM, Skeans MA, et al. OPTN/SRTR 2018 annual data report: kidney. *Am J Transplant*. 2020;20(Suppl 1):20–130. https://doi.org/10.1111/ajt.15672.

28. Kandaswamy R, Stock PG, Gustafson SK, et al. OPTN/SRTR 2018 annual data re-port: pancreas. *Am J Transplant*. 2020;20(Suppl s1):131–192. https://doi.org/10.1111/ajt.15673.

29. Gruessner AC, Gruessner RW. Pancreas transplantation of US and non-US cases from 2005 to 2014 as reported to the United Network for Organ Sharing (UNOS) and the International Pancreas Transplant Registry (IPTR). *Rev Diabet Stud*. 2016;13(1):35–58. https://doi.org/10.1900/RDS.2016.13.35.

30. Guidance on the benefits of pancreas after kidney (PAK) transplantation. OPTN/UNOS; 2017. https://optn.transplant.hrsa.gov/media/2226/pancreas_pcguidance_201707.pdf, accessed on February 29th 2024.

31. Boggi U, Vistoli F, Marchetti P, Kandaswamy R, Berney T, World Consensus Group on Pancreas Transplantation. First world consensus conference on pancreas transplanta-tion: part I—methods and results of literature search. *Am J Transplant*. 2021;21(Suppl 3):1–16. https://doi.org/10.1111/ajt.16738.

32. Boggi U, Vistoli F, Andres A, et al. First world consensus conference on pancreas transplantation: part II—recommendations. *Am J Transplant*. 2021;21(Suppl 3):17–59. https://doi.org/10.1111/ajt.16750.

33. Sutherland DE, Goetz FC, Rynasiewicz JJ, et al. Segmental pancreas transplan-tation from living related and cadaver donors: a clinical experience. *Surgery*. 1981;90(2):159–169.

34. Boggi U, Amorese G, Marchetti P, Mosca F. Segmental live donor pancreas transplan-tation: review and critique of rationale, outcomes, and current recommendations. *Clin Transplant*. 2011;25(1):4–12. https://doi.org/10.1111/j.1399-0012.2010.01381.x.

35. Sutherland DE, Radosevich D, Gruessner R, Gruessner A, Kandaswamy R. Pushing the envelope: living donor pancreas transplantation. *Curr Opin Organ Transplant*. 2012;17(1):106–1015. https://doi.org/10.1097/MOT.0b013e32834ee6e5.

36. Sung RS, Zhang M, Schaubel DE, Shu X, Magee JC. A reassessment of the survival advantage of simultaneous kidney-pancreas versus kidney-alone transplantation. *Transplantation*. 2015;99(9):1900–1906. https://doi.org/10.1097/TP.0000000000000663.

37. Rayhill SC, D'Alessandro AM, Odorico JS, et al. Simultaneous pancreas-kidney transplantation and living related donor renal transplantation in patients with dia-betes: is there a difference in survival? *Ann Surg*. 2000;231(3):417–423. https://doi.org/10.1097/00000658-200003000-00015.

38. Mohan P, Safi K, Little DM, et al. Improved patient survival in recipients of simulta-neous pancreas-kidney transplant compared with kidney transplant alone in patients with type 1 diabetes mellitus and end-stage renal disease. *Br J Surg*. 2003;90(9):1137–1141. https://doi.org/10.1002/bjs.4208.

39. Lindahl JP, Hartmann A, Aakhus S, et al. Long-term cardiovascular outcomes in type 1 diabetic patients after simultaneous pancreas and kidney transplantation compared with living donor kidney transplantation. *Diabetologia*. 2016;59(4):844–852. https://doi.org/10.1007/s00125-015-3853-8.

40. Reddy KS, Stablein D, Taranto S, et al. Long-term survival following simultaneous kidney-pancreas transplantation versus kidney transplantation alone in patients with type 1 diabetes mellitus and renal failure. *Am J Kidney Dis.* 2003;41(2):464–470. https://doi.org/10.1053/ajkd.2003.50057.
41. Bunnapradist S, Cho YW, Cecka JM, Wilkinson A, Danovitch GM. Kidney allograft and patient survival in type I diabetic recipients of cadaveric kidney alone versus simultaneous pancreas kidney transplants: a multivariate analysis of the UNOS database. *J Am Soc Nephrol.* 2003;14(1):208–213. https://doi.org/10.1097/01.asn.0000037 678.54984.41.
42. Knoll GA, Nichol G. Dialysis, kidney transplantation, or pancreas transplantation for patients with diabetes mellitus and renal failure: a decision analysis of treatment options. *J Am Soc Nephrol.* 2003;14(2):500–515. https://doi.org/10.1097/01.asn.000 0046061.62136.d4.
43. Israni AK, Feldman HI, Propert KJ, Leonard M, Mange KC. Impact of simultaneous kidney-pancreas transplant and timing of transplant on kidney allograft survival. *Am J Transplant.* 2005;5(2):374–382. https://doi.org/10.1111/j.1600-6143.2004.00688.x.
44. Huang E, Wiseman A, Okumura S, Kuo HT, Bunnapradist S. Outcomes of preemptive kidney with or without subsequent pancreas transplant compared with preemptive simultaneous pancreas/kidney transplantation. *Transplantation.* 2011;92(10):1115–1122. https://doi.org/10.1097/TP.0b013e31823328a6.
45. Wiseman AC, Huang E, Kamgar M, Bunnapradist S. The impact of pre-transplant dialysis on simultaneous pancreas-kidney versus living donor kidney transplant outcomes. *Nephrol Dial Transplant.* 2013;28(4):1047–1058. https://doi.org/10.1093/ndt/gfs582.
46. Stratta R, Coffman D, Jay C, et al. Does dialysis modality or duration influence outcomes in simultaneous pancreas-kidney transplant recipients? Single center experience and review of the literature. *Clin Transplant.*11 May 2023. https://doi.org/10.1111/ctr.15009
47. Kleinclauss F, Fauda M, Sutherland DE, et al. Pancreas after living donor kidney transplants in diabetic patients: impact on long-term kidney graft function. *Clin Transplant.* 2009;23(4):437–446. https://doi.org/10.1111/j.1399-0012.2009.00998.x.
48. Sucher R, Rademacher S, Jahn N, et al. Effects of simultaneous pancreas-kidney transplantation and kidney transplantation alone on the outcome of peripheral vascular diseases. *BMC Nephrol.* 2019;20(1):453. https://doi.org/10.1186/s12882-019-1649-7.
49. Rajkumar T, Mazid S, Vucak-Dzumhur M, Sykes TM, Elder GJ. Health-related quality of life following kidney and simultaneous pancreas kidney transplantation. *Nephrology (Carlton).* 2019;24(9):975–982. https://doi.org/10.1111/nep.13523.
50. Gruessner AC. 2011 update on pancreas transplantation: comprehensive trend analysis of 25,000 cases followed up over the course of twenty-four years at the International Pancreas Transplant Registry (IPTR). *Rev Diabet Stud.* 2011;8(1):6–16. https://doi.org/10.1900/RDS.2011.8.6.
51. Troxell ML, Koslin DB, Norman D, Rayhill S, Mittalhenkle A. Pancreas allograft rejection: analysis of concurrent renal allograft biopsies and posttherapy follow-up biopsies. *Transplantation.* 2010;90(1):75–84. https://doi.org/10.1097/TP.0b013e318 1dda17e.
52. Redfield RR, Kaufman DB, Odorico JS. Diagnosis and treatment of pancreas rejection. *Curr Transplant Rep.* 2015;2(2):169–175. https://doi.org/10.1007/s40 472-015-0061-x.

53. Parajuli S, Arpali E, Astor BC, et al. Concurrent biopsies of both grafts in recipients of simultaneous pancreas and kidney demonstrate high rates of discordance for rejection as well as discordance in type of rejection—a retrospective study. *Transpl Int.* 2018;31(1):32–37. https://doi.org/10.1111/tri.13007.

54. Uva PD, Odorico JS, Giunippero A, et al. Laparoscopic biopsies in pancreas transplantation. *Am J Transplant.* 2017;17(8):2173–2177. https://doi.org/10.1111/ajt.14259.

55. Klassen DK, Drachenberg CB, Papadimitriou JC, et al. CMV allograft pancreatitis: diagnosis, treatment, and histological features. *Transplantation.* 2000;69(9):1968–1971. https://doi.org/10.1097/00007890-200005150-00042.

56. Ward C, Odorico JS, Rickels MR, et al. International survey of clinical monitoring practices in pancreas and islet transplantation. *Transplantation.* 2022;106(8):1647–1655. https://doi.org/10.1097/TP.0000000000004058.

57. Yoo A, Riedel A, Qian I, et al. An initial analysis of the baseline levels of Dd-cfDNA after pancreas transplantation: a prospective study from high-volume centers in the United States. *Transplant Direct.* 2023;9(4):e1459. https://doi.org/10.1097/TXD.0000000000001459.

58. Gruessner RW, Gruessner AC. The current state of pancreas transplantation. *Nat Rev Endocrinol.* 2013;9(9):555–562. https://doi.org/10.1038/nrendo.2013.138.

59. Parajuli S, Aziz F, Garg N, et al. Frailty in pancreas transplantation. *Transplantation.* 2021;105(8):1685–1694. https://doi.org/10.1097/TP.0000000000003586.

60. Ziaja J, Bozek-Pajak D, Kowalik A, Krol R, Cierpka L. Impact of pancreas transplantation on the quality of life of diabetic renal transplant recipients. *Transplant Proc.* 2009;41(8):3156–3158. https://doi.org/10.1016/j.transproceed.2009.07.101.

61. Bozek-Pajak D, Ziaja J, Kowalik A, et al. Past cardiovascular episodes deteriorate quality of life of patients with type 1 diabetes and end-stage kidney disease after kidney or simultaneous pancreas and kidney transplantation. *Transplant Proc.* 2016;48(5):1667–1672. https://doi.org/10.1016/j.transproceed.2015.10.085.

62. Chen M, Dunn TB. Pancreas transplant for combined pancreatic endocrine and exocrine insufficiency. *Curr Transpl Rep.* 2022;9:108–113. https://doi.org/10.1007/s40472-022-00361-6.

16

Transplantation in Children

Raja S. Dandamudi, Britta Höcker, and Vikas Dharnidharka

Learning about kidney transplantation in children!!

Introduction

Kidney transplantation (KT) is the treatment of choice for children with end-stage kidney disease (ESKD), providing a significant survival advantage over dialysis.[1] The field of pediatric KT continues to evolve, with improvements in management strategies including immunosuppression and antiviral therapies. The etiology of ESKD, donor-recipient size mismatch, post-transplant complications, medication nonadherence, growth and neurocognitive development, social issues, and comorbidities associated with the lower urinary tract are unique challenges in pediatric KT and are addressed in this chapter.

Scope of Transplantation in Children

Incidence and Prevalence of ESKD in Children

The incidence and prevalence of ESKD are increasing in adults and in contrast, in the United States the number of children with incident ESKD decreased between 2010 (13 per million population, 925 patients) and 2020 (11 per million population, 806 patients). But the adjusted prevalence of ESKD among children increased from 72 per million population in 2010 to 76 per million population in 2020.[2] According to the European Registry Annual (ERA) 2020 Report, the prevalence of ESKD in Europe is around 60.1 per million age-related population with an incidence of 8.4 per million age-related population.[3] There was a stable incidence and increasing prevalence of European children on kidney replacement therapy during 2007–2016.[4] In Australia and New Zealand, the incidence is about 9 per million age-related population with a prevalence of 55 per million age-related population (0–17 years between 2007 and 2018).[5]

In Latin America, the provision of pediatric renal replacement therapy is also variable (prevalence from 10 per million age-related population in Paraguay to 40 per million age-related population in Argentina).[6] The data from the low-middle- and low-income countries is sparse due to the lack of national registries for ESKD. There is a large unmet need for renal replacement therapy in developing regions like India, China, Pakistan, South Asia, and Sub-Saharan Africa. In Europe, rates of pediatric KT range from 0 to 13.5 per million children population depending on the per capita income and accessibility to transplant. There is a paucity of data from middle- and low-income countries, but reports suggest that the rates of transplantation are less than 4 per million children population.[7]

Causes of ESKD in Children, Number of Pediatric Transplants Done in United States

According to the United States Renal Data System (USRDS) database, congenital anomalies of the kidney and urinary tract (CAKUT) are the most common cause of incident ESKD among children younger than 1 year (51.1%) and become less common with advancing age, down to 20.4% in the age group 13–17 years.[2] Similar trends were observed in Australia New Zealand Data (ANZDATA). In contrast, ERA data suggests CAKUT as the etiology of ESKD in 35% of cases in the 15–19 years age group versus 20% in the 0–4 years age group.[3] In the United States combined primary and secondary glomerulonephritis as the cause of incident ESKD increases with age, from 6.3% of children aged less than 1 year to 36.0% of children aged 13–17 years.

Prevalence of ESKD

African American children had the highest prevalence of ESKD. The prevalence of ESKD was nearly 50% higher in boys, probably related to obstructive uropathies.[2] In 2020 KT is the initial treatment in children with ESKD in about 14% of patients.[2] In the United States, the number of prevalent ESKD pediatric candidates on the wait list for transplant (listed <18 years) is steadily increasing and reached 2,637 in 2020 (1,083 were added to the list in 2020). Children in the age group 12–17 years account for the largest proportion on the waiting list (59.5%) in 2020, compared with those 6–11 years (19.4%), and 0–6 years (21.1%). There is a steady decrease in the proportion of pediatric candidates waiting for retransplant over the decade (26.7% in 2010 to 12.7% in 2020). By race, White candidates accounted for the largest group (42.9%) on the wait list in 2020, followed by Hispanic (27.8%), Black (19.6%), and Asian candidates (6.0%). Over the past decade, the proportion of White (37.1% to 44.7%) and Asian (3% to 6.7%) transplant candidates has increased, while the proportion of Black (26.5% to 17.8%) and Hispanic (31.8% to 27.1%) candidates has decreased.[8]

According to the analysis of the North American Pediatric Renal Transplant Cooperative Studies (NAPTRS) database spanning 30 years from 1987 to 2017, the following trends were observed as shown in Figure 16.1. A decline was noted in the proportion of white recipients. The 13- to 17-year age group continued to be the most prevalent age group throughout the years. The percentage of Living Donor (LD) transplants reached a peak of 64% in 2001 but subsequently showed a gradual decrease, falling to only 31.5% by 2017.[9]

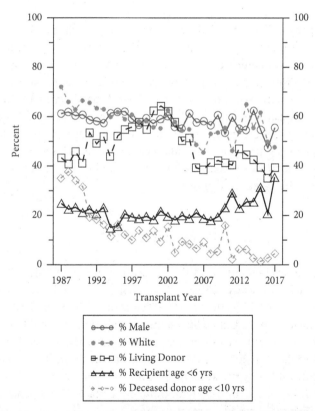

Figure 16.1 Trends in kidney disease among children in the United States from 1987 showing slight decline in the prevalence among Whites and decreasing number of LD kidney transplants.[1]

Insert Figure 16.1. herePreemptive Kidney Transplant

A preemptive KT is defined as transplantation prior to the initiation of dialysis, thereby avoiding the morbidity and mortality associated with dialysis. In the United States, 22% of incident ESKD patients 0–17 years received a preemptive KT compared to 6% in the 18–44 age group, 4% in the 46–64 year group, and 2% in the 65–74 year group (Figure 16.2).[2]

There is a wide disparity in European countries in their overall rates of pre-emptive KT ranging from less than 5% to more than 60%.[10] Analysis of the ERA registry suggested several advantages to preemptive KT. Preemptive transplants have a higher acute rejection-free proportion at 3 years post-transplant (52% vs. 37%) and improved 6-year patient survival when compared to dialysis patients (82% vs. 69%).[11] A recent meta-analysis that included 22 studies (N = 22,622) noted a reduction in overall graft loss by 43% (relative risk [RR] 0.57, 95% confidence interval [CI]: 0.49–0.66) and acute rejection by 19% (RR 0.81, 95% CI 0.75–0.88) in preemptive KT compared to transplantation after dialysis.[12] But socioeconomic factors that prevent preemptive KT may confound the long-term results. From patient management and policy matters it is important to develop pathways that can improve options for pediatric preemptive KT.

Long-Term Outcome

Improvements in Survival

The last few decades in pediatric KT witnessed significant improvement in immunosuppression protocols and patient care, which led to significant

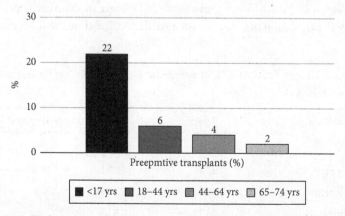

Figure 16.2 Higher proportion of preemptive transplants in children.

improvement in both allograft and patient survival. Analysis of the US Scientific Registry of Transplant Recipients (SRTR) showed significant improvements in graft survival over the years: 1-year graft survival for transplants performed in 1987 versus 2010 (81% vs. 97%), 5-year graft survival for transplants performed in 1987 versus 2006 (59% vs. 78%), and 10-year graft survival for transplants performed in 1987 versus 2001 (47% vs. 60%)[13] Comparing deceased donor (DD) versus living donor (LD) recipients,1- year graft survival of DD recipients was comparable with LD recipients (96.7% vs. 97%), but 5-year graft survival for LD recipients (92.4%) is still higher than DD recipients (83.1%)[8] (Table 16.1).

Estimated Glomerular Filtration Rate

Estimated glomerular filtration rate (eGFR) at 12 months is an early surrogate allograft outcome and in the year 2019, 70% of DD recipients and 67% of LD recipients had eGFR of at least 60 mL/min/1.73 m^2 at 1 year post-transplant.[2] But the adolescent age group has worse 5-year graft survival compared to pediatric recipients under the age of 10 years[14]

Organ Source

In the United States, the Organ Procurement and Transplantation Network (OPTN) implemented the Kidney Allocation System (KAS) in December 2014. The Kidney Donor Profile Index (KDPI) was inducted into the KAS to estimate graft longevity based on donor factors. Under the new policy, if the KDPI is <35%, pediatric candidates (<18 years at the time of listing) receive preference, after multiorgan candidates, highly sensitized candidates (calculated panel reactive antibody [cPRA] >98%), and former LD. There is no pediatric prioritization for the allocation of kidneys with a KDPI >35%. Before the KAS, under the

Table 16.1 Kidney Transplant Graft Survival at 1-, 5-, and 10-Year Post-Transplant in Children (USA)

Graft survival	1 year	5 years	10 years
1987	81%	59%	47%
Recent Era	97%	78%	60%
LD transplant	97%	92.4%	-
DD transplants	96.7%	83.1%	-

previous Share 35 policy pediatric candidates received priority for all kidneys from DD under the age of 35 years.

Globally other allocation policies prioritize pediatric patients— Eurotransplant, for pediatric patients (<16 years at the time of listing in Europe, <18 years in Germany) the points for human leukocyte antigen (HLA) mismatches are doubled and they receive bonus points for waiting time, Scandiatransplant prioritizes pediatric recipients when the donor is less than 40 years old, and in the Swiss Organ Allocation System, ABO-compatible pediatric patients (<20 years) receive preference from DD <60 years.[15] Because of the longevity of children undergoing KT, most pediatric recipients will inevitably develop graft failure, requiring a return to dialysis or a second transplant.

Kidney Transplant Wait Time

The median survival of the allograft is around 12–14 years.[16] Therefore, most pediatric recipients require retransplantation. The median waiting time for DDKT for children in the United States is around 200 days as compared to more than 40 months in individuals over 18 years of age.[2] The sequencing of a DDKT and a LDKT is a point of discussion. Because of pediatric preference in allocation systems children could receive good-quality organs in a relatively short period. Contrary arguments are based on the superior long-term graft survival of a LD graft compared to a DD graft, and on the possibility that the potential donor may be ineligible for donation when retransplantation is considered. The sequence of DD followed by LD or vice versa doesn't affect the cumulative graft survival.[17] In Eurotransplant, a recipient who is reregistered for a KT with one or more immediate previous LDKTs having failed, requiring maintenance dialysis is eligible for the return of all the waiting time.

Immunosuppression

Immunosuppressive protocols evolved over the last decade to improve outcome. Post-transplant immunosuppression includes two phases:

1. Induction immunosuppression, in the perioperative period to prevent early rejection; and
2. Maintenance immunosuppression during the perioperative period and continuing indefinitely to promote long-term graft survival.

Induction therapy depletes or modify T cells prior to donor antigen presentation and the agents are:

- Polyclonal lymphocyte-depleting antibodies:
  o Thymoglobulin: polyclonal antibody generated in rabbits using human thymocytes.
  o ATGAM: purified gamma globulin generated from horses with human thymocytes.
- Monoclonal antibody:
  o Alemtuzumab is a humanized anti-CD52 pan lymphocytic (both B and T cells) monoclonal antibody (Campath 1H)
  o IL-2 receptor antagonist—a chimeric monoclonal antibody (basiliximab).

Induction

Typically, induction protocols use a combination of corticosteroids along with one of the induction agents. The choice of the immunosuppression regimen is determined by the patient's risk of rejection. There is no standardized international consensus and immunosuppression protocols are mostly center-dependent. In the United States 94.3% of pediatric KT recipients reported some induction use in 2020. T-cell-depleting agent usage steadily increased, reaching 63.6% in 2018, and IL-2-RA therapy remained stable at 35.1%.[8] However, in European countries reporting to the Cooperative European Pediatric Renal Transplant Initiative (CERTAIN), induction therapy is used in only approximately 50% of patients and IL-2 RA therapy is the most common induction agent.[18] According to American Society of Transplantation, Kidney Disease Improving Global Outcomes (KDIGO) 2009 guidelines, young recipient age, older donor age, high HLA mismatch, Black race, PRA greater than 0, DSA, cold ischemia time of more than 24 hours, ABO incompatibility, and delayed graft function are considered as high risk.[19] For patients who are at low immunologic risk of acute rejection either basiliximab or rATG-Thymoglobulin is a reasonable induction therapy agent. For patients at high immunologic risk of acute rejection, induction therapy with rATG-Thymoglobulin is recommended.

Maintenance Immunosuppression

Usually, a combination of a calcineurin inhibitor (CNI) and an antiproliferative agent, with or without corticosteroids, is used as maintenance immunosuppression. In 2018, 57.8% of pediatric recipients in the United States received tacrolimus, mycophenolate mofetil (MMF), and steroids, and 37.5% received tacrolimus and MMF for maintenance immunosuppression.[8] Although there is a variation in immunosuppressive regimens and the number of medications, triple therapy with CNI, antiproliferative drugs, and corticosteroids was the most common immunosuppressive regimen used in KT recipients in Europe.

Pediatric-Specific Clinical Trials for Induction Immunosuppression

Basiliximab induction decreased the rate of acute rejection without an increase in postoperative infections when compared to patients with no induction[20] in an ANZDATA pediatric registry study. There was a 40% reduction in the incidence of acute rejection at 6 months post-transplant with basiliximab compared with no induction.[20] In a multicenter, open-label prospective study, the use of basiliximab induction with dual maintenance immunosuppression (cyclosporine and corticosteroids) was associated with a highly favorable safety and efficacy profile in pediatric de novo recipients of DDKT or LDKT.[21] Clark, et al. compared Thymoglobulin versus basiliximab (sample size: 42 patients in each group) and demonstrated a lower acute rejection rate in the basiliximab group (45% vs. 62%, $p < 0.05$) and lower rates of cytomegalovirus (CMV) disease in CMV-positive recipients.[22] Several studies have evaluated the effectiveness of glucocorticoid-sparing protocols in pediatric KT patients. The available evidence suggests that this approach does not increase the risk of rejection or worsen graft survival.[23-26] Khositseth et al. studied a retrospective cohort comparing ATGAM ($n = 127$) versus Thymoglobulin ($n = 71$) and showed that Thymoglobulin induction was associated with a less incidence of acute rejection and an increased incidence of Epstein-Barr virus (EBV) infection.[27] Ashoor et al. in a retrospective multicenter study demonstrated low rATG induction dose of 4.5 mg/kg or less provided safe and effective outcomes in low immunologic risk pediatric cohort.[28]

Pediatric Trials in Maintenance Immunosuppression

A multicenter study (18 centers from nine European countries, $n = 196$) compared cyclosporine and tacrolimus administered concomitantly with azathioprine (AZA) and steroids. The outcomes, incidence of acute rejection (36.9% vs. 59.1% in tacrolimus group vs. cyclosporine group) and mean GFR (mL/min/

1.73^2) at 1 year (62 in tacrolimus vs. 56 in cyclosporine group).[29] The North American Pediatric Transplant Collaborative Study (NAPRTCS) data analysis of 986 pediatric KT recipients treated with either cyclosporine, MMF, and steroids or tacrolimus, MMF, and steroids found no difference in 1-year patient and graft survival, but a significantly higher mean GFR at 1 year in patients treated with tacrolimus.[30] The largest pediatric study of 140 patients comparing MMF versus AZA found a higher 5-year graft survival with MMF (90.7% vs. 68.5%; $p < .001$).[31] Because of significant, dose-related side effects including osseous, cardiovascular, and metabolic complications, and growth retardation in children different steroid-discontinuing strategies were utilized across various centers: rapid discontinuation of steroids (within 1 week post-transplant), early withdrawal (steroid withdrawal within 7–14 days post-transplant), and late withdrawal (withdrawal within the 1st year), and some centers continue steroids indefinitely. The Organ Procurement and Transplantation Network (OPTN) database showed that the use of steroid minimization protocols increased from 8.7% in 2002 to 37% in 2009.[32] Studies comparing maintenance immunosuppression regimens with and without steroids showed no difference in terms of patient and graft survival.[24,33,34] Meta-analysis showed an increase in height-standardized Z-scores but no increase in acute rejection with steroid-avoidance/withdrawal regimens compared with steroid-based regimens. The magnitude of post-transplant growth in the prepubertal recipients was greater than that in the pubertal recipients.[35]

Age-Related Differences in Immune Function

Since birth, the immune system constantly transforms, increasing alloreactivity. The naive T cell pool in children changes to memory T cells due to thymic atrophy. In contrast to adults, children have low expression of the CD40-ligand (CD40-L/CD154), fewer antigen-specific CD8(+) T cells, and lower titers of anti-HLA antibodies prior to transplantation.[36]

Infections

Immunosuppressed children are more susceptible to infections (EBV, CMV, BK virus [BKV]), potentially triggering the immune response leading to transplant rejection. The immune response after infections has different clinical manifestations like a low-grade fever, significant lymphopenia, higher gastrointestinal symptoms, higher fatality, and prolonged viremia compared to the general population. Immediately post-transplant there is an increased incidence of wound, nosocomial, and urinary tract infections. Donor-derived infections also happen in the first few weeks post-transplant. Opportunistic infections such as CMV, EBV, and BKV, may start to occur after 1-month post-transplant. Following 6 months, the risk of late opportunistic infections remains high. The Immune Development in Pediatric Transplantation (IMPACT) study identified that 73% of patients developed viral DNAemia (EBV, 34%; CMV, 23%; BKV, 23%; and JC virus, 21%).[37]

Urinary tract infections are a common infectious complication in the renal transplant population with the highest risk within the first 6 months post-transplant and in patients with congenital anomalies of the kidney and urinary tract. Post-transplant asymptomatic bacteriuria is more common in those with pretransplant bacteriuria and in those with underlying genitourinary abnormalities including neurogenic bladders.

Children are at increased risk for viruses such as CMV and EBV in the intermediate and late transplant periods, often due to lack of infection prior to transplant, receipt of an organ from a seropositive donor, or reactivation of latent infection.

Clinically, CMV infection can be asymptomatic or present as CMV disease. Patients may have low-grade fevers, pneumonitis, diarrhea, or hepatitis; and severe infections can be fatal. In a report of the NAPTRCS, the incidence of CMV infection–related hospitalization in children was 5.6%.[38] The KDIGO recommends prophylaxis for 6 months in adult KT recipients who are CMV seropositive or who have received an organ from a CMV-seropositive donor (CMV D+/R+, D-/R+, D+/R-) in the setting of anti-T-cell antibody immunosuppression.[39-41] The International CMV consensus guidelines recommend 3–6 months of prophylaxis with valganciclovir for pediatric kidney allograft recipients with a CMV D+/R- serostatus. In CMV-positive pediatric recipients, either antiviral prophylaxis or preemptive therapy is recommended. An alternative for these patients is the so-called hybrid strategy consisting of short-term prophylaxis with surveillance after prophylaxis.[42]

EBV is an oncogenic herpes virus that primarily infects most people in early childhood and thereafter remains a latent infection. Acute infection can be either asymptomatic or can manifest as an uncomplicated mononucleosis syndrome with fever, leukopenia, and atypical lymphocytosis. Reactivation of latent infection and chronic active EBV infection can lead to persistent EBV DNAemia and lymphoproliferative disorders.

Initial treatment consists of EBV DNAemia post-transplant consists of decreasing immunosuppression, and in those who do not respond to immunosuppression reduction, some centers will treat with antiviral agents such as valganciclovir despite guideline recommendations that there are insufficient data for benefit.[43] Where PTLD occurs, additional options include cessation of antimetabolites or all immunosuppression, administration of anti–CD-20 monoclonal antibody, and potentially chemotherapy.

In pediatric KT recipients, BKV replication can cause BK nephropathy (elevated serum creatinine, interstitial inflammation) and renal allograft loss.[44] A NAPRTCS registry analysis suggested a 5% incidence of BKV-associated nephropathy.[45] The identified risk factors for BK nephropathy include BK seronegativity at the time of transplant, ureteral stents post-transplant, HLA mismatch, a higher net state of immunosuppression, tacrolimus-based immunosuppression, younger recipient age, and obstructive uropathy as primary renal disease.[46] Decreasing immunosuppression is the cornerstone of the management of BK nephropathy. Management of persistent viral replication after decreasing immunosuppression is not well defined. Intravenous immune globulin (IVIG), leflunomide, cidofovir, and quinolone antibiotics are all used with variable success, none with rigorous evidence.[47,48]

Immunizations

Compared to the general population, transplant candidates exhibit a suboptimal immune response following vaccination; however, their immune response is superior to that of patients who have undergone transplantation. Cooperative European Pediatric Renal Transplant Initiative analysis of vaccination titers pre- and post-transplant showed that there is a low percentage of patients who have positive vaccination titers prior to transplantation. Additionally, after transplantation, there is a low rate of revaccination, and even if revaccinated, the patient's antibody response is limited. Moreover, there is a high rate of vaccination titer losses observed in such patients.[49]

All potential transplant candidates should receive standard immunizations using age-appropriate guidelines. Live vaccines should be administered at least 6–8 weeks prior to transplant.[50]

Because of the risk of active disease postvaccination, live-attenuated vaccines, including varicella and measles-mumps-rubella (MMR) should be administered pretransplant. MMR and varicella are normally given at 12 months of age but can be administered to children as young as 6 months.[51] Inactivated polio vaccine is indicated, rather than oral polio vaccine. Children should receive immunization for pneumococcal infection, with the 13-valent vaccine followed by the 23-valent vaccine at a minimum of 8 weeks interval.[52] Patients with ESKD do not develop or even lose their vaccination titer. Surveillance of titers and booster vaccinations are recommended.[49] We recommend routinely providing an annual influenza vaccine to children with transplants and their family and/or household contacts. Inactivated influenza vaccine can safely be given as early as

1 month post-transplantation. KT recipients should receive a 9-valent HPV vaccine (types 6, 11, 16, 18, 31, 33, 45, 52, and 58) a three-dose series separated by 0, 1, and 6 months.[53]

Recurrent Disease

Recurrence of primary kidney disease post-transplant is the involvement of the renal allograft with the original disease that caused ESKD. The clinical spectrum of recurrence depends on the primary disease, and it can range from the recurrence of the full disease to the recurrence of some features of the disease. Clinical features of the recurrent disease include elevated creatinine, hematuria, and/or proteinuria. Recurrence can occur at any time post-transplant and accounts for approximately 7%–8% of all graft loss.[54]

Primary glomerulonephritis, secondary glomerulonephritis, and inherited metabolic diseases are the three major disease categories that can recur in renal allografts. Primary focal segmental glomerulosclerosis (FSGS), C3 glomerulopathy (formerly MPGN type 1 and 2), and immunoglobulin A nephropathy (IgAN) are the most common primary glomerular diseases that can recur. Lupus nephritis, Henoch-Schonlein nephritis, small vessel vasculitis, and hemolytic uremic syndrome are the most common secondary glomerular and vascular diseases that can recur. Primary hyperoxaluria, Fabry disease, methylmalonic acidemia, and adenine phosphoribosyl-transferase deficiency are some of the inherited metabolic disorders that can recur post-transplant. The 5-year graft losses were significantly higher for children with glomerular pathology FSGS (25.7%) MPGN (32.4%) when compared to children with CAKUT (14.4%) as the primary diagnosis.[55] The risk of FSGS recurrence post-transplant in children is around 14%–50%[56] and in adults after renal transplant is reported to be 20%–50% in first-time allograft recipients[57] and up to 80% in retransplants if recurrence occurred in the first allograft.[58] The pretransplant characteristics such as rapid progression of primary FSGS with the time interval between diagnosis and ESKD of less than 3 years, age of onset of FSGS in native kidneys between 6 and 15 years, and diffuse mesangial proliferation on native biopsy are considered to be high risk for post-transplant relapse. Early-onset post-transplant nephrotic range proteinuria is an important surrogate marker for the recurrence of FSGS.

The management of post-transplant FSGS includes plasma exchange with or without rituximab and lipid apheresis. No well-designed clinical trials compare the various reported regimens. Angiotensin-converting enzyme inhibitors and angiotensin 2-receptor blockers partially reduce proteinuria without significantly improving graft survival.

The recurrence rate of IgAN is not well documented. The recurrence rate reported in a large ANZDATA analysis was 5.4% and 10.8% at 5 and 10 years, respectively, with a median time to recurrence of 4.63 [Inter Quartile Range (IQR), 2.12–8.66] years and no increased risk of recurrence in a second graft.[59] The risk of IgAN recurrence is not associated with donor status, recipient age, race, gender, or immunosuppression.[60] Management of disease recurrence after pediatric KT made some progress in recent years owing to emerging therapies. International registries and prospective multicenter collaborative studies are needed to optimize pretransplantation risk evaluation and post-transplantation management.

Tumors

Post-transplant lymphoproliferative disease (PTLD) is the most common malignancy complicating KT in children with a relatively low incidence of 1%–3% in pediatric KT recipients.[61] Active replication of EBV after either primary infection or reactivation of latent infection plays a major role in the development of EBV-positive PTLD. Even though most B-cell lymphomas are associated with EBV infection, EBV-negative PTLD may be a late serious complication of organ transplantation. Recipient EBV seronegativity, the higher degree of immunosuppression, allograft type, host genetic variations, and especially high-level EBV DNAemia are well-recognized risk factors.[62] In solid organ transplantation, EBV-naive patients have a much higher risk of developing PTLD than patients who are EBV-seropositive at the time of transplantation. More recently, specific mutations in LMP1 increase the risk of PTLD.[63] The clinical presentation is highly variable and depends on the dysfunction of the involved organs. Nonspecific constitutional symptoms such as fever, weight loss, and fatigue are common. EBV infection and/or reactivation can be detected as increasing copy numbers of EBV DNA in the peripheral blood. The KDIGO recommended regular monitoring of EBV viral load in the high-risk EBV donor/recipient D+/R-sero mismatch, at least every 1 week in the first 3 months after transplantation, at least monthly for 3–6 months, and then every 3 months for the rest of the first year.[19]

The primary goal in the treatment of PTLD is the cure, and a concomitant objective should be the preservation of the allografted organ. Reduction of immunosuppression, immunotherapy with the CD20 monoclonal antibody rituximab, chemotherapy, radiation therapy, or a combination of these agents are employed, based on institutional protocols.

Post pediatric KT, the cumulative absolute risk of any type of cancer is approximately 35%, corresponding to a fourfold increase in the relative risk of developing cancer compared to the general population.[64] In a Dutch study, there is at least one malignancy in 41% of patients who had 30 years of follow-up starting from the first transplantation.[65] Nonmelanomatous skin cancer (squamous and basal cell) and human papillomavirus (HPV)–associated anogenital and gynecological carcinomas are the most common nonlymphoproliferative malignancies in pediatric patients receiving KT.

Growth

Growth failure is a very common complication of chronic kidney disease (CKD). When compared to age-matched controls, children with CKD have suboptimal prepubertal and pubertal growth. Children with ESKD revealed shunting of leg growth and preserved trunk growth resulting in disproportionate stunting. Various factors like resistance to growth, insulin-like growth factor-1 (IGF-1) malnutrition, anemia, and metabolic acidosis all play a role in CKD-related growth retardation.[66] Longitudinal growth post-transplant is affected by: age at transplantation (prepubertal vs. pubertal), allograft function, and corticosteroid exposure.

Although successful KT typically restores normal function of the GH/IGF-1 axis, catch-up growth post-transplant is generally not enough to compensate for the deficit that happened pretransplant. Around 30% of pediatric renal transplant recipients do not achieve a normal adult height.[67]

Early/intermediate steroid withdrawal and complete steroid avoidance are associated with improved growth outcomes after transplant in younger children.[34] Poor allograft function (GFR <50 mL/min per 1.73 m^2 in the 1st year post-transplant) hampers catch-up growth post-transplant. Catch-up growth and total height gain post-transplant correlate positively with GFR.

Post-transplant catch-up growth patterns are different among age groups. Children younger than 6 years have greater post-transplant height increase and attained normal height. Children who were 6–12 years of age showed very limited catch-up growth, and those older than 12 years at the time of transplant experienced no increase or even a slight decrease in height standard deviation.[68]

Recombinant human growth hormone is indicated in cases of persistent growth failure after the 1st year post-transplant (height less than the third percentile for age and sex, and a height velocity below the 25th percentile). Long-term follow-up demonstrated no apparent increase in the risk of malignancy or allograft rejection episodes.[69,70]

Neurocognitive Development

Children with CKD are at higher risk of abnormal neurodevelopment, with deficits in intellectual functioning and executive functions. Earlier onset ESKD(<5 years of age) and prolonged dialysis prior to transplant increase this risk. KT results in improved neurocognitive function but does not normalize developmental status or intellectual functioning compared to healthy controls. Pediatric KT recipients have higher rates of depression and anxiety (17%–36.4%), attention-deficit/hyperactivity disorder (ADHD; 22.5%), and post-traumatic stress symptoms (PTSS, 65%) in comparison to healthy peers.[71,72] Pretransplant and regular post-transplant neuropsychological testing is essential for guiding interventions, academic accommodations, and cognitive interventions.

Bone Disease

Mineral and bone disorders (MBD) can cause growth failure, bone pain, fractures, and ectopic calcification. Bone loss, with osteopenia or osteoporosis, is associated with an increased risk of fractures and reflects the imbalance between bone formation and bone resorption. Preexisting renal osteodystrophy and cardiovascular changes at the time of transplantation, immunosuppression (steroids, CNIs), hypomagnesemia, and reduced graft function all contribute to post-transplant mineral and bone disease.

Pediatric KT patients have a high burden of skeletal morbidity. Bartosh et al. showed a 41% prevalence of bone-joint abnormalities and a 23% prevalence of fractures.[73]

Calcium, phosphate, magnesium, alkaline phosphatase (ALP), PTH, and 25(OH) D levels should be regularly monitored post-transplant. KDIGO and the Spanish Society of Nephrology guidelines recommend evaluating bone volume through the measurement of bone mineral density using dual X-ray absorptiometry.[74]

General lifestyle changes including a healthy diet, regular physical activity, sodium restriction, and avoidance of smoking are advocated. KDIGO guidelines recommend vitamin D analogs to treat MBD in children with an eGFR above 30 mL/min/1.73 m^2 during the first 12 months post-transplant. There is no evidence to recommend bisphosphonates treatment. Hypophosphatemia and hypomagnesemia are corrected with supplements.

Nonadherence

Adherence is defined as the magnitude to which a patient/caregiver follows the agreed recommendations of a healthcare provider. Nonadherence is thus an important risk factor for worse allograft survival in adolescence and early adulthood. Studies have shown that about 40% of adolescent patients are nonadherent. This leads to rejection in 20% and graft loss in 16% of patients.[75] Data from the USRDS and the SRTR in some groups of recipients showed that the age group 17–24 years is at high risk of nonadherence and graft failure.[76] Patient-related factors (such as knowledge and understanding of disease and medications, cognitive functioning), socioeconomic factors (socioeconomic status, family support, race/cultural background), condition-related factors (duration of illness, health beliefs, time since transplant), therapy-related factors (side effects, number of medications and doses per day, complexity of medication regimen, and cost of medication), and healthcare factors (insurance and relationship between physician and patient) all impact adherence.

Options for adherence assessment include using self-report tools, variability in trough levels of tacrolimus, and electronic monitoring. The Teen Adherence in KT Effectiveness of Intervention Trial used a combination of electronic monitoring with feedback, text message dose reminders, identification of personal barriers, problem-solving, and action planning in addition to social support to improve adherence in adolescent patients.[77]

A multidisciplinary team with doctors, nurses, surgeons, psychologists, social workers, and dietitians should work with patients and families to identify the barriers to adherence and implement interventions to improve adherence.

The Transition of Care from Pediatric to Adults

Transition is defined as the phased preparation and movement of adolescents and young adults with chronic medical problems from a pediatric-centered to an adult-centered healthcare system. Transition protocols and recommendations for transition clinics with pediatric and adult healthcare personnel have been recommended.[78] There are no universal guidelines and a variety of care models exist. There are several milestones to be achieved for a successful transition. The first milestone is to recognize their disease process, the reason for transplant, the short-term and long-term impact of the disease, and graft failure. The second milestone is self-autonomy with supervision, where the patient is learning the names and doses of the immunosuppression, learns how to communicate with their healthcare team, self-advocate, and drug refill. The third final milestone is the phase of autonomy with support as needed. This involves achieving educational and vocational goals, establishing healthy lifestyle choices, and transferring to an adult transplant center. Studies demonstrated specialized transition clinics help with the preparation for the transfer of care and reduce the risk of rejection and graft loss. Prestidge et al. noticed that there are no graft failures within 2 years of transfer after the inception of the transition clinic as opposed to

24% graft failure rates before the inception.[79] Lower rates of nonadherence were noted (12.5% vs. 42.8%) among patients attending a transition clinic.[80]

Causes of Late Allograft Loss or Patient Death after Childhood Kidney Transplant

The success of KT in children with ESKD now results in 10-year patient survival of 90%–95%. Long-term graft survival is affected by several factors including the quality of the donated kidney, recipient characteristics, and post-transplant complications. Some of the factors impacting graft survival rate are:

- LD versus DD (better graft survival in LD)
- histocompatibility matching (superior HLA matching improved allograft outcomes)
- donor age and comorbidities
- delayed graft function
- recurrence of primary disease
- acute and chronic rejections
- viral infections and reactivation of latent infections
- recipient race and age.

Cardiometabolic Comorbidities

Even though there is improvement in the cardiovascular risk factors post-KT, cardiovascular disease remains one of the most common causes of death in children and young adults. Subclinical cardiovascular changes start at the pediatric age and are pronounced in post-transplant patients. Arterial stiffness, increased pulse wave velocity, and endothelial dysfunction are common in pediatric KT recipients.[81] Post-transplant new-onset diabetes mellitus with an incidence rate of about 8% can cause a risk of cardiovascular events leading to patient mortality.[82] The prevalence of new-onset diabetes mellitus is lower in pediatric recipients than that in adults. Steroid exposure, tacrolimus usage, obesity, African American race, and hypomagnesemia are recognized risk factors for the development of diabetes.[83] In contrast to adult data, an OPTN/UNOS and USRDS database analysis did not identify any association between new-onset diabetes post-transplantation and graft failure in children.[84]

Children experience weight gain after transplant with the greatest increase in BMI happening during the 1st year post-transplant. Obesity and metabolic syndrome increase the risk of cardiovascular mortality, but the studies done to evaluate the effects of obesity on allograft function have conflicting results.[85,86]

Hypertension post-transplant is very common and has variable incidence depending on the method used for blood pressure (BP) measurement and diagnostic criteria for hypertension. A Sinha, et al. study identified prevalence rates of post-renal transplant hypertension in the United Kingdom at 66.4%, 61.0%, 56.4%, and 55.9% of patients were hypertensive at 6 months, 1, 2, and 5 years, respectively. Seeman, et al. reported that children who remained hypertensive had significantly decreased graft function after 2 years compared with those who reached normal BP levels.[87]

Pediatric renal transplant recipients with optimal allograft function have lower levels of arterial hypertension and have their circadian blood pressure rhythm restored through the normalization of nocturnal blood pressure dipping, and mitigation of cardiovascular risk factors after steroid withdrawal.[88,89]

Pediatric death with functioning graft rates remained unchanged over the decades and remains a major factor contributing to static long-term outcomes. Infection, cardiopulmonary disease, and malignancy are the primary causes of death with functioning grafts. Leading causes for death-censored graft failure are alloimmunity, viral infections, and glomerular diseases, which improved significantly over the last few decades.

Sexual Health, Reproduction, Raising a Family, Getting a Job

Pediatric KT recipients are encouraged to resume normal activities and return to school after a waiting period of 2–3 months post-transplant. Sexual and reproductive dysfunction is common among patients with CKD and ESKD. The data are very limited in adolescent patient groups. Prevention of sexually transmitted diseases and family planning education should be part of transplant clinic visits. Adolescent patients may safely initiate treatment with progestin pills, progestin implants, and progestin injections. The teratogenic potential of immunosuppressant medications (notably MMF) and antihypertensive medications (e.g., ACE inhibitors) should be explained to the adolescent and family.

Conclusion

Pediatric KT recipients are unique by their inherent different causes for primary kidney diseases, the differences in immunosuppression protocols, viral infections, and reactivations, the potential for developmental sequelae of kidney failure, and the need for many decades of graft function. Major advances in immunosuppression, medical management of post-transplant complications including prevention and treatment of infections and changes in organ allocation policies have contributed to improved pediatric KT outcomes since the first transplant in 1960.

References

1. Gillen DL, Stehman-Breen CO, Smith JM, et al. Survival advantage of pediatric recipients of a first kidney transplant among children awaiting kidney transplantation. *Am J Transplant.* 2008;8:2600–2606.
2. https://usrds-adr.niddk.nih.gov/2022/end-stage-renal-disease/8-esrd-among-children-and-adolescents. 2022.
3.. ERA-Registry-Annual-Report2020.pdf. era-online.org. 2020.
4. Bonthuis M, Vidal E, Bjerre A, et al. Ten-year trends in epidemiology and outcomes of pediatric kidney replacement therapy in Europe: data from the ESPN/ERA-EDTA registry. *Pediatr Nephrol.* 2021;36:2337–2348.
5. Harada R, Hamasaki Y, Okuda Y, et al Epidemiology of pediatric chronic kidney disease/kidney failure: learning from registries and cohort studies. *Pediatr Nephrol.* 2022;37:1215–1229.
6. Rosa-Diez G, Gonzalez-Bedat M, Ferreiro A, et al. Burden of end-stage renal disease (ESRD) in Latin America. *Clin Nephrol.* 2016;86:29–33.
7. Harambat J, Ekulu PM. Inequalities in access to pediatric ESRD care: a global health challenge. *Pediatr Nephrol.* 2016;31:353–358.
8. OPTN/SRTR 2020 Annual data report: preface. *Am J Transplant.* 2022;22(Suppl 2):1–10.
9. Chua A, Cramer C, Moudgil A, et al. Kidney transplant practice patterns and outcome benchmarks over 30 years: the 2018 report of the NAPRTCS. *Pediatr Transplant.* 2019;23:e13597.
10. Harambat J, van Stralen KJ, Schaefer F, et al. Disparities in policies, practices and rates of pediatric kidney transplantation in Europe. *Am J Transplant.* 2013;13:2066–2074.
11. Cransberg K, Smits JM, Offner G, Nauta J, Persijn GG. Kidney transplantation without prior dialysis in children: the Eurotransplant experience. *Am J Transplant.* 2006;6:1858–1864.
12. Rana Magar R, Knight S, Stojanovic J, et al. Is preemptive kidney transplantation associated with improved outcomes when compared to non-preemptive kidney transplantation in children? A systematic review and meta-analysis. *Transpl Int.* 2022;35:10315.
13. Van Arendonk KJ, Boyarsky BJ, Orandi BJ, et al. National trends over 25 years in pediatric kidney transplant outcomes. *Pediatrics.* 2014;133:594–601.
14. Anand A, Malik TH, Dunson J, et al. Factors associated with long-term graft survival in pediatric kidney transplant recipients. *Pediatr Transplant.* 2021;25:e13999.
15. Weitz M, Sazpinar O, Schmidt M, et al. Balancing competing needs in kidney transplantation: does an allocation system prioritizing children affect the renal transplant function? *Transpl Int.* 2017;30:68–75.
16. Winterberg PD, Garro R. Long-term outcomes of kidney transplantation in children. *Pediatr Clin North Am.* 2019;66:269–280.

17. Van Arendonk KJ, James NT, Orandi BJ, et al. Order of donor type in pediatric kidney transplant recipients requiring retransplantation. *Transplantation*. 2013;96:487–493.
18. Pape L. State-of-the-art immunosuppression protocols for pediatric renal transplant recipients. *Pediatr Nephrol*. 2019;34:187–194.
19. Eckardt KW, Kasiske BL, Zeier MG. Kidney disease: improving global outcomes transplant work, G. KDIGO clinical practice guideline for the care of kidney transplant recipients. *Am J Transplant*. 2009;9(Suppl 3):S1–155.
20. Mincham CM, Wong G, Teixeira-Pinto A, et al. Induction therapy, rejection, and graft outcomes in pediatric and adolescent kidney transplant recipients. *Transplantation*. 2017;101:2146–2151.
21. Offner G, Broyer M, Niaudet P, et al. A multicenter, open-label, pharmacokinetic/pharmacodynamic safety, and tolerability study of basiliximab (Simulect) in pediatric de novo renal transplant recipients. *Transplantation*. 2002;74:961–966.
22. Clark G, Walsh G, Deshpande P, Koffman G. Improved efficacy of basiliximab over antilymphocyte globulin induction therapy in paediatric renal transplantation. *Nephrol Dial Transplant*. 2002;17:1304–1309.
23. Warejko JK, Hmiel SP. Single-center experience in pediatric renal transplantation using Thymoglobulin induction and steroid minimization. *Pediatr Transplant*. 2014;18:816–821.
24. Tsampalieros A, Knoll GA, Molnar AO, Fergusson N, Fergusson DA. Corticosteroid use and growth after pediatric solid organ transplantation: a systematic review and meta-analysis. *Transplantation*. 2017;101:694–703.
25. Grenda R, Watson A, Trompeter R, et al. A randomized trial to assess the impact of early steroid withdrawal on growth in pediatric renal transplantation: the TWIST study. *Am J Transplant*. 2010;10:828–836.
26. Höcker B, Weber LT, Feneberg R, et al. Prospective, randomized trial on late steroid withdrawal in pediatric renal transplant recipients under cyclosporine microemulsion and mycophenolate mofetil. *Transplantation*. 2009;87:934–941.
27. Khositseth S, Matas A, Cook ME, Gillingham KJ, Chavers BM. Thymoglobulin versus ATGAM induction therapy in pediatric kidney transplant recipients: a single-center report. *Transplantation*. 2005;79:958–963.
28. Ashoor IF, Beyl RA, Gupta C, et al. Low-dose antithymocyte globulin has no disadvantages to standard higher dose in pediatric kidney transplant recipients: report from the Pediatric Nephrology Research Consortium. *Kidney Int Rep*. 2021;6:995–1002.
29. Trompeter R, Filler G, Webb NJ, et al. Randomized trial of tacrolimus versus cyclosporin microemulsion in renal transplantation. *Pediatr Nephrol*. 2002;17:141–149.
30. Neu AM, Ho PL, Fine RN, Furth SL, Fivush BA. Tacrolimus vs. cyclosporine A as primary immunosuppression in pediatric renal transplantation: a NAPRTCS study. *Pediatr Transplant*. 2003;7:217–222.
31. Jungraithmayr TC, Wiesmayr S, Staskewitz A, et al. Five-year outcome in pediatric patients with mycophenolate mofetil–based renal transplantation. *Transplantation*. 2007;83:900–905.
32. Nehus E, Goebel J, Abraham E. Outcomes of steroid-avoidance protocols in pediatric kidney transplant recipients. *Am J Transplant*. 2012;12:3441–3448.
33. Webb NJ, Douglas SE, Rajai A, et al. Corticosteroid-free kidney transplantation improves growth: 2-year follow-up of the TWIST randomized controlled trial. *Transplantation*. 2015;99:1178–1185.

34. Sarwal MM, Ettenger RB, Dharnidharka V, et al. Complete steroid avoidance is effective and safe in children with renal transplants: a multicenter randomized trial with three-year follow-up. *Am J Transplant.* 2012;12:2719–2729.
35. Zhang H, Zheng Y, Liu L, et al. Steroid avoidance or withdrawal regimens in paediatric kidney transplantation: a meta-analysis of randomised controlled trials. *PLoS ONE.* 2016;11:e0146523.
36. Dharnidharka VR, Fiorina P, Harmon WE. Kidney transplantation in children. *N Engl J Med.* 2014;371:549–558.
37. Ettenger R, Chin H, Kesler K, et al. Relationship among viremia/viral infection, alloimmunity, and nutritional parameters in the first year after pediatric kidney transplantation. *Am J Transplant.* 2017;17:1549–1562.
38. Bock GH, Sullivan EK, Miller D, et al. Cytomegalovirus infections following renal transplantation—effects on antiviral prophylaxis: a report of the North American Pediatric Renal Transplant Cooperative Study. *Pediatr Nephrol.* 1997;11:665–671.
39. Humar A, Michaels M, Monitoring, A.I.W.G.o.I.D. American Society of Transplantation recommendations for screening, monitoring and reporting of infectious complications in immunosuppression trials in recipients of organ transplantation. *Am J Transplant.* 2006;6:262–274.
40. Kotton CN, Kumar D, Caliendo AM, et al. Updated international consensus guidelines on the management of cytomegalovirus in solid-organ transplantation. *Transplantation.* 2013;96:333–360.
41. Chapman JR. The KDIGO clinical practice guidelines for the care of kidney transplant recipients. *Transplantation.* 2010;89:644–645.
42. Kotton CN, Kumar D, Caliendo AM, et al. The third international consensus guidelines on the management of cytomegalovirus in solid-organ transplantation. *Transplantation.* 2018;102:900–931.
43. Green M, Squires JE, Chinnock RE, et al. The IPTA Nashville consensus conference on post-transplant lymphoproliferative disorders after solid organ transplantation in children: II—consensus guidelines for prevention. *Pediatr Transplant.,* 2022;e14350.
44. Dharnidharka VR, Abdulnour HA, Araya CE. The BK virus in renal transplant recipients—review of pathogenesis, diagnosis, and treatment. *Pediatr Nephrol.* 2011;26:1763–1774.
45. Smith JM, Dharnidharka VR, Talley L, Martz K, McDonald RA. BK virus nephropathy in pediatric renal transplant recipients: an analysis of the North American Pediatric Renal Trials and Collaborative Studies (NAPRTCS) registry. *Clin J Am Soc Nephrol.* 2007;2:1037–1042.
46. Höcker B, Schneble L, Murer L, et al. Epidemiology of and risk factors for BK polyomavirus replication and nephropathy in pediatric renal transplant recipients: an International CERTAIN Registry Study. *Transplantation.* 2019;103:1224–1233.
47. Sawinski D, Goral S. BK virus infection: an update on diagnosis and treatment. *Nephrol Dial Transplant.* 2015;30:209–217.
48. Saleh A, El Din Khedr MS, Ezzat A, Takou A, Halawa A. Update on the management of BK virus infection. *Exp Clin Transplant.* 2020;18:659–670.
49. Höcker B, Aguilar M, Schnitzler P, et al. Vaccination titres pre- and post-transplant in paediatric renal transplant recipients and the impact of immunosuppressive therapy. *Pediatr Nephrol.* 2018;33:897–910.
50. Neu AM, Fivush BA. Recommended immunization practices for pediatric renal transplant recipients. *Pediatr Transplant.* 1998;2:263–269.

51. Rubin LG, Levin MJ, Ljungman P, et al. 2013 IDSA clinical practice guideline for vaccination of the immunocompromised host. *Clin Infect Dis.* 2014;58:309–318.

52. Nuorti JP, Whitney CG, Centers for Disease Control and Prevention. Prevention of pneumococcal disease among infants and children: use of 13-valent pneumococcal conjugate vaccine and 23-valent pneumococcal polysaccharide vaccine—recommendations of the Advisory Committee on Immunization Practices (ACIP). *MMWR Morb Mortal Wkly Rep.* 2010;59:1–18.

53. Robinson CL, Romero JR, Kempe A, Pellegrini C, Advisory Committee on Immunization Practices Child/Adolescent Immunization Work Group. Advisory committee on immunization practices recommended immunization schedule for children and adolescents aged 18 years or younger—United States, 2017. *MMWR Morb Mortal Wkly Rep.* 2017;66:134–135.

54. Cochat P, Fargue S, Mestrallet G, et al. Disease recurrence in paediatric renal transplantation. *Pediatr Nephrol.* 2009;24:2097–2108.

55. Van Stralen KJ, Verrina E, Belingheri M, et al. Impact of graft loss among kidney diseases with a high risk of post-transplant recurrence in the paediatric population. *Nephrol Dial Transplant.* 2013;28:1031–1038.

56. Baum MA, Ho M, Stablein D, Alexander SR, North American Pediatric Renal Transplant Cooperative Study. Outcome of renal transplantation in adolescents with focal segmental glomerulosclerosis. *Pediatr Transplant.* 2002;6:488–492.

57. Kaplan-Pavlovcic S, Ferluga D, Hvala A, Chwatal-Lakic N, Bren AF, Vizjak A. et al. Recurrent focal segmental glomerulosclerosis after renal transplantation: is early recurrent proteinuria always a surrogate marker for recurrence of the disease? *Transplant Proc.* 2002;34:3122–3124.

58. First MR. Living-related donor transplants should be performed with caution in patients with focal segmental glomerulosclerosis. *Pediatr Nephrol.* 1995;9(Suppl):S40–42.

59. Jiang SH, Kennard AL, Walters GD. Recurrent glomerulonephritis following renal transplantation and impact on graft survival. *BMC Nephrol.* 2018;19:344.

60. Chandrakantan A, Ratanapanichkich P, Said M, Barker CV, Julian BA. Recurrent IgA nephropathy after renal transplantation despite immunosuppressive regimens with mycophenolate mofetil. *Nephrol Dial Transplant.* 2005;20:1214–1221.

61. Dharnidharka VR, Tejani AH, Ho PL, Harmon WE. Post-transplant lymphoproliferative disorder in the United States: young Caucasian males are at highest risk. *Am J Transplant.* 2002;2:993–998.

62. Al-Mansour Z, Nelson BP, Evens AM. Post-transplant lymphoproliferative disease (PTLD): risk factors, diagnosis, and current treatment strategies. *Curr Hematol Malig Rep.* 2013;8:173–183.

63. Martinez OM, Krams SM, Robien MA, et al. Mutations in latent membrane protein 1 of Epstein-Barr virus are associated with increased risk of posttransplant lymphoproliferative disorder in children. *Am J Transplant.* 2023;23(5):611–618.

64. Francis A, Johnson DW, Craig JC, Wong G. Incidence and predictors of cancer following kidney transplantation in childhood. *Am J Transplant.* 2017;17:2650–2658.

65. Ploos van Amstel S, Vogelzang JL, Starink MV, Jager KJ, Groothoff JW Long-term risk of cancer in survivors of pediatric ESRD. *Clin J Am Soc Nephrol.* 2015;10:2198–2204.

66. Tonshoff B, Kiepe D, Ciarmatori S. Growth hormone/insulin-like growth factor system in children with chronic renal failure. *Pediatr Nephrol.* 2005;20:279–289.

67. Fine RN, Ho M, Tejani A, North American Pediatric Renal Transplant Cooperative Study. The contribution of renal transplantation to final adult height: a report of the North American Pediatric Renal Transplant Cooperative Study (NAPRTCS). *Pediatr Nephrol.* 2001;16:951–956.
68. Smith JM, Stablein DM, Munoz R, Hebert D, McDonald RA. Contributions of the transplant registry: the 2006 annual report of the North American Pediatric Renal Trials and Collaborative Studies (NAPRTCS). *Pediatr Transplant.* 2007;11:366–373.
69. Longmore DK, Conwell LS, Burke JR, McDonald SP, McTaggart SJ. Post-transplant lymphoproliferative disorder: no relationship to recombinant human growth hormone use in Australian and New Zealand pediatric kidney transplant recipients. *Pediatr Transplant.* 2013;17:731–736.
70. Wu Y, Cheng W, Yang XD, Xiang B. Growth hormone improves growth in pediatric renal transplant recipients—a systemic review and meta-analysis of randomized controlled trials. *Pediatr Nephrol.* 2013;28:129–133.
71. McCormick King ML, Mee LL, Gutiérrez-Colina AM, Eaton CK, Lee JL, Blount RL. Emotional functioning, barriers, and medication adherence in pediatric transplant recipients. *J Pediatr Psychol.* 2014;39:283–293.
72. Dobbels F, Decorte A, Roskams A, Van Damme-Lombaerts R. Health-related quality of life, treatment adherence, symptom experience and depression in adolescent renal transplant patients. *Pediatr Transplant.* 2010;14:216–223.
73. Bartosh SM, Leverson G, Robillard D, Sollinger HW. Long-term outcomes in pediatric renal transplant recipients who survive into adulthood. *Transplantation.* 2003;76:1195–1200.
74. Ketteler M, Block GA, Evenepoel P, et al. Executive summary of the 2017 KDIGO chronic kidney disease-mineral and bone disorder (CKD-MBD) guideline update: what's changed and why it matters. *Kidney Int.* 2017;92:26–36.
75. Dobbels F, Ruppar T, De Geest S, et al. Adherence to the immunosuppressive regimen in pediatric kidney transplant recipients: a systematic review. *Pediatr Transplant.* 2010;14:603–613.
76. Van Arendonk KJ, King EA, Orandi BJ, et al. Loss of pediatric kidney grafts during the "high-risk age window": insights from pediatric liver and simultaneous liver-kidney recipients. *Am J Transplant.* 2015;15:445–452.
77. Foster BJ, Pai ALH, Zelikovsky N, et al. A randomized trial of a multicomponent intervention to promote medication adherence: the Teen Adherence in Kidney Transplant Effectiveness of Intervention Trial (TAKE-IT). *Am J Kidney Dis.* 2018;72:30–41.
78. Bell LE, Bartosh SM, Davis CL, et al. Adolescent transition to adult care in solid organ transplantation: a consensus conference report. *Am J Transplant.* 2008;8:2230–2242.
79. Prestidge C, Romann A, Djurdjev O, Matsuda-Abedini M. Utility and cost of a renal transplant transition clinic. *Pediatr Nephrol.* 2012;27:295–302.
80. McQuillan RF, Toulany A, Kaufman M, Schiff JR. Benefits of a transfer clinic in adolescent and young adult kidney transplant patients. *Can J Kidney Health Dis.* 2015;2:45.
81. Borchert-Mörlins B, Thurn D, Schmidt BMW, et al. Factors associated with cardiovascular target organ damage in children after renal transplantation. *Pediatr Nephrol.* 2017;32:2143–2154.
82. Chanchlani R, Kim SJ, Dixon SN, et al. Incidence of new-onset diabetes mellitus and association with mortality in childhood solid organ transplant recipients: a population-based study. *Nephrol Dial Transplant.* 2019;34:524–531.

83. Al-Uzri A, Stablein DM, R AC. Posttransplant diabetes mellitus in pediatric renal transplant recipients: a report of the North American Pediatric Renal Transplant Cooperative Study (NAPRTCS). *Transplantation.* 2001;72:1020–1024.

84. Kuo HT, Poommipanit N, Sampaio M, Reddy P, Cho YW, Bunnapradist S. Risk factors for development of new-onset diabetes mellitus in pediatric renal transplant recipients: an analysis of the OPTN/UNOS database. *Transplantation.* 2010;89:434–439.

85. Ladhani M, Lade S, Alexander SI, et al. Obesity in pediatric kidney transplant recipients and the risks of acute rejection, graft loss and death. *Pediatr Nephrol.* 2017;32:1443–1450.

86. Dick AAS, Hansen RN, Montenovo MI, Healey PJ, Smith JM. Body mass index as a predictor of outcomes among pediatric kidney transplant recipient. *Pediatr Transplant.* 2017;21(6):e12992.

87. Seeman T, Simková E, Kreisinger J, Vondrák K, et al. Improved control of hypertension in children after renal transplantation: results of a two-yr interventional trial. *Pediatr Transplant.* 2007;11:491–497.

88. Hocker B, Weber LT, Feneberg R, et al. Improved growth and cardiovascular risk after late steroid withdrawal: 2-year results of a prospective, randomised trial in paediatric renal transplantation. *Nephrol Dial Transplant.* 2010;25:617–624.

89. Hocker B, Weber LT, John U, et al. Steroid withdrawal improves blood pressure control and nocturnal dipping in pediatric renal transplant recipients: analysis of a prospective, randomized, controlled trial. *Pediatr Nephrol.* 2019;34:341–348.

17

Management of Patients with Failing and Failed Kidney Transplant

Sandesh Parajuli and Gaurav Gupta

Assisting failing and failed kidney transplant—an ignored entity!

Introduction

For patients with advanced chronic kidney disease (CKD) or end-stage kidney disease (ESKD), kidney transplantation remains the best treatment modality. Kidney transplantation as opposed to long-term dialysis offers longer life expectancy with better quality of life and is cost-effective. There is an effort to offer kidney transplantation as the preferred modality to many recipients. In 2019, the president of United States of America signed an Executive Order, "Advancing American Kidney Health," intending to facilitate and promote kidney transplantation.[1] In 2021, a total of 24,670 kidneys were transplanted, which was a record high despite being in the midst of the COVID-19 pandemic (Figure 17.1 left).[2] The number of patients with functioning kidney transplants continues to increase. In the United States, 239,413 patients had a functional kidney transplant (KT) in 2019, which had doubled in 20 years from 1999 (Figure 17.1 right).[3] The largest population with functional kidney are patients aged 45–64 years.[3] It is expected that many of these patients would eventually have irreversible graft failure requiring repeat transplant or long-term dialysis treatment. It is prudent to know how best to manage patients with failing transplants. In this chapter, we address various clinical aspects of failing and failed kidney transplants.

Failing Kidney Transplant

Epidemiology

The rate of death-censored graft failure in KT recipients has decreased over the last two decades, due to major improvements in 1st-year and progressive

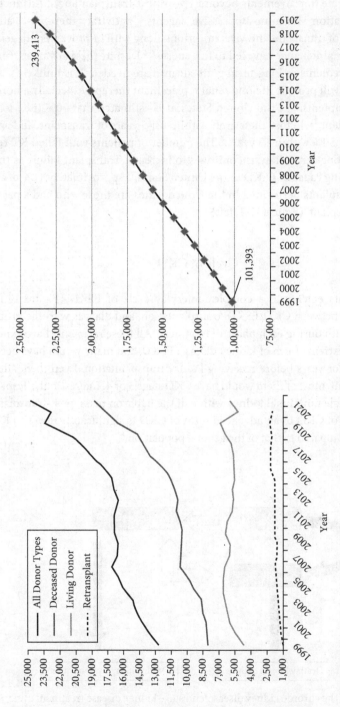

Figure 17.1 Total number of kidney transplants [left panel] in the United States increases from 1999 to 2020 (data from SRTR), largely from increasing deceased donor transplants. The number of recipients with a functional kidney allograft [right panel] also increased from 1999 to 2019 (data from USRDS).

mild-moderate improvements beyond 1 year post-transplantation. Advances in combination immunosuppressive agents, antiviral therapies, and monitoring of transplant and viral infections along with improvement in general health maintenance have led to this success.[4] Despite these advances, further improvements in long-term graft survival are needed. It is unlikely that a single KT will provide lifelong renal replacement therapy, especially among younger recipients.[5] In the United States, it is estimated that 20% (i.e., 1 in 5) KT recipients will lose their graft within just 5 years of transplant, and approximately 50% within 10 years.[6] The number of patients with failed KT returning to long-term dialysis continues to increase. Transplant failure is the fourth-leading cause of ESKD in the United States.[7] Approximately 12% of all kidney transplants performed in the United States are those who had a prior kidney transplant. (Figure 17.1, left).

Cycle of CKD

KT recipients enter into a complex interplay cycle of ESKD (Figure 17.2) surrounded between CKD/ESKD, transplantation, and dialysis with the probability of death during each phase of treatment. All these recipients have experienced an extreme form of kidney disease, ESKD, and many would have been on dialysis for years before receiving kidney transplantation. Even then, after the transplant, most of them would have CKD stage 3 or 4. Interestingly, despite having a single functional kidney with half the nephron mass, post-transplant progression of CKD to an advanced form of CKD is significantly lower in KT recipients compared to that of the general population.[8]

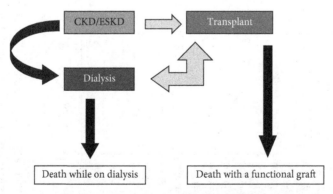

Figure 17.2 The chronic kidney disease/end stage kidney disease treatment cycle.

Definition of Failing Kidney

Due to a lack of consensus, there are variations of definitions and criteria used to define a failing kidney transplant.[9] A recent proposal through the American Society of Transplantation (AST) Kidney and Pancreas Community of Practice (KPCOP) workgroup proposed failing kidney transplants as those with:

1. Stable but low transplant function;
2. Declining function, with anticipated transplant failure within 1 year, and
3. Return to renal replacement therapy.[9]

For this chapter, we consider failing transplants as recipients with low transplant function or declining function. Return to renal replacement therapy either with long-term dialysis or repeat transplantation is considered a failed graft.

Causes of Kidney Transplant Failure

Premature death with a functioning transplant is the most important reason for kidney transplant failure. However, causes of death-censored graft failure are heterogeneous, multifactorial, and time-dependent. Even in the current era, acute and chronic T cell and antibody rejections are the most common causes of death-censored graft failure both early and late post-transplant.[10] However, nonalloimmune injury to the transplant also contributes significantly to transplant failure as well.[11] Common causes of graft failure include:

1. Chronic active T-cell-mediated rejection
2. Chronic active antibody-mediated rejection
3. Recurrent and de novo diseases
4. Early or late BK virus nephropathy
5. Deceased donor kidney with minimal reserves, including high Kidney Donor Profile Index (KDPI) score
6. Obstructive uropathy
7. Recurrent or severe acute kidney injuries (e.g., from volume depletion, drug/contrast toxicity, heart failure, sepsis, COVID, etc.)

Both immunological and nonimmunological causes lead to tubular atrophy and interstitial fibrosis (IF/TA), and glomerulosclerosis, classical findings of progressive nephron loss. Thus, renal transplant scarring, a multifactorial nonspecific pathological finding in kidney biopsies, reflects the final common pathway toward terminal KT failure. Nephron damage leads to compensatory hyperfiltration and glomerular hypertension in the remaining functioning nephrons, initiating apoptosis, inflammation, and fibrosis that gradually increase, in glomeruli, tubules, and interstitium, leading to progressive further renal functional deterioration.[11,12]

In the past, calcineurin nephrotoxicity was considered an important nonimmunological cause of progressive IF/TA after transplantation. However, studies of minimizing or avoiding calcineurin inhibitors (CNIs), have not shown to benefit, but rather have led to the development of immunological injury including the development of donor-specific antibodies leading to chronic active antibody-mediated rejection and chronic active T-cell-mediated rejection.[13,14] However, all of these studies were done before the approval of belatacept (costimulation blockade). To the best of our knowledge, we are not aware of any published studies looking at the impact of belatacept in the failing graft, although recently one trial was concluded (clinicaltrial.gov:NCT01921218). With this, weighing risks and benefits, we believe a continuation of CNI is beneficial to preserve kidney graft function.

Various important aspects of graft failure are recurrence of glomerulonephritis, BK virus nephropathy, diabetes mellitus (pretransplant or new onset), intercurrent medical and surgical illnesses unrelated to the transplant, and many more.[11] These topics are discussed in other chapters. There is no definite therapeutic intervention among these recipients with failing transplants to avoid or defer the need for renal replacement therapy. Therapeutic strategies are mainly evidence-based and particularly extrapolated from nontransplant patients with CKD and ESKD, including both through pharmacological and nonpharmacological interventions such as weight control, smoking cessation, better blood pressure and blood sugar control, management of proteinuria, volume control, and many more.

Management of Failing Kidney Transplant

Management of recipients with stable transplant graft function with estimated glomerular filtration rate (eGFR) around 20 mL/min/1.73 m^2 or more, should continue the same standard of care management as other kidney transplant recipients. However, recipients with declining eGFR to values lower than 20 mL/min/1.73 m^2 need careful attention and aggressive intervention, especially if the recipient is a candidate for retransplantation.[9] This is summarized in Table 17.1. Briefly, if the recipient is considered to be a suitable candidate for retransplant, the option for relisting and encouragement to identify living donors should be discussed when eGFR is less than 20 mL/min. However, in certain countries patients can be listed for repeat transplantation only after the

Table 17.1 Proposed Management of Failing Kidney Transplant

Patient suitable for repeat transplant	Patient not suitable for repeat transplant
Early Referral for relisting for transplantation when eGFR approaches <20 mL/min or after starting dialysis-based local listing criteria	Transition of care to general nephrology
Encourage identifying living donor	Establish vascular access
Discuss options for decreasing time to transplantation: e.g., higher KDPI kidney, hepatitis C-positive donor	Coordinate reduction in immunosuppression over time
Consider reduction in immunosuppression (antimetabolites and CNI) after weighing risk and benefit	Monitor for graft intolerance syndrome (graft pain, hematuria, refractory anemia, and graft infection)
Maintain CNI trough levels in the low range	Optimize CKD management (BP, anemia, bone disease)
Obtain baseline PRA level	Involve palliative care, if the patient not considering long-term dialysis treatment option
Involve general nephrology for preparation of dialysis	
Optimize CKD management (BP, anemia, bone disease)	

initiation of long-term dialysis. The 2014 British Transplant Society "Guidelines for the Management of Failing Kidney Transplant" recommend that patients suitable for retransplantation be evaluated for repeat transplantation when graft survival is anticipated to be less than 1 year as a 1B recommendation.[15] The timely early referral is prudent, as the wait time for retransplantation may be longer due to sensitization from the previous KT. The general guidelines for immunosuppression management among these recipients with failing grafts include:

1. Avoid high doses and levels of immunosuppressive agents.
2. Avoid total withdrawal of immunosuppressive agents to prevent symptomatic rejection and increase risk of sensitization for repeat transplantation.
3. Avoid initiation of mammalian target of rapamycin (mTOR)-based therapy for those with proteinuria and low GFR.
4. Avoid full doses of mycophenolic acid due to higher bioavailability with low GFR.

CKD Management

Kidney transplant recipients and patients with native CKD have almost the same complications associated with CKD. Despite that, CKD management among KT recipients is suboptimal.[16] A cross-sectional study among patients with CKD 4 and 5 compared kidney transplant recipients and native CKD on various aspects of CKD. Parameters such as the use of angiotensin receptor blockade, phosphorus binders, and referral to the vascular access for dialysis or access ready dialysis, higher serum phosphorus levels, and other complications of CKD were similar.[16] In an analysis of 16,728 previous KT recipients with failed transplants and who initiated dialysis between January 2006 and September 2011, 65% initiated dialysis with a central venous catheter.[17] This is likely due to the complexity of the other medical problems associated with transplants: CKD management is sometimes disregarded and it needs more attention. Other medical issues, including addressing issues of depression due to failing graft, frailty, blood pressure and proteinuria control, use of sodium-glucose cotransporter-2 inhibitors in an appropriate patient along with calcium/phosphorus management, and anemia management, should also get priority in this population.

Failed Kidney, Now on Dialysis

The number of patients with KT failures who are back in dialysis is rising. In the United States, in 2018 alone more than 7,000 recipients returned to dialysis after failed transplants.[18,19] The optimal management of immunosuppressants after failed KT is controversial, with wide variation in clinical practice. The risk and benefits of continuation versus tapering off immunosuppression should be balanced between the risk of symptomatic rejection, graft intolerance syndrome, and development of anti–human leukocyte antigen (HLA) antibodies versus the risk of infection, cardiovascular disease, and malignancies.[18] In one prospective study from Canada, authors report the continuation of immunosuppressants beyond the 1st year of graft failure is associated with a lower risk for death, without increased risk of infection-associated hospitalization.[18] There is no evidence to guide the optimal method for tapering and withdrawing immunosuppression following KT failure. However, the approach depends mainly on the timing of the transplant failure and candidacy for repeat transplant. In general, recipients with graft failure within the 1st year of transplant and those with symptoms of graft rejection usually undergo nephrectomy followed by immediate withdrawal of immunosuppressive medications after nephrectomy. However, there are no definite guidelines and some centers continue immunosuppression for a few months after nephrec-tomy to reduce the risk of sensitization, in case the patient is a candidate for retransplantation. Reported rates of transplant nephrectomy after graft failure vary from center to center and range from 9% to 74%.[20,21] Other common indications for graft nephrectomy include:

1. Symptomatic rejection [(pain, hematuria, chronic anemia)
2. Transplant infection—recurrent pyelonephritis
3. Bleeding from kidney transplant (gross hematuria)
4. Hydronephrosis

Among recipients with late transplant failure, that is, more than 1 year post-transplant, the approach differs depending on whether the patient is likely to receive another kidney transplant within 1 year. Among patients anticipated to get another transplant within a year, usually, antimetabolite is discon-tinued immediately after graft failure but CNI is continued at a lower dose (usually once a day), along with maintenance prednisone until the time of transplant. If there is no well-defined plan for another transplant and the anticipated wait time is more than a year, usually antimetabolite is withdrawn immediately, followed by a lower dose (approximately half or one-fourth of the regular dose] of CNI for 6–12 months. Also, prednisone is tapered and discontinued. All patients who are undergoing withdrawal from their immu-nosuppression should be closely monitored for complications of withdrawal, such as symptomatic rejection, adrenal insufficiencies, and loss of residual renal function.

Repeat Kidney Transplantation

The outcomes of patients with a history of transplant failure who return to dial-ysis remain poor. If suitable, preemptive transplantation is the preferred repeat transplant. However, optimal timing among recipients with early graft failure (<1 year post-transplant) is controversial and some suggest a brief period of dial-ysis before retransplant.[22,23] We believe each case should be assessed individually among patients with early graft failure. It is reasonable to wait and re-evaluate medical, psychosocial, and other issues among recipients who had early graft failure due to noncompliance and acute rejection. Patients who had graft failure due to BK virus nephropathy can undergo successful repeat transplantation after the resolution of BK viremia. Patients who had aggressive early recurrent dis-ease (FSGS, aHUS, C3GN) and graft failure should be counseled about high rates of recurrence and can be considered for repeat transplantation with appropriate preventive and treatment strategies. Patients who had graft failure mainly due to technical issues should be offered repeat transplants as soon as possible if available, when the patient is ready both physically and emotionally. Factors to consider for repeat transplant include:

1. Medically suitable (age, cardiac, pulmonary, liver, nutrition, vascular disease, functional status)
2. Immunologically suitable (PRA, preferably HLA mismatch from the previous donor)
3. Prior infection (BK virus infection, cytomegalovirus [CMV] infection, fungal, other)
4. Presence of active malignancy (other than skin)
5. Social determinants (socioeconomic status, support system)

Despite inferior graft survival outcomes in second KT recipients compared to the primary transplant, transplantation is associated with a clinically similar reduction in the risk of death compared with treatment with dialysis in patients with and without a prior history of transplant failure.[24] This is true even among recipients receiving 3rd or 4th kidney transplants and the elderly.[25]

Future Directions and Summary

There has been continuous improvement in long-term kidney graft survival outcomes in the recent era. Median graft survival for deceased donor transplants increased from 8.2 years in 1995–1999 to 11.7 years in the most recent era of 2014–2017.[26] Similar positive effects have been noted among living donor recipients too and have increased from 12.1 years to 19.2 years during the same time frame.[26] There are many reports from various centers about multiple patients with kidney graft survival for more than 25 years.[27,28] The number of transplants has also increased along with the total number of recipients with a functional transplant. These recipients are always under the threat of increased risk of graft failure. So, our first goal should be to preserve their graft functions as much as possible. Once graft function starts to deteriorate, interventions to prevent the progression of CKD, CKD management, and timely referral for repeat transplant remain the key. Multidisciplinary approaches involving the participation of a general nephrologist, primary care provider, and counselors are needed to provide optimal care to the growing population of failing kidney transplants.

References

1. Thomas E, Milton J, Cigarroa FG. The advancing American kidney health executive order: an opportunity to enhance organ donation. *JAMA*. 2019;322(17):1645–1646.
2. Organ Procurement and Transplantation Network. 2022. https://optn.transplant. hrsa.gov/data/view-data-reports/national-data/#.
3. United States Renal Data System. *2021 USRDS Annual Data Report: Epidemiology of kidney disease in the United States*. National Institutes of Health, National Institute of Diabetes and Digestive and Kidney Diseases, Bethesda, MD, 2021.
4. Loupy A, Lefaucheur C, Vernerey D, et al. Complement-binding anti-HLA antibodies and kidney-allograft survival. *N Engl J Med*. 2013;369(13):1215–1226.
5. Marcen R, Teruel JL. Patient outcomes after kidney allograft loss. *Transplant Rev (Orlando)*. 2008;22(1):62–72.
6. Davis S, Mohan S. Managing patients with failing kidney allograft: many questions remain. *CJASN*. 2022;17(3):444–451.
7. Sellares J, de Freitas DG, Mengel M, et al. Understanding the causes of kidney transplant failure: the dominant role of antibody-mediated rejection and nonadherence. *Am J Transplant*. 2012;12(2):388–399.
8. Djamali A, Kendziorski C, Brazy PC, Becker BN. Disease progression and outcomes in chronic kidney disease and renal transplantation. *Kidney Int*. 2003;64(5):1800–1807.
9. Lubetzky M, Tantisattamo E, Molnar MZ, et al. The failing kidney allograft: a review and recommendations for the care and management of a complex group of patients. *Am J Transplant*. 2021;21(9):2937–2949.
10. Parajuli S, Aziz F, Garg N, et al. Histopathological characteristics and causes of kidney graft failure in the current era of immunosuppression. *World J Transplant*. 2019;9(6):123–133.
11. Van Loon E, Bernards J, Van Craenenbroeck AH, Naesens M. The causes of kidney allograft failure: more than alloimmunity: a viewpoint article. *Transplantation*. 2020;104(2):e46–e56.
12. Yang B, El Nahas AM, Thomas GL, et al. Caspase-3 and apoptosis in experimental chronic renal scarring. *Kidney Int*. 2001;60(5):1765–1776.
13. Sharif A, Shabir S, Chand S, Cockwell P, Ball S, Borrows R. Meta-analysis of calcineurin-inhibitor-sparing regimens in kidney transplantation. *JASN*. 2011;22(11):2107–2118.
14. Lim WH, Eris J, Kanellis J, et al. A systematic review of conversion from calcineurin inhibitor to mammalian target of rapamycin inhibitors for maintenance immunosuppression in kidney transplant recipients. *Am J Transplant*. 2014;14(9):2106–2119.
15. Management of the Failing Kidney Transplant. 2014. https://bts.org.uk/wp-content/uploads/2016/09/13_BTS_Failing_Graft-1.pdf.
16. Akbari A, Hussain N, Karpinski J, Knoll GA. Chronic kidney disease management: comparison between renal transplant recipients and nontransplant patients with chronic kidney disease. *Nephron Clin Pract*. 2007;107(1):c7–13.
17. Chan MR, Oza-Gajera B, Chapla K, et al. Initial vascular access type in patients with a failed renal transplant. *CJASN*. 2014;9(7):1225–1231.
18. Knoll G, Campbell P, Chassé M, et al. Immunosuppressant medication use in patients with kidney allograft failure: a prospective multicenter Canadian cohort study. *Journal of the American Society of Nephrology: JASN*. 2022;33(6):1182–1192.

19. United States Renal Data System. *2022 USRDS Annual Data Report: Epidemiology of kidney disease in the United States.* National Institutes of Health, National Institute of Diabetes and Digestive and Kidney Diseases, Bethesda, MD, 2022.
20. Johnston O, Rose C, Landsberg D, Gourlay WA, Gill JS. Nephrectomy after transplant failure: current practice and outcomes. *Am J Transplant.* 2007;7(8):1961–1967.
21. Mazzucchi E, Nahas WC, Antonopoulos IM, Piovesan AC, Ianhez LE, Arap S. Surgical complications of graft nephrectomy in the modern transplant era. *J Urol.* 2003;170(3):734–737.
22. Wong G, Chua S, Chadban SJ, et al. Waiting time between failure of first graft and second kidney transplant and graft and patient survival. *Transplantation.* 2016;100(8):1767–1775.
23. Goldfarb-Rumyantzev AS, Hurdle JF, Baird BC, et al. The role of pre-emptive re-transplant in graft and recipient outcome. *Nephrol Dial, Transplantation.* 2006;21(5):1355–1364.
24. Clark S, Kadatz M, Gill J, Gill JS. Access to kidney transplantation after a failed first kidney transplant and associations with patient and allograft survival: an analysis of national data to inform allocation policy. *Clinical Journal of the American Society of Nephrology: CJASN.* 2019;14(8):1228–1237.
25. Sandal S, Ahn JB, Segev DL, Cantarovich M, McAdams-DeMarco MA. Comparing outcomes of third and fourth kidney transplantation in older and younger patients. *Am J Transplant.* 2021;21(12):4023–4031.
26. Poggio ED, Augustine JJ, Arrigain S, Brennan DC, Schold JD. Long-term kidney transplant graft survival—making progress when most needed. *Am J Transplant.* 2021;21(8):2824–2832.
27. Kettler B, Scheffner I, Bräsen JH, et al. Kidney graft survival of >25 years: a single center report including associated graft biopsy results. *Transpl Int.* 2019;32(12):1277–1285.
28. Parajuli S, Mandelbrot DA, Aziz F, et al. Characteristics and outcomes of kidney transplant recipients with a functioning graft for more than 25 years. *Kidney Dis (Basel).* 2018;4(4):255–261.

18

Tolerance after Kidney Transplantation

Natasha M. Rogers and Angus W. Thomson

"Tolerence" the ultimate Holy Grail for transplantation!

Introduction

Despite major advances in understanding of how alloimmunity is regulated and how transplant tolerance can be induced at the pre-clinical (small animal) models, transplant patients remain highly-dependent on life-long costly immunosuppressive (IS) drug therapy. Moreover, the half-life of human kidney grafts (10–14 years) has slightly improved in recent years, but toxic effects of conventional immunosuppression (IS) (calcineurin inhibition; CNI) and failure of IS agents to control late graft failure (chronic rejection) remains a hurdle for better long-term outcome. In mice, experimental therapies such as combined (CD28/CD40) co-stimulation blockade induce tolerance to fully allogeneic, highly immunogenic skin grafts and inhibit chronic vascular rejection of organ allografts[1]. However, development of a therapeutic regimen(s) that can safely induce transplant tolerance, particularly within the first several years post-transplant, has remained elusive. In addition, there are no reliable/robust laboratory markers that are predictive of/correlate with a state of immune status and IS drug-free tolerance. For more than six decades, since (skin) allograft tolerance was first demonstrated in mice[2], the induction of tolerance (the so-called "holy grail" of transplantation immunology) has been regarded as the logical solution which could eliminate all the adverse effects associated with long-term IS therapy in patients. It will remain the optimal approach to minimize the risk of chronic allograft rejection and failure as well.

Definition of Tolerance

Transplantation tolerance may be defined as the specific absence of a destructive immune response to a foreign, HLA-incompatible organ or tissue, without ongoing exogenous IS. Conventionally, clinical "operational" tolerance is deemed to exist if all IS therapy has been stopped for at least one year, with stable graft function in the absence of biopsy-proven evidence of rejection. Additional considerations include:

I)   Absence of donor-specific alloantibodies,
II) Absence of destructive (as opposed to presumptive regulatory) lymphocytic infiltrates in graft biopsies,
III) Evidence of donor-specific unresponsiveness, with preservation of third-party responses in functional in vitro assays (systemic tolerance) and
IV) Demonstration of possible molecular signatures of tolerance.

Such definitions may also take account the deletion of damaging donor alloreactive immune effector cells, as well as the (non-exclusive) role of immune regulatory mechanisms in the induction/maintenance of tolerance. Notably, transplant tolerance (particularly of liver, but also of kidney grafts) can occur "spontaneously" across MHC barriers and without any IS therapy in rodents. Spontaneous transplant tolerance, physician-directed withdrawal of all immunosuppression occurs clinically in select liver transplant recipients, but rarely among kidney recipients.

Aims of this chapter

Our aim is to provide a concise understanding of the state of organ transplant tolerance (spontaneous and induced) and underlying mechanisms. We will consider how this information is being applied in efforts to develop clinically acceptable, safe, and generalizable regimens that can potentially promote IS drug minimization/donor-specific kidney transplant tolerance (KT) in appropriate patient cohorts. We discuss candidate biomarkers and signatures of tolerance, risk/benefit assessment, which patients to be considered for enrollment in tolerance trials, issue surrounding funding of such trials, patient's and physician's perspectives, and potential novel strategies for tolerance induction.
Spontaneous KT tolerance and underlying mechanisms in preclinical models

Russell et al demonstrated 'spontaneous' acceptance of kidney allografts in certain MHC mis-matched mouse strain combinations, in the absence of any IS therapy[3]. Significantly, this phenomenon appeared to be both species- and organ-specific. Thus, kidney allografts in other species, as well as mouse heart allografts were rejected rapidly under the same conditions. In the DBA/2 to C57BL/6 strain KT model, allograft acceptance was associated with regulated T cell-mediated immunity, i.e. transforming growth factor beta (TGFβ)-mediated inhibition of donor-reactive T cell responses[4]. Subsequently, evidence was reported that mouse spontaneous kidney allograft acceptance was dependent on the development of donor-specific regulatory T cells (Treg)[5], and periarterial Treg-rich organized lymphoid structures (TOLS) within the grafts[6]. Moreover, Tregs isolated from accepted renal allografts could transfer tolerance of skin grafts to naïve recipients[7]. However, while early acceptance of mouse kidney allografts was shown to be Treg-dependent, their long-term survival was associated with a progressive increase in intra-graft indoleamine dioxygenase (IDO) gene expression, likely mediated by regulatory dendritic cells (DCreg)[8] that may have provided more robust regulation. Recently, Oh et al[9] have shown that mouse spontaneous kidney allograft tolerance correlates with induction of Tregs by non-conventional plasmacytoid DC that is dependent on strain and MHC class II disparity.

Reduction/withdrawal of immunosuppression in kidney transplant patients

A reduction in IS that facilitates development of kidney allograft tolerance is much more difficult to achieve in kidney allograft compared to the quintessentially tolerated liver allograft [10]. Prior to molecular typing techniques, particularly monitoring of post-transplant alloimmunity, calcineurin inhibitor (CNI) withdrawal universally resulted in increased acute rejection rates[11-13] and no clear benefit in terms of allograft function or survival. However, sub-cohort analyses suggested a potentially permissive recipient phenotype that could identify individuals capable of tolerating CNI withdrawal. A subsequent study again focused on CNI withdrawal in immunologically quiescent recipients resulted in acute rejection and development of *de novo*, donor-specific antibodies[14], prompting premature termination. A recent Cochrane Systematic Review that assessed >80 studies and >16,000 renal transplant recipients[15] confirmed that CNI withdrawal – regardless of IS substitution with mechanistic target of rapamycin inhibition (mTORi) – was associated with increased acute rejection. These results are confounded by the lack of long-term follow-up in this patient population.

In recent years, the quest for IS reduction and tolerance has focused on the use of alternative drug regimens, particularly conditioning treatments pre-transplant, combined with adjuvant cellular therapy to modify the recipient immune response to the persistent presence of alloantigens. Despite a plethora of potential biomarkers related to tolerance, the major caveat is that these strategies have been explored in small numbers of patients (typically <50, often <20), which limits biological replicates and rigorous bioinformatics testing through the need for validation and testing cohorts.

Cell-based biomarkers of operational tolerance

Biomarkers that have been evaluated in kidney transplant tolerance and their significance are summarized in Table 18.1.

Cellular markers of operational tolerance have been extensively explored by the Institut National de la Santé et de la Recherche Médicale (INSERM) group in Nantes, France.[19, 23, 30-34] Albeit in small numbers of patients, they identified changes in the T-cell receptor (TCR) Vbeta usage and transcript accumulation (excluding pro-inflammatory cytokines)[30]. They found that the altered TCR profile was enriched in CD8+ T cells, with increased central memory and decreased effector cell populations[31], particularly profiles of CD8+CD28- T cells, which was thought to reflect suppression of cytotoxicity. Levels of CD25hiCD4+ T cells and contained FOXP3 transcripts were similar between operationally tolerant recipients and healthy controls[32, 35]. Later work[26] observed higher proportions of CD4+ T cells with demethylated FOXP3, and specific expansion of CD4+ CD45RA-Foxp3hi memory cells, with concurrent CD39 and glucocorticoid-induced TNF-related receptor (GITR) levels.

Humoral responses to vaccination of operationally tolerant individuals were also found to be heterogeneous[36]. The advent of gene sequencing provided additional supportive data, with a tolerance blood-based footprint of 49 genes[19], that included reduced immune activation (including costimulatory gene expression and T cell activation) and signal transduction, but increased regulation of cell cycle processes. Expansion of the tolerant patient group across continents facilitated creation of validation and testing cohorts for phenotyping (B and NK cell expansion, fewer activated CD4+ T cells, and donor-specific CD4+ T cell hyporesponsiveness including lower IFN-γ ELIspot responses) and gene sequencing studies (B cell-related pathways)[18]. Increased B cell numbers are associated with enhanced expression of co-stimulatory (CD80, CD40 and CD62L) and memory (CD19, IgD-, CD38+/-, CD27+) molecules with no cytokine polarization[23]. Additional inhibitory signalling moieties were described, including increased B-cell scaffold protein with ankyrin repeats 1 (BANK1), CD1d and CD5 expression, as well as decreased Fc gamma RIIA/IIB ratio. The microRNA miR-142-3p has also been shown to be overexpressed in B cells from operationally tolerant patients, modulating many genes previously identified as functionally relevant[22].

T follicular helper (Tfh) cells play a crucial role in B cell differentiation, and tolerant patients also display reduced Tfh subsets that also fail to synthesize IL-21[37], potentially creating a feedback loop that increases B cell activation and simultaneously facilitates immunoregulation. Three particular genes with high positive and negative predictive value have been shown to distinguish tolerant from non-tolerant individuals: immunoglobulin (Ig) kappa variable cluster

Table 18.1 Biomarkers in kidney transplant tolerance

Biomarker	Molecular significance	Clinical significance in tolerant patients
B cells (well-reviewed in [16] Peripheral blood microarray: ITN: 23 genes, 77% specific for B cells[17] IOT*: 10 genes, 60% specific for B cells[18] Nantes: 49 genes including CD19, CD20, CD79A[19] Combined analysis (Nantes, IOT, ITN): 35 genes, 69% specific for B cells[20, 21]	IOT signature: CD79B*, TCL1A*, HS3ST1, SH2D1B*, MS4A1*, TLR5, FCRL1*, PNOC, SLC8A1, FCRL2* *denotes B cell related genes ITN: IGKV1D-13, IGKV4-1, IGLL1[21] AKR1C3, CD40*, CTLA4, ID3, MZB1*, TCL1A miRNA-142-3p[22] Upregulation of BANK1 in PBMC (reduced alloresponse), downregulation CD32a/CD32b transcripts (lower B cell activation)[23]	Percentage and/or absolute number of B cells is increased in peripheral blood CD86+CD19+ B cells CD19+CD27+IgM+IgD+ memory B cells[23] T1+T2 transitional B cells expressing IL-10 (ITN results) IgD-CD38+/-CD80+ memory B cells[23]
NK cells		Increased percentage of CD56+ CD3- NK cells[18]
T cells	Downregulated - T cell activation genes (CD69, TACTILE, LAG3, SLAM) - cytotoxicity genes (granzyme A perforin, fas, granulysin)[19] Upregulated GATA3 (transcription factor for Th2 cells)[24], not verified[25] but demonstrated decreased RORC and ERK2	Decreased percentage of CD3+ T cells[18] Fewer activated CD4+ T cells Lower frequency of anti-donor IFN-γ CD4+ T cell response Donor-specific hyporesponsiveness Decreased Th17 cells[25] Expansion of CD4+CD45RA-Foxp3hi memory Tregs, increased Foxp3 TSDR demethylation, higher CD39/GITR expression[26] Increase Foxp3/α-1-2 mannosidase ratio[18]
Urine		elevated CD20 by qPCR in urinary sediment[17] versus no difference[27] Increased Foxp3 mRNA[28] Decreased CD25, trends to decreased CD3ε, IP-10, granzyme B, CD103[27]

See also[29], *IOT, indices of tolerance

(IGKV)4-1, Ig lambda-like polypeptide 1 (IGLL1) and Ig kappa variable 1D-13 (IGKVID-13), - the latter two are robustly stable over time[38]. The ARTIST study [21, 39] classified potentially tolerant renal allograft recipients based on IGKV4-1 and IGKVID-13 expression. Interestingly, the presence of IS did not affect development of this B cell signature and was greatest in those receiving CNI-based treatment.

Liquid biopsy samples for detecting immunological tolerance

Urine remains the ideal compartment for prediction and monitoring of tolerance, and discharge of graft-infiltrating or parenchymal cells into the urine provides a non-invasive method for distinguishing recipient phenotypes. More than 2 decades ago, increased mRNA levels of molecules biologically relevant to activated T cells (including granzyme B, perforin, and FOXP3) and dendritic cells (CD103) were used to diagnose acute rejection[40-42], and shown to be predictive in a multicentre trial[43], even with modest sensitivity and specificity. Urinary chemokines, particularly CXCL10[44] and CXCL9[45], can identify patients at risk of AR, or indeed those who are immunologically quiescent. Most studies have used urine to diagnose AR [46]). More recently, urinary Proteobacteria diversity has also been associated with minimal IS and operational tolerance[47], as has kynurenic acid and tryptamine[48]. Metabolomic profiling of any liquid sample is an exciting development in identifying relevant metabolic pathways implicated in immune regulation.

Patient selection for tolerance trials

Strict criteria must be met for patients to reach the definition of operational tolerance: there must be measurable evidence of prolonged allograft survival in the absence of IS, normal graft histology, and clear donor-specific hyporesponsiveness, with retention of 3rd party alloreactivity. Cessation of IS rarely results in successful and prolonged long-term allograft function. Of a select population of 48 transplant recipients who discontinued IS, only 25% and 12.5% maintained good graft function at 1 and 3-years respectively [49]. A recent summary suggests there are <250 tolerant patients who have been extensively studied over the last 4 decades[50]. Most tolerant patients are discovered serendipitously, as patients who have independently and gradually weaned IS. Identifying a biomarker is associated with several substantial methodological issues: the first is the rarity of patients and the capacity to recruit sufficient numbers (although the DESCARTES European Renal Association-European Dialysis and Transplant Association working group are supporting these efforts through the TOMOGRAM transcriptomic study) [51]; the second is the lack of an appropriate control population as healthy volunteers and stable graft recipients on IS will have a number of factors that affect transcriptomic signatures and downstream products. Similarly, studies designed to provide conditioning regimens conducive to operational tolerance have so far recruited highly selected, unsensitised recipients. Patients with high levels of sensitisation (donor specific antibodies) are already at significant risk of T-cell and antibody-mediated rejection, current drug regimens fail to eliminate niches of long-lived memory (T and B) cells, and even strict adherence to IS can fail to avert chronic allograft injury. For the foreseeable future, it is likely that tolerance regimens in kidney transplant recipients will be exclusively for those without a potential memory response.

To date, only a few transplant centres have successfully developed robust treatment protocols that facilitate kidney transplant tolerance across a variety of HLA barriers. These protocols are based on extensive pre-clinical work in small animals and non-human primates but require traditional conditioning therapies including myeloablation and concurrent donor hematopoietic cell transplantation (HCT). They are summarized in Table 18.2. The goal is development of chimerism [55, 56], which may be mixed or complete, transient, or permanent. The induction of mixed chimerism is accompanied by the risk of graft-versus-host-disease (GVHD), which is unacceptable in the quest for tolerance in patients. Studies to date, however, have shown a very low risk, particularly in the context of transient mixed chimerism.

Investigators at the Massachusetts General Hospital[57, 58] were the first to conduct clinical trials for the induction of renal allograft tolerance. In the first report[59] a patient with multiple myeloma and concurrent ESKD was treated with a concurrent ABO-compatible, HLA-identical bone marrow and renal transplant. Chimerism was demonstrated over the first 9 weeks post-transplant, and 2 decades later the patient remains off IS with normal renal function[60]. The protocol was based on a previously successful study[61] of 5 patients with refractory non-Hodgkin's lymphoma who underwent bone marrow transplantation from haplo-identical donors and in whom the generation of mixed lymphohematopoietic chimerism limited development of GVHD, but was also able to provide sufficient graft-versus-lymphoma effects.

For patients without concurrent malignancy and non-HLA matched donors, the pre-conditioning regimen consisted of cyclophosphamide, anti-CD2 antibody, and thymic irradiation, followed by kidney transplantation and IV infusion of freshly-isolated donor bone marrow. Cyclosporin A (CSA) monotherapy was commenced and then tapered over several months. The first modification of the protocol occurred with the 3rd enrolled recipient, adding rituximab

Table 18.2 Chimerism-based kidney transplant tolerance trials

Site	Protocol	Additional protocol information	Reported outcomes and refs
MGH (Boston)	**Original protocol:** Cyclophosphamide 60mg/kg Day -5, -4 Humanized anti-CD2 Ab (0.6mg/kg) Day -2, -1, 0 CSA (5mg/kg) Day -1 Thymic irradiation (7 Gy) Day -1 Unprocessed donor marrow infusion (2-3x10e8 mononuclear cells/kg) CyA 8-12mg/kg/d **Modification 1:** Rituximab 375mg/m2/dose Day -7, -2 Prednisone 2mg/kg/d (taper over 10 days) **Modification 2:** Rituximab 375mg/m2/dose Day 5,12 Prednisolone to Day 20 Tac, weaned over 8 months		12 patients: 2 graft losses (AKI with ABMR and AKI with tacrolimus-induced TMA) (Longest time off IS: 13 years) 1 with acute rejection, 2 with chronic rejection Compared to 31 live donor KTR on conventional IS - less HT - no PTDM - no dyslipidemia - no malignancy Better overall health [52]

	Protocol	Prophylaxis / Criteria	Outcomes
Stanford	**HLA matched:** rATG day (1.5mg/kg) Day 0-4 TLI (80-120 cGy) Day 0-4, 7-11 HCT infusion Day 11, CD34+ cells 10x10e6/kg CD3+ cells 1x10e6/kg Tapering steroids: Day 0-10 CyA: 6-12 months from day 0 MMF: commences Day 11, for 1 month **HLA mismatched:** rATG day (1.5mg/kg) Day 0-4 TLI (80-120 cGy) Day 0-4, 7-11 HCT infusion Day 11, CD34+ cells 10x10e6/kg CD3+ cells 3-100x10e6/kg Tapering steroids: Day 0-30 Tac: 12-15 months from day 0 MMF: commences Day 0, 9-12 months	Nystatin: 1 month Trimethoprim-sulphamethoxazole: 1 year Valganciclovir: 3-6 months Acyclovir: post valganciclovir prophylaxis for 18 months BKV monitoring month 1-6, 9, 12 DSA monitoring: months 6, 8, 12, 18 (HLA MM trial only) Exclusion criteria: high risk of recurrent disease (primary FSGS, MCGN, aHUS), increased risk PTLD (EBV positive donor/negative recipient), age >65 years (HLA matched) or >60 y (HLA MM)	29 patients At least 4x10e6 CD34+ cells/kg 27 received 1x10e6 CD3+ T cells/kg (Longest survival: 13 years) 5 patients displayed chimerism < 6 months, not candidates for IS withdrawal 10 patients had persistent chimerism 19 lost chimerism 3 patients died – unrelated to treatment 2 graft losses – kidney disease, no evidence of rejection 4 patients IS drugs resumed (3 with kidney disease, 1 with rejection) Average duration off IS drugs: 48 mo[53]
Northwestern (Chicago)	Fludarabine 30mg/kg Day -4, -3, -2 Cyclophosphamide 50mg/kg Day -3, +3 TBI 200cGy Day -1 FCRx infusion Day +1 Tac from Day -2, trough level 8-12ng/ml for 12 months MMF from Day -2 discontinue at 6 months	PRA>20% Female-to-male donor-recipient living unrelated pairs (minimize risk of GVHD) Avoid myelotoxic agents including ganciclovir	42 patients enrolled, 37 transplants 30 with chimerism 23 with durable chimerism 22 patients off IS Deaths – 1 with CMV/GVHD, 1 with lung Ca Graft losses – within 1 year secondary to opportunistic infection GVHD-2[54]

See also: Sykes M et al, Meeting Report: The Fifth Samuel Strober Workshop on clinical transplant tolerance. Transplantation (2023), in press and a tapering dose of prednisone. Further modification replaced CSA with tacrolimus. Acute kidney rejection occurring 10-20 days after transplantation and likely secondary to cyclophosphamide was experienced by many recipients (an effect not seen in non-human primate studies). This effect was associated with loss of chimerism, and renal histology was consistent with endothelial injury secondary to capillary-based immune cell infiltration.

The Stanford University protocol[62, 63], implemented in 2000, uses rabbit antithymocyte globulin and total lymphoid irradiation (TLI) following kidney transplantation, allowing its implementation in living and deceased donor recipients. To date however, it has only been used in living donor transplantation. TLI, compared to total body irradiation (TBI), only targets primary (thymus) and secondary lymphoid organs (lymph nodes, spleen) using multiple small doses, and is used to limit the risk of GVHD after donor HCT. It also depletes naïve T cells, changing the balance of (radiation-resistant) regulatory and immunologically-active cells and favouring a tolerogenic milieu characterised by suppressive cytokines (IL-4, IL-10, arginase, IDO). Living donors are treated with granulocyte-colony-stimulating factor (G-CSF) and then undergo leukapheresis to enrich for CD34+ cells. CD3+ (donor) T cells are added in limited quantities to the cell preparation to facilitate engraftment by eliminating host (recipient) T cells. Macrochimerism is typically seen within 2 weeks, and if persisting after 6-9 months, IS drug tapering is performed. Surveillance biopsies are used to reduce the risk of subclinical rejection. Loss of chimerism results in cessation of drug taper. This protocol has been successfully transferred to 3 patients in Europe who received a kidney transplant from HLA-identical siblings[64]. Reports of adverse events were not significant, with no pancytopenia related to TLI, no infectious complications requiring hospital admission and no GVHD. Engraftment syndrome with early (<2 weeks) loss of chimerism was only seen in 1 patient.

Investigators at Northwestern University have used a CD8+TCR- facilitating cell (FC) population[65] that is phenotypically similar (but functionally more potent) than pre-plasmacytoid DCs. The αβTCR is replaced by a FCp33-TCRβ heterodimer[66, 67]. Multiple pre-clinical studies support the utility of FCs in establishing donor-specific tolerance following solid organ or HSC transplantation[65, 66]. In the first clinical report of 8 HLA-mismatched KT recipients[68], patients underwent conditioning with fludarabine, TBI and cyclophosphamide followed by mycophenolate mofetil and tacrolimus IS which was eventually weaned. No engraftment syndrome or GVHD was noted. Five patients developed durable chimerism, donor-specific hyporesponsiveness and immunocompetence, and were weaned from IS. An additional 2 patients exhibited transient chimerism and were maintained on tacrolimus monotherapy. In 2018, 42 subjects were enrolled in this program, with 37 transplants. Thirty (out of 31 patients) demonstrated donor stem cell engraftment, with durable donor chimerism in

23 patients, and 22 patients weaned off IS [54, 69]. Measurement of immune reconstitution in these patients has demonstrated a rapid return of CD4+ and CD8+ central and effector memory cells, and most thymic emigrant cells are chimeric. Ratios of CD4+CD25+ regulatory/effector T cells also increased early in patients with either stable or transient chimerism. There was evidence of retention of immunologic memory and response to vaccination. Randomized controlled studies of this approach are awaited with great interest.

Emerging strategies for promotion of kidney transplant tolerance.

Promising approaches include adoptive regulatory immune cell therapy designed to take advantage of the cells' tolerogenic properties. In the recent ONE Study, 40% of living donor KT recipients that did not receive induction therapy, but were given polyclonal Tregs, regulatory DCs or regulatory macrophages, were weaned successfully to tacrolimus monotherapy over 60 weeks post-transplant. A favourable safety profile and fewer infections were reported compared with a standard-of-care reference group given basiliximab[70]. To date, evidence of Treg efficacy has been limited to a single uncontrolled trial in liver transplantation. More potent Ag-specific suppression can potentially be achieved using autologous Tregs transduced to express a chimeric Ag receptor (CAR). Such CAR Tregs are very effective in enhancing allograft survival in preclinical models. A first-in-human clinical trial of CAR Tregs in kidney transplantation has been instigated with the aim of inducing tolerance after HLA-A2-mismatched renal transplantation[71]. Selective stimulation of Treg expansion *in vivo* is an alternative approach to adoptive Treg therapy. Thus, clinical testing of an IL-2 "mutein" Fc fusion protein with strong binding affinity for IL-2R alpha on Tregs, but limited binding to IL-2R beta/gamma (found on CD8 and NK cells) is also underway (in GVHD and SLE). For discussion of the topic of Treg therapy see: [72].

Conclusion

Our understanding of transplant tolerance at molecular and cellular levels has expanded significantly over the last 2 decades, particularly with advances in cell phenotyping capacity and genomic signature profiling. However, kidney allograft and patient survival over the same time has slightly improved with dependency on IS and the inability to robustly identify recipients who might safely benefit from IS withdrawal. Despite major advances in therapeutic opportunities that promote KT tolerance, their widespread clinical application is limited as the available conditioning regimens remain demanding. In addition, current protocols are unable to overcome immunologic diversity and memory responses (as in the case of sensitisation). An understanding of regulatory and/or suppressive immune mechanisms may substantially improve our capacity to induce tolerance through cell therapy. Regardless, further trials are required to fully delineate how tolerogenic regimens can be applied to the transplantable population.

REFERENCES

1. Larsen CP, Elwood ET, Alexander DZ, et al. Long-term acceptance of skin and cardiac allografts after blocking CD40 and CD28 pathways. *Nature*. May 30 1996;381(6581):434–8. doi:10.1038/381434a0
2. Billingham RE, Brent L, Medawar PB. Actively acquired tolerance of foreign cells. *Nature*. Oct 3 1953;172(4379):603–6. doi:10.1038/172603a0
3. Russell PS, Chase CM, Colvin RB, Plate JM. Induced immune destruction of long-surviving, H-2 incompatible kidney transplants in mice. *J Exp Med*. May 1 1978;147(5):1469–86. doi:10.1084/jem.147.5.1469
4. Bickerstaff AA, Wang JJ, Pelletier RP, Orosz CG. Murine renal allografts: spontaneous acceptance is associated with regulated T cell-mediated immunity. *J Immunol*. Nov 1 2001;167(9):4821–7. doi:10.4049/jimmunol.167.9.4821
5. Hu M, Wang C, Zhang GY, et al. Infiltrating Foxp3(+) regulatory T cells from spontaneously tolerant kidney allografts demonstrate donor-specific tolerance. *Am J Transplant*. Nov 2013;13(11):2819–30. doi:10.1111/ajt.12445
6. Rosales IA, Yang C, Farkash EA, et al. Novel intragraft regulatory lymphoid structures in kidney allograft tolerance. *Am J Transplant*. Mar 2022;22(3):705–716. doi:10.1111/ajt.16880
7. Miyajima M, Chase CM, Alessandrini A, et al. Early acceptance of renal allografts in mice is dependent on foxp3(+) cells. *Am J Pathol*. Apr 2011;178(4):1635–45. doi:10.1016/j.ajpath.2010.12.024
8. Cook CH, Bickerstaff AA, Wang JJ, et al. Spontaneous renal allograft acceptance associated with "regulatory" dendritic cells and IDO. *J Immunol*. Mar 1 2008;180(5):3103–12. doi:10.4049/jimmunol.180.5.3103
9. Oh NA, O'Shea T, Ndishabandi DK, et al. Plasmacytoid Dendritic Cell-driven Induction of Treg Is Strain Specific and Correlates With Spontaneous Acceptance of Kidney Allografts. *Transplantation*. Jan 2020;104(1):39–53. doi:10.1097/TP.0000000000002867
10. Massart A, Pallier A, Pascual J, et al. The DESCARTES-Nantes survey of kidney transplant recipients displaying clinical operational tolerance identifies 35 new tolerant patients and 34 almost tolerant patients. *Nephrol Dial Transplant*. Jun 2016;31(6):1002–13. doi:10.1093/ndt/gfv437
11. Ekberg H, Grinyo J, Nashan B, et al. Cyclosporine sparing with mycophenolate mofetil, daclizumab and corticosteroids in renal allograft recipients: the CAESAR Study. *Am J Transplant*. Mar 2007;7(3):560–70. doi:10.1111/j.1600-6143.2006.01645.x

12. Abramowicz D, Del Carmen Rial M, Vitko S, et al. Cyclosporine withdrawal from a mycophenolate mofetil-containing immunosuppressive regimen: results of a five-year, prospective, randomized study. *J Am Soc Nephrol.* Jul 2005;16(7):2234–40. doi:10.1681/ASN.2004100844

13. Roodnat JI, Hilbrands LB, Hene RJ, et al. 15-year follow-up of a multicenter, randomized, calcineurin inhibitor withdrawal study in kidney transplantation. *Transplantation.* Jul 15 2014;98(1):47–53. doi:10.1097/01.TP.0000442774.46133.71

14. Hricik DE, Formica RN, Nickerson P, et al. Adverse Outcomes of Tacrolimus Withdrawal in Immune-Quiescent Kidney Transplant Recipients. *J Am Soc Nephrol.* Dec 2015;26(12):3114–22. doi:10.1681/ASN.2014121234

15. Karpe KM, Talaulikar GS, Walters GD. Calcineurin inhibitor withdrawal or tapering for kidney transplant recipients. *Cochrane Database Syst Rev.* Jul 21 2017;7(7):CD006750. doi:10.1002/14651858.CD006750.pub2

16. Chesneau M, Danger R, Soulillou JP, Brouard S. B cells in operational tolerance. *Hum Immunol.* May 2018;79(5):373–379. doi:10.1016/j.humimm.2018.02.009

17. Newell KA, Asare A, Kirk AD, et al. Identification of a B cell signature associated with renal transplant tolerance in humans. *J Clin Invest.* Jun 2010;120(6):1836–47. doi:10.1172/JCI39933

18. Sagoo P, Perucha E, Sawitzki B, et al. Development of a cross-platform bio-marker signature to detect renal transplant tolerance in humans. *J Clin Invest.* Jun 2010;120(6):1848–61. doi:10.1172/JCI39922

19. Brouard S, Mansfield E, Braud C, et al. Identification of a peripheral blood tran-scriptional biomarker panel associated with operational renal allograft toler-ance. *Proc Natl Acad Sci U S A.* Sep 25 2007;104(39):15448–53. doi:10.1073/pnas.0705834104

20. Baron D, Ramstein G, Chesneau M, et al. A common gene signature across multiple studies relate biomarkers and functional regulation in tolerance to renal allograft. *Kidney Int.* May 2015;87(5):984–95. doi:10.1038/ki.2014.395

21. Roedder S, Li L, Alonso MN, et al. A Three-Gene Assay for Monitoring Immune Quiescence in Kidney Transplantation. *J Am Soc Nephrol.* Aug 2015;26(8):2042–53. doi:10.1681/ASN.2013111239

22. Danger R, Pallier A, Giral M, et al. Upregulation of miR-142-3p in peripheral blood mononuclear cells of operationally tolerant patients with a renal transplant. *J Am Soc Nephrol.* Apr 2012;23(4):597–606. doi:10.1681/ASN.2011060543

23. Pallier A, Hillion S, Danger R, et al. Patients with drug-free long-term graft function display increased numbers of peripheral B cells with a memory and inhibitory pheno-type. *Kidney Int.* Sep 2010;78(5):503–13. doi:10.1038/ki.2010.162

24. Moraes-Vieira PM, Takenaka MC, Silva HM, et al. GATA3 and a dominant regula-tory gene expression profile discriminate operational tolerance in human transplan-tation. *Clin Immunol.* Feb 2012;142(2):117–26. doi:10.1016/j.clim.2011.08.015

25. Nova-Lamperti E, Chana P, Mobillo P, et al. Increased CD40 Ligation and Reduced BCR Signalling Leads to Higher IL-10 Production in B Cells From Tolerant Kidney Transplant Patients. *Transplantation.* Mar 2017;101(3):541–547. doi:10.1097/TP.0000000000001341

26. Braza F, Dugast E, Panov I, et al. Central Role of CD45RA- Foxp3hi Memory Regulatory T Cells in Clinical Kidney Transplantation Tolerance. *J Am Soc Nephrol.* Aug 2015;26(8):1795–805. doi:10.1681/ASN.2014050480

27. Leventhal JR, Mathew JM, Salomon DR, et al. Genomic biomarkers correlate with HLA-identical renal transplant tolerance. *J Am Soc Nephrol.* Sep 2013;24(9):1376–85. doi:10.1681/ASN.2013010068

28. Nissaisorakarn V, Lee JR, Lubetzky M, Suthanthiran M. Urine biomarkers informative of human kidney allograft rejection and tolerance. *Hum Immunol.* May 2018;79(5):343–355. doi:10.1016/j.humimm.2018.01.006

29. Bontha SV, Fernandez-Pineros A, Maluf DG, Mas VR. Messengers of tolerance. *Hum Immunol.* May 2018;79(5):362–372. doi:10.1016/j.humimm.2018.01.008

30. Brouard S, Dupont A, Giral M, et al. Operationally tolerant and minimally immuno-suppressed kidney recipients display strongly altered blood T-cell clonal regulation. *Am J Transplant.* Feb 2005;5(2):330–40. doi:10.1111/j.1600-6143.2004.00700.x

31. Baeten D, Louis S, Braud C, et al. Phenotypically and functionally distinct CD8+ lymphocyte populations in long-term drug-free tolerance and chronic rejection in human kidney graft recipients. *J Am Soc Nephrol.* Jan 2006;17(1):294–304. doi:10.1681/ASN.2005020178

32. Louis S, Braudeau C, Giral M, et al. Contrasting CD25hiCD4+T cells/FOXP3 patterns in chronic rejection and operational drug-free tolerance. *Transplantation.* Feb 15 2006;81(3):398–407. doi:10.1097/01.tp.0000203166.44968.86

33. Miqueu P, Degauque N, Guillet M, et al. Analysis of the peripheral T-cell repertoire in kidney transplant patients. *Eur J Immunol.* Nov 2010;40(11):3280–90. doi:10.1002/eji.201040301

34. Brouard S, Le Bars A, Dufay A, et al. Identification of a gene expression profile associated with operational tolerance among a selected group of stable kidney transplant patients. *Transpl Int.* Jun 2011;24(6):536–47. doi:10.1111/j.1432-2277.2011.01251.x

35. Braudeau C, Racape M, Giral M, et al. Variation in numbers of CD4+CD25highFOXP3+ T cells with normal immuno-regulatory properties in long-term graft outcome. *Transpl Int.* Oct 2007;20(10):845–55. doi:10.1111/j.1432-2277.2007.00537.x

36. Ballet C, Roussey-Kesler G, Aubin JT, et al. Humoral and cellular responses to influenza vaccination in human recipients naturally tolerant to a kidney allograft. *Am J Transplant.* Nov 2006;6(11):2796–801. doi:10.1111/j.1600-6143.2006.01533.x

37. Chenouard A, Chesneau M, Bui Nguyen L, et al. Renal Operational Tolerance Is Associated With a Defect of Blood Tfh Cells That Exhibit Impaired B Cell Help. *Am J Transplant.* Jun 2017;17(6):1490–1501. doi:10.1111/ajt.14142

38. Newell KA, Asare A, Sanz I, et al. Longitudinal studies of a B cell-derived signature of tolerance in renal transplant recipients. *Am J Transplant.* Nov 2015;15(11):2908–20. doi:10.1111/ajt.13480

39. Asare A, Kanaparthi S, Lim N, et al. B Cell Receptor Genes Associated With Tolerance Identify a Cohort of Immunosuppressed Patients With Improved Renal Allograft Graft Function. *Am J Transplant.* Oc22017;17(10):2627–2639. doi:10.1111/ajt.14283

40. Li B, Hartono C, Ding R, et al. Noninvasive diagnosis of renal-allograft rejection by measurement of messenger RNA for perforin and granzyme B in urine. *N Engl J Med.* Mar 29 2001;344(13):947–54. doi:10.1056/NEJM200103293441301

41. Muthukumar T, Ding R, Dadhania D, et al. Serine proteinase inhibitor-9, an endogenous blocker of granzyme B/perforin lytic pathway, is hyperexpressed during acute rejection of renal allografts. *Transplantation.* May 15 2003;75(9):1565–70. doi:10.1097/01.TP.0000058230.91518.2F

42. Ding R, Li B, Muthukumar T, et al. CD103 mRNA levels in urinary cells predict acute rejection of renal allografts. *Transplantation.* Apr 27 2003;75(8):1307–12. doi:10.1097/01.TP.0000064210.92444.B5

43. Suthanthiran M, Schwartz JE, Ding R, et al. Urinary-cell mRNA profile and acute cellular rejection in kidney allografts. *N Engl J Med*. Jul 4 2013;369(1):20–31. doi:10.1056/NEJMoa1215555

44. Rabant M, Amrouche L, Morin L, et al. Early Low Urinary CXCL9 and CXCL10 Might Predict Immunological Quiescence in Clinically and Histologically Stable Kidney Recipients. *Am J Transplant*. Jun 2016;16(6):1868–81. doi:10.1111/ajt.13677

45. Hricik DE, Nickerson P, Formica RN, et al. Multicenter validation of urinary CXCL9 as a risk-stratifying biomarker for kidney transplant injury. *Am J Transplant*. Oct 2013;13(10):2634–44. doi:10.1111/ajt.12426

46. Lubetzky ML, Salinas T, Schwartz JE, Suthanthiran M. Urinary Cell mRNA Profiles Predictive of Human Kidney Allograft Status. *Clin J Am Soc Nephrol*. Oct 2021;16(10):1565–1577. doi:10.2215/CJN.14010820

47. Colas L, Mongodin EF, Montassier E, et al. Unique and specific Proteobacteria diversity in urinary microbiota of tolerant kidney transplanted recipients. *Am J Transplant*. Jan 2020;20(1):145–158. doi:10.1111/ajt.15549

48. Colas L, Royer AL, Massias J, et al. Urinary metabolomic profiling from spontaneous tolerant kidney transplanted recipients shows enrichment in tryptophan-derived metabolites. *EBioMedicine*. Mar 2022;77:103844. doi:10.1016/j.ebiom.2022.103844

49. Zoller KM, Cho SI, Cohen JJ, Harrington JT. Cessation of immunosuppressive therapy after successful transplantation: a national survey. *Kidney Int*. Jul 1980;18(1):110–4. doi:10.1038/ki.1980.116

50. Massart A, Ghisdal L, Abramowicz M, Abramowicz D. Operational tolerance in kidney transplantation and associated biomarkers. *Clin Exp Immunol*. Aug 2017;189(2):138–157. doi:10.1111/cei.12981

51. Viklicky O, Klema J, Mrazova P, et al. Operational tolerance in kidney transplant recipients: Tomogram Transcriptomic Study. *Am J Transplant*. 2020;20 (suupl 3)

52. Madariaga ML, Spencer PJ, Shanmugarajah K, et al. Effect of tolerance versus chronic immunosuppression protocols on the quality of life of kidney transplant recipients. *JCI Insight*. Jun 2 2016;1(8)doi:10.1172/jci.insight.87019

53. Busque S, Scandling JD, Lowsky R, et al. Mixed chimerism and acceptance of kidney transplants after immunosuppressive drug withdrawal. *Sci Transl Med*. Jan 29 2020;12(528)doi:10.1126/scitranslmed.aax8863

54. Leventhal JR, Ildstad ST. Tolerance induction in HLA disparate living donor kidney transplantation by facilitating cell-enriched donor stem cell Infusion: The importance of durable chimerism. *Hum Immunol*. May 2018;79(5):272–276. doi:10.1016/j.humimm.2018.01.007

55. Starzl TE, Demetris AJ, Murase N, Ildstad S, Ricordi C, Trucco M. Cell migration, chimerism, and graft acceptance. *Lancet*. Jun 27 1992;339(8809):1579–82. doi:10.1016/0140-6736(92)91840-5

56. Starzl TE, Demetris AJ, Trucco M, et al. Systemic chimerism in human female recipients of male livers. *Lancet*. Oct 10 1992;340(8824):876–7. doi:10.1016/0140-6736(92)93286-v

57. Kawai T, Sachs DH, Sykes M, Cosimi AB, Immune Tolerance N. HLA-mismatched renal transplantation without maintenance immunosuppression. *N Engl J Med*. May 9 2013;368(19):1850–2. doi:10.1056/NEJMc1213779

58. Kawai T, Cosimi AB, Spitzer TR, et al. HLA-mismatched renal transplantation without maintenance immunosuppression. *N Engl J Med*. Jan 24 2008;358(4):353–61. doi:10.1056/NEJMoa071074

59. Spitzer TR, Delmonico F, Tolkoff-Rubin N, et al. Combined histocompatibility leukocyte antigen-matched donor bone marrow and renal transplantation for multiple myeloma with end stage renal disease: the induction of allograft tolerance through mixed lymphohematopoietic chimerism. *Transplantation*. Aug 27 1999;68(4):480–4. doi:10.1097/00007890-199908270-00006

60. Spitzer TR, Tolkoff-Rubin N, Cosimi AB, et al. Twenty-year Follow-up of Histocompatibility Leukocyte Antigen-matched Kidney and Bone Marrow Cotransplantation for Multiple Myeloma With End-stage Renal Disease: Lessons Learned. *Transplantation*. Nov 2019;103(11):2366–2372. doi:10.1097/TP.0000000000002669

61. Sykes M, Preffer F, McAfee S, et al. Mixed lymphohaemopoietic chimerism and graft-versus-lymphoma effects after non-myeloablative therapy and HLA-mismatched bone-marrow transplantation. *Lancet*. May 22 1999;353(9166):1755–9. doi:10.1016/S0140-6736(98)11135-2

62. Scandling JD, Busque S, Dejbakhsh-Jones S, et al. Tolerance and chimerism after renal and hematopoietic-cell transplantation. *N Engl J Med*. Jan 24 2008;358(4):362–8. doi:10.1056/NEJMoa074191

63. Scandling JD, Busque S, Dejbakhsh-Jones S, et al. Tolerance and withdrawal of immunosuppressive drugs in patients given kidney and hematopoietic cell transplants. *Am J Transplant*. May 2012;12(5):1133–45. doi:10.1111/j.1600-6143.2012.03992.x

64. Fehr T, Hubel K, de Rougemont O, et al. Successful Induction of Specific Immunological Tolerance by Combined Kidney and Hematopoietic Stem Cell Transplantation in HLA-Identical Siblings. *Front Immunol*. 2022;13:796456. doi:10.3389/fimmu.2022.796456

65. Kaufman CL, Colson YL, Wren SM, Watkins S, Simmons RL, Ildstad ST. Phenotypic characterization of a novel bone marrow-derived cell that facilitates engraftment of allogeneic bone marrow stem cells. *Blood*. Oct 15 1994;84(8):2436–46.

66. Fugier-Vivier IJ, Rezzoug F, Huang Y, et al. Plasmacytoid precursor dendritic cells facilitate allogeneic hematopoietic stem cell engraftment. *J Exp Med*. Feb 7 2005;201(3):373–83. doi:10.1084/jem.20041399

67. Schuchert MJ, Wright RD, Colson YL. Characterization of a newly discovered T-cell receptor beta-chain heterodimer expressed on a CD8+ bone marrow subpopulation that promotes allogeneic stem cell engraftment. *Nat Med*. Aug 2000;6(8):904–9. doi:10.1038/78667

68. Leventhal J, Abecassis M, Miller J, et al. Chimerism and tolerance without GVHD or engraftment syndrome in HLA-mismatched combined kidney and hematopoietic stem cell transplantation. *Sci Transl Med*. Mar 7 2012;4(124):124ra28. doi:10.1126/scitranslmed.3003509

69. Leventhal JR, Miller J, Mathew JM, et al. Updated follow-up of a tolerance protocol in HLA-identical renal transplant pairs given donor hematopoietic stem cells. *Hum Immunol*. May 2018;79(5):277–282. doi:10.1016/j.humimm.2018.01.010

70. Sawitzki B, Harden PN, Reinke P, et al. Regulatory cell therapy in kidney transplantation (The ONE Study): a harmonised design and analysis of seven non-randomised, single-arm, phase 1/2A trials. *Lancet*. May 23 2020;395(10237):1627–1639. doi:10.1016/S0140-6736(20)30167-7

71. Schreeb K, Culme-Seymour E, Ridha E, et al. Study Design: Human Leukocyte Antigen Class I Molecule A(*)02-Chimeric Antigen Receptor Regulatory T Cells in Renal Transplantation. *Kidney Int Rep*. Jun 2022;7(6):1258–1267. doi:10.1016/j.ekir.2022.03.030

72. Pilat N, Steiner R, Sprent J. Treg Therapy for the Induction of Immune Tolerance in Transplantation-Not Lost in Translation? *Int J Mol Sci*. Jan 16 2023;24(2). doi:10.3390/ijms24021752

19

Long-term Care of Kidney Transplant Patients—Conclusion

Hamid Rabb

The Finale!

Kidney transplantation has been one of the most effective and dramatic medical advances over the last 70 years. Fundamental developments in immunology, surgical techniques, dialysis treatment, and medical ethics fueled the first wave of progress. The more recent advances have had pronounced impact on extending the lives of allografts and patients. Long-term care of the kidney transplant patient is both an art and a science and has led to a new subspecialty field of medicine, nursing, and administration. In this context, the current book by the renowned transplant nephrologist Sundaram Hariharan and his team of expert international authors is a timely contribution to the field. Despite the current medical education trend away from textbooks toward short snippets of information from internet sources of variable credibility, the current book succinctly addresses a panorama of key aspects of long-term kidney transplant care in a compact but very readable fashion.

One must start with the numbers, which Chapter 1 nicely provides for the impact and successes of long-term kidney transplant (KT) care. This has been well highlighted recently.[1] Chapter 2, on the post-transplant phases, gives a dynamic view of the patient care journey. Chapter 3, on wellness, is refreshing and in step with the modern approach to holistic patient care. No solid guide to kidney transplant care can be without the key chapter on transplant immunosuppression. An excellent historic timeline of key immunosuppression studies is provided in Chapter 4. We continue to learn and evolve about both immunologic and nonimmunologic factors determining allograft outcome, well highlighted in Chapter 5. It is important to note that long-term outcomes are heavily influenced by the original quality of the allograft, and expanding the deceased donor pool has both pros and cons.[2] Chapters 6 and 7, on T- and B-cell-mediated kidney rejection, address both the better studied early post-transplant phase and then the less clear but nonetheless important late allograft rejections. Chapters 8, 9, and 10, on cardiovascular diseases, infections, and cancers, cover the very important major determinants of the patients' lifespan. Recurrent disease is incompletely understood and hard to treat; it is discussed directly in Chapter 11. The increasingly well recognized impact of psychosocial, behavioral, and social determinants of the health of the kidney transplant patient are highlighted as well in Chapters 12 and 13. Dual-organ transplants are becoming more common, traditionally with kidney and pancreas, and now increasingly kidney with liver and even with heart and lung transplants. These are discussed in Chapters 14 and 15. Kidney transplantation in children has unique features, ably discussed in Chapter 16. Management of the failing kidney transplant is described in Chapter 17. This is increasingly important given the increasing number of kidney transplants globally, and management of these patients sometimes gets insufficient attention and poorly studied. Finally, no transplant book could be complete without an up-to-date discussion on the "Holy Grail" of transplantation: tolerance, discussed in Chapter 18. This book on long-term management of patients provides instructions on comprehensive care and balances the difficult goals of breadth and depth.

There are additional topics that transplant professionals and patients deal with that are not covered in detail in this volume. The unique regulatory aspects of kidney transplantation, with many common aspects like patient and graft outcome, have many nuances depending on country and even region. Emerging infections like COVID have heavily impacted long-term kidney transplant care, and management approaches are changing almost too rapidly to put in a book. Organ utilization and wastage is another important issue and has not been tackled. Pre- and post-transplant bone disease has not been well studied but is likely to be particularly important especially for the pediatric and geriatric populations. Also, live donors need long-term attention given risk of CKD.

This excellent book has chapters that are neither short and superficial, nor too long and difficult for a reader to read at one glance. I highly recommend this book for everyone associated with care of KT patients—nephrologists, surgeons, and basic scientists along with key associates such as nurse coordinators, pharmacists, psychologists, and social workers. On a personal level, I learned a lot reading it, which will help me provide better patient care and teaching.

This book marvelously takes us in various chapters from the past to the present. However, where do we go from here? The monumental breakthroughs of dialysis and transplantation were made over 70 years ago. We are overdue for more disruptive game-changers that will transform the lives of our patients. There are many exciting avenues, including the following four (Figure 19.1).[3] They are as follows:

A. The implantable bioartificial kidney and wearable artificial kidney. Each has the potential to maintain homeostasis and provide continuous dialysis.

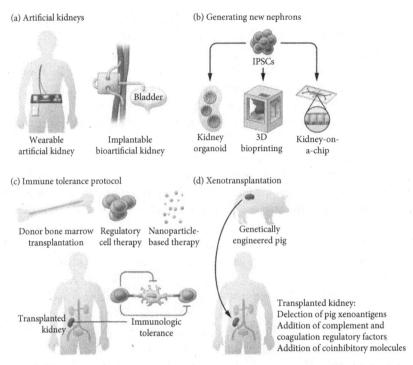

(a) Artificial kidneys

Wearable
artificial kidney

Implantable
bioartificial kidney

(b) Generating new nephrons

IPSCs

Kidney
organoid

3D
bioprinting

Kidney-on-
a-chip

(c) Immune tolerance protocol

Donor bone marrow
transplantation

Regulatory
cell therapy

Nanoparticle-
based therapy

Transplanted
kidney

Immunologic
tolerance

(d) Xenotransplantation

Genetically
engineered pig

Transplanted kidney:
Delection of pig xenoantigens
Addition of complement and
coagulation regulatory factors
Addition of coinhibitory molecules

Figure 19.1 Next-generation approaches for end stage renal disease beyond current dialysis and transplant. (A) The automated wearable artificial kidney is designed to perform continuous dialysis throughout the day with increased portability. The implantable bioartificial kidney is a surgically implanted device that mimics a native kidney. (B) The 3D cell bioprinting technique allows layer-by-layer stacking of cells and facilitates further development of both kidney organoid and kidney-on-a-chip technologies. (C) Clinical transplantation tolerance trials using chimerism induction approaches have made substantial progress with safety. (D) Pigs that have been genetically engineered, including by deletion of pig xenoantigens and insertion of protective human transgenes to induce immunologic tolerance, are currently available.[3]

Early data demonstrates that the wearable kidney is favorably received by patients, and the bioartificial kidney was safe and effective in canines.

B. Kidney on a chip is an approach where tubules and glomeruli can be placed on chips with a microfluidic system to mimic kidney physiology. The next steps would include development of chips that can generate an entire functional nephron. Growing a new kidney using organoids derived from pluripotent stem cells. 3-D printing can assist in tissue development in a spatial and automated fashion. A major challenge is to recapitulate the entire mature kidney.

C. Novel immune tolerance protocols are being developed. Transplant tolerance induction by developing mixed chimerism with donor bone marrow transplantation or donor-derived hematopoietic stem cell transplantation is being tested in a number of centers. Use of regulatory cell-based therapy or nanoparticle therapy is also being tested in clinical trials.

D. Xenotransplantation using genetically modified pigs lacking major xenoantigens has received a lot of recent public and scientific attention. Short-term viability of these pig-to-human kidney and heart transplants has energized this field of research.

Time will reveal the feasibility of these novel approaches to replace conventional approaches to manage ESKD and whether they will dramatically change how we manage KT patients. In the meantime, the current book will likely be the gold-standard manual for long-term KT care around the world.

References

1. Hariharan S, Israni AK, Danovitch G. Long-term survival after kidney transplantation. *N Engl J Med*. 2021;385(8):729–743.
2. Tullius SG, Rabb H. Improving the supply and quality of deceased-donor organs for transplantation. *N Engl J Med*. 2018;378(20):1920–1929.
3. Rabb H, Lee K, Parikh CR. Beyond kidney dialysis and transplantation: what's on the horizon? *J Clin Invest*. 2022;132(7):e159308.

Index